Textbook of
Pharmacognosy and
Phytochemistry I

As per the latest syllabus prescribed by
Pharmacy Council of India
for Bachelor of Pharmacy Course

Textbook of
Pharmacognosy and Phytochemistry I

**As per the latest syllabus prescribed by
Pharmacy Council of India
for Bachelor of Pharmacy Course**

AN Kalia PhD
Former
Professor and Head
Department of Pharmaceutical Sciences
Maharshi Dayanand University
Rohtak, Haryana

Director
Herbal Drug Research
ISF College of Pharmacy, Moga, Punjab

Director-Principal
Sri Sai College of Pharmacy
Badhani, Pathankot, Panjab

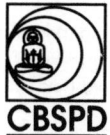

CBSPD

CBS Publishers & Distributors Pvt Ltd

New Delhi • Bengaluru • Chennai • Kochi • Kolkata • Lucknow • Mumbai
Gujarat • Hyderabad • Jharkhand • Nagpur • Patna • Pune • Uttarakhand

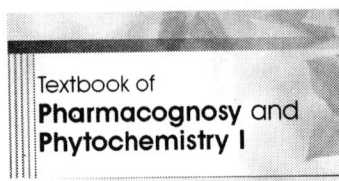

Textbook of
Pharmacognosy and
Phytochemistry I

ISBN: 978-93-89688-62-7

First Edition: 2021

   Reprint: 2023, **2026**

Published by **Satish Kumar Jain** and produced by **Varun Jain** for

CBS Publishers & Distributors Pvt Ltd

4819/XI Prahlad Street, 24 Ansari Road, Daryaganj, New Delhi 110 002, India
Ph: 011-23289259, 23266838   Website: www.cbspd.com
        e-mail: delhi@cbspd.com

Corporate Office: 204 FIE, Industrial Area, Patparganj, Delhi 110 092
Ph: 011-4934 4934   Fax: 011-4934 4935   e-mail: publishing@cbspd.com; publicity@cbspd.com

Branches

- **Bengaluru:** Seema House 2975, 17th Cross, K.R. Road, Banasankari 2nd Stage, Bengaluru 560 070, Karnataka, India
  Ph: +91-80-26771678/79   Fax: +91-80-26771680   e-mail: bangalore@cbspd.com

- **Chennai:** 18/8B, Subbarayan Street, Shenoy Nagar, Chennai 600 030, Tamil Nadu, India
  Ph: +91-44-42032115, 26681266   e-mail: chennai@cbspd.com

- **Kochi:** 42/1325, 1326, Power House Road, opposite KSEB, Power House, Ernakulam 682 018, Kochi, Kerala, India
  Ph: +91-484-4059061-65   Fax: +91-484-4059065   e-mail: kochi@cbspd.com

- **Kolkata:** 147, Hind Ceramics Compound, 1st Floor, Nilgunj Road, Belghoria, Kolkata 700 056, West Bengal, India
  Ph: +91-33-25633055-56   e-mail: kolkata@cbspd.com

- **Lucknow:** Basement, Khushnuma Complex, 7-Meerabai Marg (behind Jawahar Bhawan), Lucknow 226 001, UP, India
  Ph: +91-522-4000032   e-mail: tiwari.lucknow@cbspd.com

- **Mumbai:** PWD Shed. Gala No. 25/26, Ramchandra Bhatt Marg, Next to JJ Hospital Gate No. 2, Opposite Union Bank of India Noorbaug
  Mumbai 400 009, Maharashtra, India
  Ph: +91-22-66661880/89   e-mail: mumbai@cbspd.com

Representatives

- **Gujarat**   • **Hyderabad**   • **Jharkhand**   • **Nagpur**   • **Patna**   • **Pune**   • **Uttarakhand**

For trade terms please contact customercare@cbspd.com

For general enquiries please contact info@cbspd.com

Printed at Rashtriya Printers, Dilshad Garden, Delhi, India

Preface

The syllabus of this book is newly introduced course for B Pharmacy students of semester IV, under the revised syllabus recommended by Pharmacy Council of India (PCI), New Delhi, under Bachelor of Pharmacy Course Regulation 2014. It is effective throughout India from the academic year 2016–17.

The Council has recommended the division of the course contents into five units with the certain scope and objective:

Scope: The subject involves the fundamentals of pharmacognosy like, classification of crude drugs, their identification and evaluation, phytochemicals present in them and their medical properties.

Objective: Upon completion of the course. The student shall be able to: (i) Know the techniques in cultivation and production of crude drugs, (ii) Know the crude drugs their uses and chemical nature, (iii) Know the evaluation techniques for herbal drugs, and (iv) Cary-out the microscopic and morphological evaluation of crude drugs.

With an extensive experience in the field of teaching in pharmaceutical sciences at different levels such as B Pharm, M Pharm and PhD in the subject of pharmacognosy and after attaining the popularity from wide acceptance of my previous book *Textbook of Industrial Pharmacognosy* by the students and teachers community aimed to write this *Textbook of Pharmacognosy and Phytochemistry I* for B Pharm students of semester IV.

Therefore this book is divided into five units:

Unit I provides a general introduction to pharmacognosy to cover the objective, the text is discussed under subheading (a) Definition, history scope and development. (b) Organised and unorganised drugs with examples as per recommendation; classification of drugs and quality control of drugs of natural origin with respect to adulteration evaluation by physical, chemical, microscopic and biological methods and properties.

Unit II provides the knowledge of cultivation, collection, processing and storage of drugs of natural origin as well as conservation of medicinal plants.

Unit III explains the development and applications of plant tissue culture in pharmacognosy as well the edible vaccines.

Unit IV discusses the role of pharmacognosy in various system of medicines (Ayurveda, Sidha, Unani and Homeopathy) and also the introduction of secondary metabolites of plants useful in medicines.

Unit V provides the knowledge about the biological source, chemical nature and uses of drugs of natural origin with examples such as fibers, hallucinogens, teratogens, natural allergens and primary metabolites such as carbohydrates, proteins and enzymes; lipids (waxes fats and fixed oils) and the novel medicinal agents from marine source.

The information cited in this book are procured from published books, scientific periodicals, websites of government agencies like AYUSH, WHO; internet and current science. To acknowledge for thanks all the information sources have been given as bibliography. My aim of compiling the information in the form of textbook is for easy access of students at one place to achieve the objective of Pharmacy Council of India's recommendation for semester IV.

I am highly grateful to my daughters, Dr Aparna and Dr. Vandana and son-in-law's Dr Ajay and Dr Mahendera for their generous help in the preparation of this book.

I would like to thank CBS Publishers & Distributors Pvt. Ltd., New Delhi for their cooperation in the publication of this book.

I will be grateful to have any criticism and suggestion from readers for further improvement of the book.

ANKalia

Contents

UNIT III
Plant Tissue Culture

UNIT IV
Pharmacognosy in Various Systems of Medicines

UNIT V
Study of Biological Sources, Chemical Nature and Uses of Plant Products

9. Primary Metabolites

10. Marine Pharmacognosy (Novel Medicinal Agents from Marine Source)

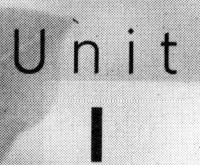

Unit
I

Introduction to Pharmacognosy Definition, History, Scope and Development in Pharmacognosy

Introduction to Pharmacognosy

The pharmacognosy is the subject which deals with crude drugs, phytopharmaceuticals, excipients, surgical dressings, filtering aids and support media for the production and discovery of drugs from natural sources.

Crude drugs: The word crude drug is used for those natural products (plant or parts of plant, extracts and exudates) which are not processed. Most of crude drugs are obtained from plants. Few are obtained from animals or insects origin (lard, beeswax, honey, etc.) and from the marine origin.

HISTORY

Dioscorides, A Greek physician, who lived in first century A.D. wrote 'De Materia Medica' in 78 A.D. in which he described about 6000 plants having medicinal properties out of which large number of plants are still in use in modern medicine. Aloe, belladonna, colchicum, ergot, hyoscyamus, and opium are few of them which are still in use in the same manner.

Galen (131–200 A.D.) a Greek pharmacist-physician who lived in Rome, described methods of preparing the formula containing plants and animal drugs. As a tribute to his accuracy in recording his observations the term 'galenical' pharmacy originated.

The term materia medica, meaning medicinal materials, was synonymous with the substances and products derived from natural sources and was employed by the physician in that era.

The term pharmacognosy first appears to have its origin in the 18th century by John Adam Schmidt (1759–1809), Professor of General Pathology, Therapeutics, Materia Medica at the Medicosurgical Joseph Academy in Vienna founded in 1785. The term was found in his 'Lehrbuch der Materia Medica' published posthumously in Vienna in 1811. At that time, knowledge of drug was limited and could easily be contained in one subject.

The term pharmacognosy was finally introduced by C.A. Seydler (1815), in Germany. This name was then formed from two Greek words, 'pharmakon', drug, and 'gnosis', knowledge.

F.A. Fluckiger (1870), Professor in pharmacy in Strasburg, stated that pharmacognosy is simultaneous application of various disciplines with the object of acquiring knowledge of drugs from every point of view.

In the 18th century, Linnaeus made an important contribution to the development of pharmacognosy through the introduction of his new system of naming and classification of plants.

Though, in 1803 F.W. Serturner isolated morphine from opium and thus the era of drug discovery started in pharmacognosy but till the end of the 18th century crude drugs were still being used as powders, simple extracts or tinctures.

In nineteenth century the name pharmacognosy came into practice and expanded the arena of pharmacognosy beyond botany.

Hence, in broad sense, pharmacognosy is the knowledge of history, distribution, cultivation, collection, preparation, identification evaluation (chemical and biological), pre-servation and use of drugs and economic substances that affect health of man and animals.

As a part of pharmaceutical curriculum pharmacognosy forms an important link between pharmacognosy and medicinal chemistry on one hand and between pharmacy and clinical pharmacy on the other hand.

SCOPE AND DEVELOPMENT

Seydler in 1815, first time defined pharma-cognosy as a pharmaceutical discipline. Alexander Tschirch (1909) gave the following definition to pharmacognosy:

'The name pharmacognosy means the science which has task to learn everything about drugs originating from plants and animals, in all aspects except physiology.'

During 19th century, it was the mother of all present day pharmaceutical disciplines. But in 1899 synthetic chemistry became more important for developing new drugs with the synthesis of aspirin (1990).

In the 19th century, microscopy was introduced for the quality control of pharma-ceutical formulations from plants but with the fast decreasing trend in herbal preparations in pharmacy, it became difficult task to maintain the prominent position in pharmaceutical curriculum in sixties and seventies.

Fortunately, in 1967, the development of thin layer chromatography (TLC) by Egon Stahl (1967) again brought the status of pharmacognosist among the pioneers in the analysis of plant materials. Thus, gas chromatography (GC), high performance liquid chromatography (HPLC) and thin layer chromatography (TLC) became the important tools in the study of active compounds. In seventies, spectrophotometric methods such as mass spectrometry (MS) and nuclear magnetic resonance spectrometry (NMR) were also introduced in their search for new biologically active compounds.

In 1999, the international scientist community had shown increasing interest in the field of a pharmacognosy and natural product research which has been illustrated from large number of scientists attending 5 yearly events. In July 1999, at Amsterdom attendance was almost double the number of previous year's meeting, the reason being the increased interest in the field of research in pharma-cognosy and natural products which is illustrated from the trend shown in the new drug discovery in the period from 1983 to 1994 from list of the approved drugs, 78% of the new antibiotics and 61% of the new antitumour drugs were natural products or natural product derivatives.

In the beginning of 20th century international scientists had shown the interest in the research in pharmacognosy and natural products, because of the following reasons:

- Search for new leads for drug development.
- Technology for the production of pharma-ceuticals.
- Health claims for food (nutraceuticals).
- Validation of traditional medicine.
- Increased interest in phytotherapy.

Currently, the following are the three hot areas of interest of pharmacognosist:

i. Study of new biologically active natural products
ii. Quality control of drugs from natural origin.
iii. Production of drug from natural origin, including new methods such as bio-technology.

Lead finding: Lead finding process has become easy with the introduction of High Throughput Screening (HTS) method. By using molecular targets, large number of samples even up to 100,000 in 24 hours can be screened for single activity. Thus, by the development of HTS large number of plant extracts could be easily fractionated for its biological activity.

Recently, high performance liquid chromatography (HPLC) method has been developed for determining biological activity.

Plant cell culture extract is another intresting option for screening as it can be made from rare plants to ensure the production for the interested activities. Lead finding for drug development using biodiversity or traditional medicine is one of the major area in which pharmacognosy can see a fast growth.

Biotechnology: Biotechnology has opened new perspectives in pharmacognosy. Traditionally, pharmacognosy focuses on plants only and little attention was paid to microorganisms as a source of drug. Plant cells biotechnology emerged as new possibility for the production of secondary metabolites. In mid-seventies, the pharmacognosists eagerly moved into this field. Genetic engineering can be used to increase the production of valuable pharmaceuticals, e.g. proteins in microorganisms (insulin in *E. coli*) or plants (human serum albumin or vaccines).

These new technologies, of course, also require a new type of pharmacists and pharmacognosists. A pharmacognosist need to have not only expertise on the botanical aspects of medicinal plants, but also on phytochemistry, advanced separation techniques, proteins and on molecular biology. In the field of protein, the proteomics is field of interest for pharmacognosist. The molecular biology technique is an important tool in quality control not only for the biotechnological products but also in characterising medicinal plants.

Health claim for food (nutraceuticals): Nutraceuticals are food or part of food that provides medical or health benefits including the prevention and treatment of diseases. Detailed knowledge of the influence of diet on human health has been increased greatly in the global community. The pharmacognosist plays a major role in the biological evaluation of herbs or botanical products and other components used in the formulation of nutraceuticals that claim to be useful in the treatment of diseases without toxicity.

Nutraceuticals on the basis of their natural source and chemical grouping, categorises into **nutrients, herbs, dietary supplements** and **dietary fibres**. The most rapidly growing segment of industry are dietary supplements (20.5%), dietary fibre and natural/herbal products (about 14.0%). Global nutraceuticals market is about 115 to 120 billion USD.

Phytotherapy: Phytotherapy was introduced in 20th century especially in developed countries like North America, Europe, Australia. Although the traditional medicine was very common in developing countries, but now it is being used worldwide by people/population of many countries especially old age people prefer to use food supplement or others herbal formulations (phytomedicine) to combat the old age problems with the belief that these natural products are safe to use. Hence it becomes challenge for health professional having insufficient knowledge about the natural products. Therefore, it is new era for pharmacognosists to provide information regarding the identification, standardisation/validation of the nutraceuticals for their potency as well as toxicity.

The last decade has seen a greater use of herbal remedies/botanical products among the members of general public through self-selection than ever before. This has greatly increased the relevance of the subject.

SOURCES OF DRUGS

Drugs are derived from minerals, plants, animals and microbes of both terrestrial and marine origin. Now, plant tissue culture (biotechnology) has also been considered to be source of drugs. Plants form an important part of everyday diet of all living being and their nutritional as well as medicinal values have been intensively explored for decades. Henkel et al, 1999 has reported that the origin of 30,000 bioactive natural products are of natural origin, which could be divided among animals (13%), bacteria (33%), fungi (26%), and plants (27%). The potential diversity of bacteria and fungi is quite large with some 5000 out of about 40,000 bacteria and only 70,000 out of about 1.5 million fungi, having been identified. Only a relatively small percentage (5–15%) of higher plants has been systematically investigated for the presence of biologically active compounds.

About 25% of the prescription drugs are obtained from plants. As per WHO; about 80% of world population depend upon plants for the maintenance and cure of general health and ailments. Plants also serve as building block for the raw material required for the synthesis of drugs and pharmaceutical products. Since ancient times plants remained the source for herbal medicines, used by indigenous systems of medicine by the traditional practitioners. Plants are the source for new chemical entities (NCE) and drugs for the newer discovery.

I. Plants as a Source of Drugs

Plants are used as therapeutic resources in several ways, as herbal teas or other home-made remedies made from medicinal plants. (Medicinal plant is any plant used in order to relieve, prevent, and cure disease or to alter any physiological and pathological process in living being or any plant used as raw material or precursor for the synthesis of medicine). They can be used as crude extracts or therapeutic fractions in pharmaceutical preparation (such as tinctures, fluid extracts, powder or pills and capsules) and they are subjected to isolation of pure compounds as a medicine. About 26% of drugs prescribed world-wide come from plants, as per WHO more than 125 such active compounds being in current use, of the 252 drugs considered as basic and essential, 11% are exclusively of plant origin and number of synthetic drugs are obtained from the precursor of plant origin. Examples of important drugs obtained from plant origin are digoxin from *Digitalis* spp., atropine from *Atropa belladonna*, ajmalicine from *Rauwolfia* spp., artemisinin from *Artemisia* spp., berberine from *Berberis hydrastis*, caffeine from *Camellia sinensis*, codeine from *Papaver somniferum*, digitoxin, digoxin and gitoxin from *Digitalis* spp., podophylotoxin from *Podophyllum peltatum*, hyoscyamine from *Hyoscyamus niger*, morphine from *Papaver somniferum*, peclitaxel from *Taxus* spp., quinine from *Cinchona ledgeriana*, reserpine from *Rauwolfia serpentina*, vincristine and vinblastine from *Catharanthus roseus* and zingiberene from *Zingiber officinalis*. It is estimated that about 60% of antitumour and anti-infectious drugs are already in the market are from the natural origin as most of them yet are not to be synthesised hence are obtained from cultivated or the wild source.

The WHO has included phytotherapy in its health programs in developing countries. Eastern countries, such as China and India have well-developed herbal medicine industries and Latin American countries have been investing in research programs in medicinal plants, standardisation and regulation of phytomedicinal products. In Germany 50% of phytomedicinal products are sold on medical prescription. In North America phytomedicinal products are sold as health foods.

The National Cancer Institute, USA (NCI) has tested more than 50,000 plant samples for anti-HIV activity and about 33,000 samples for antitumour activity.

II. Animals as a Source of Drug

A number of medicines are either contain animal products in the form of tablets, injections, capsules, creams, mixture and vaccines, e.g. **gelatin** (partially hydrolysed collagen usually obtained from bovine (beef) or porcine (pig) in origin. Gelatin is used for making the capsules shell and used as a stabilisers in pharmaceutical products such as vaccines. **Heparin**, an anticoagulant is prepared from a porcine.

Out of 252 essential chemicals selected by WHO, 8.7% are from animals, and out of 150 prescription drugs used in United States of America, 27 are from animals.

Animals used as source of drugs in therapeutics:
Thyroid-modified preparations of thyroid glands of sheep and pigs.

Conjugated oestrogens: These are amorphous preparations containing water soluble conjugated form of mixed oestrogen obtained from urine of pregnant mares, used in the treatment of menopausal systems in female and in dysmenorrhea.

Insulin-prepared from cattles and pigs:

Oxytocin: It is polypeptide hormone secreted by posterior pituitary glands.

Enzymes: Pancreatin, tryptophan, chymotrypsin, fibrinolysin, pepsin and hyallourinidase.

Animal extractive organs: Liver and stomach preparation and bile.

Natural products from insects: Antimicrobial, antifungal, antiviral, anticancer, antioxidant, anti-inflammatory and immunomodulator.

Insects used are ant, bees, wasp, bettels, cockroaches, termites, flies, true bugs and moth.

Entomotherapy (medical use of insects) is an alternative to modern therapy in the many parts of the world including Korea, India, Mexico, China, Spain, Brazil, etc.

Ants and ant by products are used throughout the globe in folk medicine. For example, in Northern India, scabies, wounds and boils are treated through topical applications of paste made from crushed black ants (*Bothroponera rufipes*).

Official Drugs Obtained from Animals

Cantharidin, cochineal, leeches, gelatin, galls, ichthammol, lactose and honey:

Cantharidin: It is obtained from dried beetle (*Lytta vesicatoria*) Latr. Family Meloidae. Major constituent is cantharidin and used for the topical medication.

Cochineal: It is dried female insect *Dactylopius coccus* costa, enclosing the numerous eggs and young larvae, family Coccidae. It contain carminic acid used as colouring agent, therapeutically used in the treatment of urine retention as renal capillary relaxation.

Leeches: *Hirudo medicinalis* Linn (Speckled leech), *Hirudo quinquestriatus* Schmarda (Australian leech), used to revive intraocular pressure in acute glaucoma and in cardiovascular diseases (chemical derived from the saliva of leech).

Gelatin: It is an animal protein obtained from the skin and bones of animals, used in the pharmaceutical preparations and in osteoarthritis and osteoporosis.

Galls (Nut gall, Aleppo galls): It is an excrescent formed on young shoot of *Quercus infectoria* Olivier family Fagaceae used as a source of tannic acid.

Ichthammol: Synonyms ammonium bituminosulfonate, it is the fossil remains of fishes and other marine animals. It is the product of natural origin obtained by dry distillation of sulfur-rich oil shale, followed by sulfonation, and subsequent-neutralisation with ammonia (*Bituminous Schists*). It is used in the treatment of eczema, psoriasis, etc. by local application.

Honey: It is the saccharine secretion deposited in the honeycomb by bee *Apis mellifera* Linn of family Apidae, used as nutrient and sweetener.

Drugs obtained from porcine: There are number of drugs obtained from porcine. For example, anticoagulant (Heparin sodium), Vaccines (rotavirus live and attenuated vaccine, Zoster virus vaccine, etc.) digestive enzymes (amylase, lipase, protease enzymes, etc.)

Bovine: Digestive supplements (*Lactobacillus acidophilus, Bovine colostrums,* etc.) plasma volume expander (polygeline), vaccines (hepatitis A vaccine, *Salmonella typhi* live vaccine, etc.) Insulin preparations (insulin, isophane, etc.) and other pharmacological preparation like collagen, haemostatic agents, etc.

Chinese Hamster Ovary (CHO) Cells: Drugs obtained are haemostatic agents, antiplastic, immunomodulator, enzyme replacement therapy, pituitary hormones, etc.

Murine (mouse): Drugs obtained are antineoplastic agents (avastin, herceptin, mabthera, etc.), immunomodifier (remicade, simulect, etc.), anticoagulant (reopro).

Eggs: Number of vaccines are obtained from eggs like influenza virus H1N1, rabies, Coxiella, a Pandemic vaccine, etc.

Equine (Horse): Drugs obtained are antivenom (antithymocyte globulin, black snake antivenom, death adder antivenom), gonadal hormones and haemostatic agents, etc.

Above all, chitin, lanolin, histoplasmin, coccidioidin, immune globulins, etc.

III. Marine Source of Drugs

Sea covers about 70% of the earth, is the promising source of new biological active compounds, because of amazing biological diversity of the sea. The rate of discovery of marine species has been higher than terrestrial since the 1950S, but only 16% of all named species on earth are marine. From the diversity point of view, the ocean is a more diverse as compared to the plant and animal on the land. Marine invertebrates such as sponges, cnidarians and ascidians constitute largest amount of biomass of marine microfauna, which is rich source of both biological and chemical diversity which has been the unique source of biological active compounds for the industrial development as pharmaceuticals, cosmetics and nutritional supplements. During the last few decades numerous novel biologically active compounds have been isolated from the marine organism such as **antibacterial, antiviral, anticoagulants, antimicrobial, antibiotics, anti-inflammatory, antianthelmintic, anticancer, antitumour** and **cardiovascular active compounds**. Marine compounds reported to act on a variety of molecular targets and thus could potentially contribute to several pharmacologic classes. Hence pharmacological research with marine chemicals continue to contribute towards potentially novel chemical leads to the ongoing global search for therapeutic agents in the treatment of number of diseases. Chemicals are polyketides, peptides, nitrogen containing compounds, terpenes, steroids, polysaccharides, etc.

IIIa. Antibiotics from Microorganisms

Fungi are best source of natural antibacterial and antifungal compounds. It has been reported that 38–59% of test extracts from marine fungi exhibited antibacterial and antifungal activities. The dominant genera in the marine fungi producing antibacterial and antimicrobial compounds are: *Aspergillus* genus (31 strains) and *Penicillium* genus (18 strains).

Examples
Nitrogen Containing Compounds

Peptides: Cyclopeptides, and desmethylisation and few novel peptides isolated from mangrove fungi *Phomopsis* spp. and *Astromyces cruciatus*.

Indole alkaloids example, Asporyzin isolated from *Aspergillus oryzae* active against Gram +ve and Gram –ve bacteria.

Cristatumins A, D and E were isolated from *Eurotium cristatum* and *E. herbariorum* active against both *E. coli* and *S. aureus*.

Pyridines and Pyridone

Isolated from *Trichoderma species* showed activities against Gram+ve *B. subtilis* and *S. epidermidis* and antifungal activity against *Candida albicans* compounds named are trichodin A to D.

Piperazine and Pyrimidine/Pyrimidinone Alkaloids

Aspergicin from *Aspergillus* species derived from mangroves epiphytic fungi.

Steroids and Terpenoids

There are number of steroids and terpenoids compounds isolated from fungi having antifungal activities against *A. niger* and *Alternaria brassicae* and also have antibacterial activities against *E. coli* and *S. aureus*. For example, penicisteroids A. About fifty compounds are reported from *Aspergillus ustus* and *Penicillium chrysogenum*.

Antibacterial sequiterpenoids isolated from *Aspergillus* species and *Leucostoma persoonii*, e.g. Aspergiterpinoids, (–) sydonol and (–) sydonic acid.

Polyketides: Quinones, anthraquinones, xanthones and quinine derivatives. Hence, there is big list of compounds reported from fungi.

More than 5,300 products are reported from sponges and algae, few of them are mentioned below:

Two quinolinols (2n-pentyl-4-quinolinol and 2n-heptyl-4-quinolinol) are isolated from yellow marine *Pseudomonas bromoutilis* of the *Altermonas* species.

A new antibiotic, aplasmomycin, active against Gram +ve bacteria including *Mycobacteria in vitro,* and plasmodia *in vivo* are reported from ss-20 strain of *Streptomyces griseus* from shallow sea.

The anticancer antibiotics has also been reported from culture broth of marine actinomycete of *Actinomadura* species, e.g. chandrananimycins A, B and C.

Antibiotics from Sponges

Sponges have greatest percentage of anti-microbial activity but are difficult to identify hence many sponges having antimicrobial activity still remained unidentified. However, caribbean sponge of the *Agelas* species reported to have remarkable antimicrobial activity against *S. subtilis, E. coli* and *P. atroventum.*

Antibiotics from Algae

Red algae of the genus *Laurencia* contain sesquiterpene phenols as their antibiotic metabolites (Laurinterol and debromo-laurinterol).

Antibiotics from Tunicate

Large quantities of geranyl hydroquinone are reported from the genus *Aplidum.*

Hence, the ocean continue to provide novel marine-derived antibiotics.

Anti-inflammatory Drugs from Marine

Sesquiterpene, diterpenes, steroids, poly-saccharides, alkaloids, fatty acids, proteins and other chemical compounds are isolated from marine organism having anti-inflammatory activities. Following are few examples:

From algae: Terpenoids (apo-9′ Fucoxanthinone, asta-Xanthin), polyketide (6 6-bieckol).

From sponges: Alkaloids (benzamide A and B), and from fungus alkaloid (Bis-N-norgliovictin).

Antituberculosis Drugs from Marine

Tuberculosis (TB), caused mainly by the *Mycobacterium tuberculosis,* is the second cause of death worldwide due to infectious disease, after human immunodeficiency virus (HIV/AIDS), In 2012 World Health Organisation (WHO, Geneva, Switzerland) reported almost nine million new cases of TB, 1.3 million deaths due to TB and 0.3 million deaths resulting from a co-infection with HIV and TB.

Marine derived natural and semisynthetic compounds examined for *in vitro* activity against *Mycobacterium tuberculosis.* Three new classes of compounds including c-19 hydroxy steroids, scalarin sesquiterpenoids and tetrabromo spiros cyclohexadienyl isoxazolines have been identified as having potential as leads for continued investigations as new tuberculosis agents.

Following is the list of compounds have already been confirmed having antituberculosis activity.

Terpenoids (asperterpenoid A, S. flava-diterpene), terpenoid glycoside (lobophorin G), alkaloid (brevianamide S) and polyketide (urdamycinone).

Antiviral Compounds

Examples of the compounds isolated from sponge, soft coral and fungus used in the treatment by human herpes simplex virus inhibition, HIV protease inhibition, HIV replication inhibition, influenza virus, neuraminidase inhibition and H1N1 influenza virus inhibition are terpenoids (L. arboreum, halistanol sulphate), terpenoid alkaloid (stachyflin), polyketide (massarilactone-H).

Cardiovascular System and Neurophysiological Agents

Lepadiformines A and B (alkaloid) cardiac inward rectifying K^+ current inhibition, zooxanthellamide (polyketide). Vasoconstriction of rat blood.

Immune System Effecting Compounds

Glycosphingolipids (demicoside), obtained from sponge, stimulate the spleen cell pro-liferation.

Laminarin (polysaccharide) obtained from algae, inhibit the lymphocyte apoptosis.

Cucumariosides (triterpene oligoglycoside), from sea cucumber, stimulates the lymphocytes and neutrophils.

Lobocrassin B (terpenoid), from soft coral, inhibits the dendritic cell activation.

Penicacid (polyketide), isolated from fungus, inhibits the T-lymphocyte proliferation.

Nervous System Affecting Compounds

Asteropsin A (peptide), isolated from sponge, effects the enhancement of neuronal Ca^{2+} influx.

C-consors peptide, isolated from cone snail, causes the muscle relaxation induction.

Convolutamydine A (alkaloid), obtained from Bryozoa (phylum of aquatic invertebrate), has anti-nociceptive activity.

Serinolamide b (alkaloid), obtained from bacterium, effects the CB_1 and CB_2 binding.

FDA Approved Marine Anti-cancer Drugs from Invertebrates

Cytarabine, also known as cytosine arabinoside, obtained from sponges is used in chemotherapy medication for the treatment of acute myeloid leukemia and non-Hodgkins lymphoma. It acts as DNA polymerase inhibitor.

Ziconotide (peptide), isolated from cone snail, is used as a modulator of neuronal calcium channels (kill pain).

Trabectedin (alkaloid), isolated from tunicate, is anti-cancer agent. It inhibit the cancer cell growth and also affect the tumor micro-environments.

Eribulin mesylata (Macrolide) isolated from sponge, is an anti-breast cancer compound.

Bren tuximab (antibody drug conjugate), obtained from Mollusk, effective in lymphoma.

IV. Plants Tissue Culture

Proved to be important source of drugs either through organogenesis or by genetic transformation. Plant tissue culture has great potential as a source of valuable secondary metabolites, used as pharmaceuticals, nutraceuticals and additives. Moreover, the production by plant tissue culture is independent of environmental conditions and quality fluctuations unlike the conventional agriculture production of secondary metabolites: alkaloids, flavonoids, terpenoids, carotenoids, saponins, steroidal alkaloids, sterols, tannins and several others components.

Since the last decade considerable success has been achieved in increasing the yield of secondary plant metabolites because of recent advances in the field of plant biotechnology by controlling the factors affecting its synthesis and/or accumulation. Examples of plant derived products of importance; ajmaline (*Rauwolfia serpentina*), camptothecin (*Camptotheca acuminate*), codeine (*Papaver somniferum*), colchicine (*Colchicum autumnale*), elipticine (*Ochorosia elliptica*), shikonin (*Lithospermum erythrorhizon*), taxol (*Taxus brevifolia*), vinblastine (*Catharanthus roseus*).

Examples of food additives from plant cell culture: Anthocyanins, crocin, carotenoids, anthraquinones and napthaquinones. Flavours (vanillin, garlic, coffee and cocoa, etc.). Pungent (capsaicin), sweetner (stevioside, glycyrrhizin).

It is also possible to increase the yield of secondary metabolites by the selection of high-yielding cell lines, e.g. Shikonin (*Lithospermum erythrorhizon*), Serpentine (*Catharanthus roseus*), Sanguinarine (*Papaver somniferum*), Anthraquinone (*Morinda citrifolia*).

To overcome the hurdles of harvesting and extraction processing, the tissue culture is the alternative method of assured regular uniform supply of the material for the whole years. Moreover most of the secondary metabolites accumulate after certain age or maturity of the plant, examples cinchona, rauwolfia, camptotheca, taxus, Ochrosia spp., etc. attain maturity in few years to accumulate the active compounds in high amounts, as well as it is difficult to increase the area of cultivation for particular species and growth of plants takes its own course of time. To meet the ever increasing demand the natural source is not sufficient, the plant cell/tissue culture is the only alternative source.

ORGANISED AND UNORGANISED DRUGS

Crude drugs are classified into two main classes:

I. Organised Drugs

As the name indicates, these drugs are cellular in nature, having definite shape and size.

These are obtained from plants/animals, as entire or parts of the plants/animals; aerial part or herbs; leaf, flowers, fruits, seeds, stem, roots, rhizomes and bulb. They can be characterised by morphological, microscopical and chemical tests.

Drugs from aerial part

These are herbaceous in nature and generally short-lived and outgrowth is rapid. They are small in size (< 2 feet), soft and short, e.g. chirayata (*Swertia chirata* Wall), brahmi (*Bacopa monnieri* Linn), pudina (*Mentha arvensis* Linn), tulsi (*Ocimum sanctum* Linn), kalmegh (*Andrographis paniculata* Burm), lajwanti (*Mimosa pudica* Linn), etc.

Leaves

Leaves arise out of the stem. They prepare food for the plant through photosynthesis and they also store some secondary metabolites. Hence they are used as drug, e.g. Deadly nightshade (*Atropa belladonna* L), Digitalis common name tilpushpi (Hindi) foxglove (English) (*Digilalis purpura* Linn), Paan patta (Betal) (*Piper betle* Linn), Chai (Tea plant) (*Camellia sinensis* Kuntze), Sanai patti (Hindi), Senna leaflet (English) *Cassia acutifolia* Delite (Botanical source).

Flowers

Flowers are the essential reproductive organ of a plant, generally coloured to attract the insects for pollination. Flowers are of great botanical importance but few of them are used as drug in pharmacy, e.g. Jasmine (*Jasminum grandiflorum* L), Chamomile (*Matricaria recutita* L), Calendula (*Calendula officinalis*), Primrose (*Primula veris* L, *P. officinalis* Linn), Rose (*Rosa damascena, R. gallica, R. alba*), hops (*Humulus lupulus* L).

Fruits and Seeds

Fruit is a matured ovary of the plant. It is the organ of plant (angiosperm) which disseminates seeds. Seeds are matured ovule.

Fruits and seeds have yielded important therapeutical drugs, e.g. Caraway (*Carum carvi* L), Fennel (*Foeniculum vulgare* Miller), Nutmeg (*Myristica fragrans* Houtt), Linseed (*Linum usitatissimum* Linn), Coriander (*Coriandrum sativum* Linn), Colchicum seed (*Colchicum luteum* Baker), Fenugreek (*Trigonella foenum-graecum* Linn), Nux vomica (*Strychnos nux-vomica* Linn), Ispaghula (*Plantago ovate* Forssk), Mustard (rai) (*Brassica juncea* Czern & Coss), white mustard (*Sinapis alba* L).

Stem

It transports water and minerals from the soil to the other part of the plant. Moreover, it supports the plant. Woody species has clear distinction between bark (outer) and wood (inner), e.g. drugs being used in medicine as stem: Ephedra (*Ephedra sinica* Stapf), liquorice (*Glycyrrhiza glabra* Linn).

Bark

Bark consists of all tissue outside the cambium. In botany, all the tissue lying outside periderm. The pharmacognostical bark consists of epidermis, primary cortex, endodermis, pericycle and phloem.

Following are medicinally important barks:

Cinchona: *Cinchona succirubra* pavon

Cascara: *Rhamnus purshiana* DC

Quillaia: *Quillaja saponaria*

Wild cherry bark: *Prunus serotina*

Cinnamon: *Cinnamomum zeylanicum*

Kurchi: *Holarrhena antidysenterica.*

Wood

Inner of the stem consisting of xylem tissue, e.g. Quassia: *Picrasma excelsa* also known as Jamaica quassia.

Sandal wood: *Santalum album.*

Root

It develops from the radicle (tap root) or its branches or adventitious. It is main organ of the plant for the uptake of water and inorganic nutrients. It generally stores secondary metabolites and surplus energy in the form of starch and roots inulin (polysaccharide).

Following are medicinally important roots:

Jalap: *Ipomoea purga*

Aconite: Dried roots of *Aconitum napellus*

Belladonna: Roots of *Atropa belladonna*

Rauwolfia: *Rauwolfia serpentina*

Senega: *Polygala senega* L

Velerian root: *Valeriana officinalis, Valeriana wallichii*

Liquorice: *Glycyrrhiza glabra* Kuth.

Rhizomes: Zinger: *Zingber officinalis*

Rhubarb: *Rheum palmatum* L

Podophyllum: *Podophyllum hexandrum*

Ipecac: *Ciphaelis ipecacuanha* (Brotero)

Sarsaparilla: *Smilax regelii* Kilip

Bulb: Scilla (Squill) *Urginea maritina*

Diascorea: *Dioscorea deltoidea* Wall

Garlic: *Allium sativum* Linn

Onion: *Allium cepa* Linn.

II. Unorganised Drugs

Unorganised drugs are solid, semisolid or liquid in nature. They do not have specific shape, size and structure and are without cellular structure.

They are obtained from plants or animals by extraction such as decoction, e.g. agar; expression, e.g. olive oil; distillation, e.g. volatile oils; incision, e.g. opium and natural secretion like resin, oleo resin; exudates, gums; dried juices, e.g. aloe.

These drugs can be identified and characterised by their colour, odour, fracture, solubilities in organic solvents (ether chloroform or alcohol) and by specific chemical tests.

Classification

1. **Dried juice,** e.g. Aloe
2. **Latex,** e.g. opium
3. **Extracts,** e.g. Catechu, agar
4. **Oil and fats,** e.g. Olive oil, cod liver oil, almond oil, lard wool fat.
5. **Gums,** e.g. Tragacanth, acacia gum.
6. **Resins,** e.g. Colophony, myrrh.
7. **Waxes:** Spermaceti, beeswax.
8. **Volatile oils:** Clove oil, cinnamon oil.
9. **Balsams:** Storax, tolu, benzoin.

- **Aloe:** It is dried form of juice. The residue obtained by evaporating the liquid to dryness, obtained by draining from the leaves cut from various species of Aloe. *Aloe ferox* Mill yield Cape aloe. *Aloe vera* Linn var. officinalis, family Liliaceae.

  Aloe contain aloin and other water-soluble components. It is an anthraquinone containing drug used as laxative, and in skin diseases and as inflammatory.

- **Latices (Latex):** Latex is the milky aqueous liquid formed in certain plants in tube-like structures which are either known as vessels or special cells called coenocytes (laticiferous cells) formed by breakdown of the dividing cell walls formed by nuclear division. Plants belonging to family Euphorbiaceae.

  Opium is the only official latex, occurs in laticiferous vessels in the walls of unripe capsules of *Papaver somniferum*, family Papaveraceae.

  Gutta-percha is the dried purified latex occurs in laticiferous vessels in the trunk of species of *Palaquium* and *Payena* tree indigenous to Sumatra, Ceylon and Peninsula.

- **Juices:** Juices are aqueous liquid containing dissolved substances occurring in specialised tissue other than laticiferous cells or vessels. Juices are obtained by incisions, e.g. dried form of juice of aloe.

- **Extracts:** Extracts are the water soluble components leftover after the evaporation. For the extraction usually decoction is employed to isolate the constituents drug, e.g. catechu and agar.

Catechu

Synonyms: Pale catechu, Gambier

Botanical source: A dried aqueous extract prepared from the leaves and young shoots of *Uncaria gambir* (Hunter) Roxb, family Rubiaceae. It contains catechin, an astringent substance.

It is available as reddish brown coloured or pale brown coloured cubes about 2–5 cm along edges. Readily broken and reduced to powder. Taste is astringent and gives positive test for tannins.

Agar

Agar is the dried, hydrophilic, colloidal substance extracted from: (i) *Gelidium cartilagineum* (Linn) Gaillon, family Gellidiaceae. (ii) *Gracilaria confervoides* (Linn) Greville, family Gracilariaceae. (iii) Red alge (class Rhodophyceae).

Agar may be light yellowish orange, yellowish grey to pale yellow to colourless, brittle, odourless with mucilaginous taste.

Chemically, it is the calcium salt of strongly ionised, acidic polysaccharides. It contains two major compounds—agarose and agropectin. Used as laxative and as suspending agent.

Exudates

* **Gums:** Gums are formed by degenerative changes in cell walls by enzyme action, the process is called **gummosis**. Gums are insoluble in alcohol and organic solvents but they swell and form mucilaginous mixture with water.

  The gums exude from tree and shrubs in tears like striated nodules or amorphous lumps. On drying they become hard, glassy, in different colours. For example:

  Gum acacia: White to pale amber.

  Karaya gum: Pale grey to dark brown.

  Tragacanth: White to dark brown.

  Gum exudes from plant by making incision, injury or stripping the bark of the tree or shrub. Excretion of exudation is affected by temperature and humidity.

  Use: They are used as thickening, emulsifying and stabilising agents, e.g. Gum acacia, Gum tragacanth.

  Gum acacia: *Synonyms:* Gum acacia; Gum arabica.

  Source: Dried gummy exudation from the stem and branches of *Acacia senegal* wild and other species of Acacia.

  Family Leguminosae: Gum acacia tears are rounded or ovoid 0.5–6.0 cm in diameter or even sometimes are angular fragments. They are colourless or pale yellow in colour but freshly broken pieces are opaque and glassy in appearance.

However, the Indian acacia tears are too dark in colour, because of tannins. Official gum acacia is native to Africa, i.e. kordofan or sudan gum, which is completely soluble in water to give mucilaginous suspension, whereas Indian gum has insoluble material in the suspension.

Used as emulsifying, suspending and binding agents.

Indian (ghatti) gum is exuded from the stem of *Anogeissus latifolia* Wallich family Combretaceae.

Tragacanth

Synonym: Gum Dragon

Source: Dried gummy exudation obtained by incision from *Astragalus gummifer* Labill and some other species of *Astragalus* (Persian tragacanth), family Leguminosae.

Indian tragacanth is obtained from *Sterculia urens* Roxb and other species of *Sterculia*. This is obtained by incision given on trees grown wild in India. It is of inferior quality.

Tragacanth appears as ribbon-like flakes about 23 × 12 mm in size usually curved and twisted.

They are white or pale yellow; more or less translucent; **Fracture** is short and horny and have no odour.

Tragacanth is partially soluble in water. The soluble portion is called **tragacanthin** and insoluble portion termed **bassorin.** Tragacanthin is a complex carbohydrate whereas the bassorin contains along with complex carbohydrate the sugars; tragacanthose and xylose.

Uses: Emulsifying, suspending and thickening agent in pharmaceutical formulation.

* **Resin, Gum resin and Oleo resin:**
  Resins used in pharmacy are obtained from living natural sources. Most of them are plant product except shellac an insect.

  Resins are solid amorphous substance obtained from plants, produced in special tubes (Resin ducts).

  Resins are insoluble in water and petroleum ether but-dissolve all most completely in alcohol, chloroform and ether. On heating they soften and finally melt. **Chemically, they are made-up of complex mixture of resin acids, alcohols (resinols) phenols (resinotannols), esters (consisting mostly of resinols and cinnamic, benzoic and ferulic acids) and also contain neutral substance known as resenes.**

A solution of resin in volatile oil, when painted on a smooth surface, they immediately evaporate leaving behind hard transparent film.

Classification of resinous exudates: The resinous exudates may contain **resin only**, e.g. benzoin.

Resin and volatile oil together, i.e. oleo resin, e.g. turpentine and copaiba, may be associated with gum and volatile oil together known as **oleo gum resin**, e.g. myrrh.

When gum resin or oleo-gum resin contains benzoin or cinnamic acid alone or combined form the resin are known as **balsams**, e.g. balsam tolu, balsam peru and storax.

Resin

Benzoin

Sumatra and Siam benzoin

Sumatra benzoin: It is obtained from incised stem of *Styrax benzoin* and *S. paralleloneurus* Perkins. In commerce known as Sumatra benzoin.

Note: Styrax is the Greek name of storax.

Family: Styraceae

Sumatra benzoin occurs as blocks or irregular masses composed of different size tears embedded in translucent or opaque matrix.

Tears are milky white and become soft on warming. The matrix is reddish or greyish brown.

Chemical composition: It contains balsamic acids (6%), triterpene acids and traces of vanillin and esters (phenylpropyl cinnamate, etc.).

Siam benzoin: It is made from hard, brittle, flattened tears, from 1 to 5 cm long, pale yellowish-brown, the fractured surface is milky white in appearance.

Chemically contain mainly coniferyl benzoate (60–70%) along with small amount of free benzoic acid (10%), triterpenes (siaresinol 6%) and traces of vanillin.

Solubility: Sumatra benzoin yields alcohol soluble extractive not <75%, whereas the Siam benzoin yields not <90% extractive.

Uses: Antiseptic, stimulant, expectorant and diuretic.

Oleo-resin

Turpentine

Turpentine (volatile oil) is collected from the long pine leaves of *Pinus palustris* Miller and from other species of *Pinus* family Pinaceae.

The oleo resin is secreted in ducts located directly beneath the cambium in the sapwood. The collected oleo resin on steam distillation yields volatile oil (turpentine oil). The product of the first year cutting is of superior quality and is known as "Virgin" turpentine. The residue left over after filtration while hot is known as rosin or colophony.

The United States of America is major producer of turpentine oil. Important constituents of turpentine oil are α-pinene (64%) and β-pinene (33%).

Uses: Used as counterirritant in the OTC drugs.

Colophony or Rosin: It is the residue left over after distilling the volatile oil from the oleo-resin collected from various species of Pinus family Pinaceae.

Major supplier south-east USA and south-west France.

Colophony usually occurs as shiny, sharp, angular fragments, translucent often covered with yellowish dust.

It is hard, brittle and easily pulverisable and soluble in alcohol, ether, benzene, carbon disulfide, acetic acid, fixed oils, volatile oil and in solution of sodium or potassium hydroxide (alkali).

Odour: Like turpentine. On heating, a sticky mass is formed.

Colophony consists of 80 to 90% anhydride of abietic acid; sylvic acid (decomposition product of abietic acid); saponic acid, pimaric acid and resene (hydrocarbon).

Uses: Used as stiffening agent in plasters and ointments. Commercially, it is used in the manufacture of varnishes and paint dryer.

Copaiba (oleo-resin)

Botanical source: It is an oleo-resin obtained from South American species of *Copaifera* Linn family Leguminosae.

The oleo-resin is formed in schizolysigenous cavities in the wood. The trees are tapped or boxed in the centre. The colour of the resin is yellow to yellowish brown depending on the varieties mixed together. *C. reticulata* (yellowish brown), *C. guianensis* (yellowish brown), *C. multijuga* (brown) and *C. officinalis* (yellowish brown).

Odour: Aromatic because of volatile content.

Taste: Bitter, acrid and persistent.

Uses: Used as genitourinary disinfectant.

Gum resins

As the name indicates it contains gum and resin but in some cases small proportion of volatile oils.

Composition of gum is also like gum acacia. Gum resins form emulsion with water, they are present in plant cells as such (emulsion) hence they exude from the plant on giving incision and dries at the surface, e.g. Asafoetida.

Oleo-gum resin

Asafoetida

Botanical source: Obtained by incision from the living roots and rhizome of *Ferula foetida* Regel and *F. rubricaulis* Boiss and other species of Ferula, family Umbelliferae.

Geographical source: Afghanistan (Distt. Karan and Chagai) and eastern Persia.

Asafoetida occurs as agglutinated tears or as separate ovoid tears (1–4 cm in diameter). Their colour is yellowish-white, when fresh but turns pinkish, violet-streaked and finally reddish brown. They are soft when fresh but become hard and brittle on drying. **Odour** is alliaceous, and **taste** is bitter or acrid.

Composition: The drug contains about 5–20% of volatile oils, 40–65% of resin and 25% of gum and small quantities of terpenes. Resin consists of asaresinotannol free or in combination with ferulic acid.

The oil contain sulphur compounds, responsible for the evil smell of asafoetida.

Contains at least 24 sesquiterpene hydrocarbons and number of diterpenes.

Uses: Used as carminative, expectorant, antispasmodic and laxative.

Myrrh

The name myrrh is derived from the Arabic 'murr', meaning bitter; 'commiphora' is Greek means gum bearing, "molmol" is the native Somali.

Botanical source: The oleo-gum resin obtained from the stem of *Commiphora molmol* Eng and other species of *Commiphora*.

Family: Burseraceae

Geographical source: Somaliland (central and western).

The myrrh exudes naturally or after the incision given in the bark of the plant. When freshly exuded it is yellowish in colour but soon becomes harder and darker in colour and then it is collected. Two varieties of myrrh are available– **Somali** (African) and **Yemen** myrrh (Arabian) but the Somali myrrh considered to be of better quality. Commercially Somali myrrh is the main supply.

Composition: Myrrh contains volatile oils responsible for the characteristic odour of myrrh, which contains eugenol, m-cresol and cuminaldehyde. On exposure to air, gets resinified.

Resin contents are about 25 to 40%; containing resin acid (α-β-commiphoric acid) resene and phenolic compounds.

Gum is about 60% consisting of soluble and insoluble portion forming mucilage with water that does not ferment readily.

Uses: Stomachic, stimulant, and as mouth wash; being astringent.

Balsams

Balsams are aromatic, oily and resinous mixtures that contain large proportions of benzoic, cinnamic or both the acids or esters of these acids.

Storax

It is the balsam obtained from the wounded trunk of *Liquidambar orientalis* Miller (Levant storx); *L. styraciflua* Linn (American storax).

Family: Hamamelidaceae.

The balsam storax is pathological product which exudes into natural pockets (new wood formed) between the bark and wood, formed by injury, in large quantity even up to 4 kg. It is scraped with a knife having small curved blade and collected into the containers. It is exported in tin cans.

The **Levant storax** is greyish to greyish-brown in colour, viscid, more or less opaque and semisolid mass. It is deposited as dark brown oleo-resin layers on standing.

The **American storax** is nearly clear yellowish brown semisolid that becomes hard, opaque and darker coloured on standing **odour:** Balsamic.

Solubility: Insoluble in water. Completely soluble is warm alcohol.

Chemistry

Storax contains cinnamic acid and their esters. Made from alcohol storesinol, partly in free state and partly in combined form. It also contains vanillin responsible for the odour.

Pharmacopoeial requirement is that storax should contain balsamic acid up to 30% with reference to the substance dried on water bath for one hour.

Uses: It is component of compound benzoin tincture and used as stimulant and expectorant.

Balsam of Tolu

Name tolu is on the name of place tolu near Cortagena.

Botanical source: Solid or semisolid resin obtained by incision from the trunk of *Myroxylon balsamum* Linn and *Myroxylon toluifera* H.B. and K.

Family: Leguminosae

Geographical source: Columbia, San Salvador (United States) gets balsam and tolu from Great Britain.

This balsam is a pathological product secreted in oleo-resin duct in the new wood, formed as a result of injury. It is obtained from trees by making V-shaped incision in the wood through bark.

Balsam tolu occurs as plastic solid that gradually hardens, becoming yellowish brown to brown. Thin layers are translucent, dried one is brittle and shows numerous crystals of cinnamic acid. **Odour** resembles vanilla; **taste** is slightly pungent.

Composition

It contain cinnamic acid 10–15%, benzoic acid 6.8%, balsamic esters 7.5% made-up of chiefly benzyl benzoate with small amount of benzyl cinnamate and resin esters (75–80%), consisting of toluresinotannol along with cinnamic acid.

Uses: Used as flavouring in medicinal syrups, confectionary and chewing gums.

Balsam of peru

Botanical source: It is obtained from the trunk of *Myroxylon pereirae* (Royl) Klostzsch, after beating and scorching the bark.

Family: Leguminosae.

Peru refers to the early importation of the balsam into Spain via Lima, Peru.

The balsam is a pathological product, produced by injury to tree. The bark of the tree is removed by beating and scorching with torch. The intermediate strips are left uninjured to save the tree from dying. After the removal of bark, trunk is wrapped in rags, the saturated rags with balsams are changed with new one. The rags are boiled with water, on cooling the balsam settles out, recovered, strained and packed.

Peruvian balsam occurs as dark brown viscid liquid. In thin layer it appears reddish brown and translucent. Its **odour** is like vanilla and taste bitter, acrid and persistent.

Balsam peru contain 60–70% balsamic ester consisting of benzyl cinnamate and benzyl benzoate); resin esters (peru resinotannol, cinnamic and benzoic acid), vanillin, and free cinnamic acid.

Uses: Local protectant, rubifacient, antiseptic in alcohol solution or in the form of an ointment.

FURTHER READING

1. Alejandro M, Mayer S, et al. Marine pharmacology in 2012–2013.
2. Bruneton J. 1999. Pharmacognosy, Phytochemistry Medicinal Plants. 2nd ed. Lavoisier Publication.
3. Chemotaxonomy and Serotaxonomy—Google Books *https://books.google.com›Science›Life Sciences› Biochemistry*
4. Cronquist A. (1981). An integrated system of classification of flowering plants. Columbia University Press, New York.
5. Divya A. Pharmacognosy: Facts and Future. Research & Reviews: Journal of Pharmacognosy and Phytochemistry. 2015;3(2):1–8.
6. Doshi, et. al. Novel Antibiotics from Marine Sources. www.reseachgate.net (pdf) Antibiotics from Marine Organism.
7. Evans WC. 2009. Trease and Evans Pharmacognosy, 16th ed., Elsevier; New York.
8. Global Tuberculosis Report 2013. http://www. who.int/tb/publication/global_report/en/
9. Kalia AN. Textbook of Industrial Pharmacogonsy. (2005). CBS Publishers and Distributors, New Delhi.
10. Kirikar KR, Basu BD. Indian Medicinal Plants Vol. 1–4. Allahabad, India 1933.
11. Namraj Dhami. Trends in Pharmacognosy: A modern science of natural medicines. Journal of Herbal Medicine. 2013;3(4):123–31.
12. Quality control methods for herbal material— WHO, updated edition of quality control methods for medicinal plant materials, 1998. Through www.who.int
13. Rotblatt M, Ziment I, eds. 2002. Evidence-Based Herbal Medicine. Philadelphia: Hanley & BelfusInc.
14. Satyajit D Sarker. Pharmacog may in modern pharmacy curricula. Pharmacogn Mag. 2012; 8(30): 91–2.
15. Serotaxonomy/Encyclopedia.com https:// www.encyclopedia.com›science›serotaxonomy
16. Serotaxonomy: Definition, History and Roles/ Plant Taxonomy www.biologydiscussion.com› plant-taxonomy›serotaxonomy-definition
17. SMK. Rates Plants as source of Drugs Review. Toxicon. 2001;39:603–13.
18. Stuessy T. (1990). Plant Taxonomy. Columbia, NY.
19. Takhtazan AL. Outline of the classification of flowering plants (Magnoliophya). Bot Rev. 1980;46(3):225–359.
20. Thorne RF. Phytochemistry and angiosperm phylogeny: a summary statement. In: Young DA, Seigler DS (eds) Phytochemistry and angiosperm phylogeny. Praeger, New York, 1981;233–95.
21. Tyler VE, Brady LR, Robbers JE. 1988. Pharmacognosy, 9th Edition-Leo and Fabiger. Philadelphia.
22. Wallis TE. Textbook of pharmacognosy. CBS Publishers and Distributors, New Delhi, 2005; 68–101.
23. Wilson JE, Metzger KL. Trends in Taxonomy revealed by the published literature. Bio Science. 1998;48:121–8.

Chapter 2

Classification of Drugs

It is the arrangement of natural drugs into a sequence/group, based on their similarity in one of the following characters/category for study or research purpose.

Following are the different methods of drugs classification: Alphabetical, morphological, taxonomical, chemical, pharmacological, and serotaxonomical.

ALPHABETICAL

In this system of classification drugs are arranged in accordance with their first letter of the name (Latin/English) of drug/s in alphabetical order.

Merits

It is very simple and widely followed/accepted method of arranging the drugs moreover easy to introduced or delete any drug without much disturbance in the order/sequence.

Demerits

Main drawback of the system is the lack of differentiation between the sources of drug (plants/animals or mineral) origin. It is also not able to differentiate between organised or unorganised drugs.

This system is being followed by some Pharmacopoeias, monographs and reference books, e.g. European pharmacopoeia vol. I-III 1969–1975 (Latin titles), British pharmacopoeia vol, 11 1988 (English). British pharmaceutical codex 1979 reprinted in 1988 (English title). United States Dispensatory 1973 (English titles), British Herbal Pharmacopoeia 1983 (English titles), Indian Pharmacopoeia 1955 (Latin), Indian Pharmacopoeia 1966 (English).

For examples, acacia, aconite root, agar, agave, alaxander senna, atropa, balsam peru balsam tolu, belladonna, benzoin, capcicum, clove, cassia caraway, cinchona, digitalis, datura, ephedra, ergot, eucalyptus, fennel, fennugreek, garlic, gentian, ginger, honey, hyoscyamus, ipecac, ispaghula, jalap, jatropha, jute, kurchi, lard, lemon peel, liquorice, lobelia, mentha, menthol, myrrh, myrstica, nutmeg, nux vomica, olive oil, plantago, podophylum, quassia, rauwolfia, rhubarb, saffron, theobroma, cocoa, valerian, vinca, wallnut, woolfat, yeast, and yew.

MORPHOLOGICAL BASIS OF CLASSIFICATION

In this system of classification the drugs are classified on the basis of source of drug: Part of plant or animal having pharmacologically active compound(s).

For examples:

Leafy drugs: Belladonna, buchu, cocoa, digitalis hyoscyamus, stramonium, vasaka, etc.

Flowers: Clove chamomile, pyrethrum, artemesia, rose, saffron, (*Crocus sativus*) viola, etc.

Seeds: Cardamom, colchicum, nux vomica, nutmeg, strophanthus, psyllium, linseed, ispaghula, etc.

Fruits: Bael, senna pods, tamarind, dill, caraway, capsicum, colocynth, coriander, gokhru, etc.

Bark: Arjuna, ashoka cinnamon, cinchona, cascara, pacific yew, quillaia, kurchi, wild cherry, etc.

Wood: Quassia, sandalwood

Roots: Aconite, belladonna, ipecac, liquorice senega, valerian, gentian, rauwolfia, jalap (tuberous root), ipomea.

Subterrarian drugs

Rhizomes: Indian podophyllum, liquorice, malefern, rhubarb, ginger (*zingiber*).

Bulb: Scilla, garlic, onion.

Corm: Colchicum

Entire plant: Chirata, chondrus, Indian hemp, ephedra, lobelia, savin, etc.

Hairs/fibres: Cotton, hemp, jute, flax and silk.

Plants/animals secretions

Gums: Acacia, tragacanth, guargum

Resin: Balsams, colophony, benzoin, storax, etc.

Animal secretions: Venoms, honey, beeswax, gelatin.

Example of textbooks following this system: Wallis TE. (1967) Text Book of Pharmacognosy; Denston, TC (Revised Edition 2012) Text Book of Pharmacognosy.

Merits

Easy to identify for practical purpose.

Demerits

Lack in differentiation for the purpose of pharmacological evaluation.

TAXONOMICAL

In this system of classifications, drugs are arranged into phylum, class, order, family, genera and species.

Phylum or division: The plants are classified into six parts. Thallophytes; Bryophytes; Pteridophytes; Gymnosperms; Angiosperms (Dicotyledons and monocotyledons) (Flowchart 2.1).

Following are some of the families of pharmaceutical interest (Table 2.1).

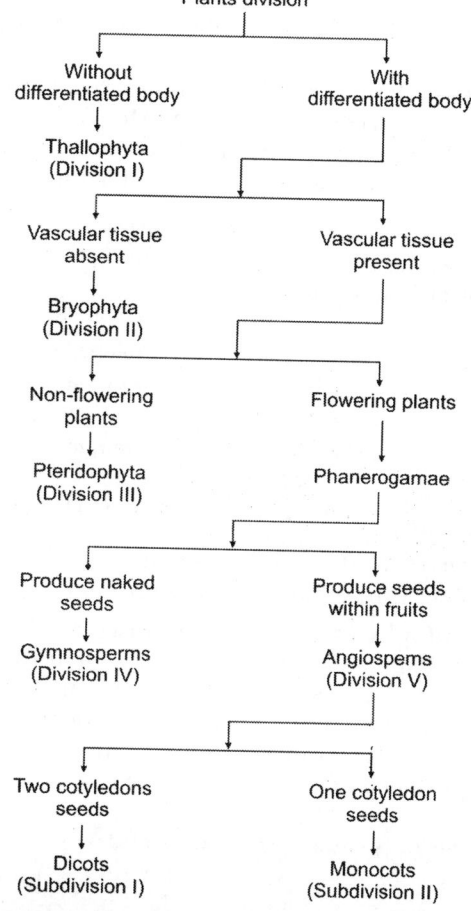

Flowchart 2.1: Plants division

Table 2.1: Thallophytes			
Phyla	*Order*	*Family*	*Drugs*
Bacteriophyta	Eubacteriales	Rhizobiaceae micrococcaccae	Rhizobium Spp.
Chrysophyta (Diatomeae)	Discales pennatales	Actinodiscaceae, Fragilariaceae Naviculariaceae	Japanese agar
Phaeophytas (Brown Algae)	Laminariales, Fucales	Laminariaceae Fucaceae Sargassaceae	Laminaria Spp. Fucus Sargassaceae Spp.
Rhodophyta (Red algae)	Galidales, Gigartinales	Galidaceae Gracilariaceae Gigartinaceae	Agar British Agar Carageen or Irish moss

Thallophytes (thalloid plants) relatively simple or 'lower plants', include fungi, lichens and algae usually found in moist or wet places and are autotrophic in nature. True roots and vascular system are absent.

Bryophytes and Pteridophytes

Both these phyla are not of much pharmaceutical interest:

Bryophyllum: The phylum is further divided into classes liverworts (Hepaticae) and Mosses (Musci).

Following is the division of bryophyte orders, families and genera of the interest of research:

Class	Order	Genera
Liverworts (Hepaticae)	Jungermaniinales Solenostoma	Bazzania
		Diplophyllum
	Jubulineales	lunularia
	Sphagnales (336 Spp)	Sphagnum
Mosses (Musci)	Dicranales (52 Spp)	Dicranum
	Funariales	Funaria (117 Spp)

Liverworts: It is a leaf-like thallus
Mosses (Musci) leafy plant with stem.

Pteridophytes: These are the vascular plants, that disperses spores but—they have roots, stems and leaves but lacking flowers and seeds. It comprise of ferns, horsetails and club mosses.

Classification of few of the medical importance pteridophyte (Table 2.2).

Gymnosperms are a group of naked seeds producing plants that includes conifers, cycads, ginkgo and gnetophytes.

Following is the list of a few orders of medical importance, as per the Engler's classification (Table 2.3).

Angiosperms: Plants of large group having about 13,164 genera and 369,000 known species) comprising flowering plants producing seeds enclosed within a carpel, include herbaceous plants, shrubs, grasses and most trees.

Angiosperm phylum is further subdivided into two division based on the number of cotyledons (dicotyledons and monocotyledon).

Angiosperm Dicotyledons

The dicotyledons are herbs, shrubs or trees. The seeds of which have two cotyledons—bearing leaves usually reticulately veined and typical stem structure with rings of open vascular bundles.

Dicotyledons plants include more than 250,000 species of herbs, shrubs and trees. Engler has divided the dicotyledons into two groups—Archichlamydeae and Sympetalae.

Archichlamydae: It contains those families, the flowers of which have either no perianth or a perianth that is differentiated into sepals and petals. It comprise of 37 orders and about 226 families.

Examples of few of them.

Table 2.2: Classification of pteridophytes			
Class	Order	Families	Genera
Filices	Filicales	Polypodiaceae (divided into many sub families)	Polypodium (about 50 Spp) Dryopteris (about 150 Spp) Pteris (280 Spp) Pteridium (1 Spp) Onychium (6 Spp) Dennstaedtia (70 Spp) Adiantum (about 200 Spp) Athyrium (180 Spp) Asplenium (300 Spp)
Articulatae	Equisetales	Equisetaceae	Equisetum (about 32 Spp)
Lycopsida	Lycopodiales	Lycopodiaceae	Lycopodium (about 450 Spp)

Table 2.3: Classification of order

Orders	Families	Genera
Cycadales	Cycadaceae	Cycas Spp.
Ginkolide	Ginkgoaceae	Ginkgo biloba
Comiferal	Pinaceae Taxodiaceae	Pinus Spp.
	Cupressaceae	Juniperus Spp
	Araucariaceae	Araucaria Spp
	Podocarpaceae	Podocarpus Spp
	Cephalotaxaceae	Cephalotaxus
Taxales	Taxaceae	Taxus Spp.
Gnetales	Ephedraceae	Ephedra

Order	Families	Genera
Cactales	Cactaceae	Cactus
Ranunculales	Ranunculaceae, Berberidaceae Menispermaceae	Aconitum Podophyllum Calumba
Papaverales	Papaveraceae Capparaceae Cruciferae	Argemone Capperis Brassica
Rosales	Hamamelidaceae Rosaceae Saxifragaceae Leguminosae Krameriaceae	Hamamelis Prumus Saxifrage Trigonella Krameria

Sympetalae: This subclass consist of 11 orders and 63 families, as the name indicate the fact that their petals are fused.

For example, are mentioned below.

Order	Families	
Primulales	Myrsinaceae, Primulaceae	Primula
Oleales	Oleaceae	Olea spp.
Tubiflorae	Convolvulaceae Labiateae, Solanaceae	Ipomoea Mentha Datura
Tubiflorae	Scrophulariaceae Bignoniaceae Acanthaceae, Gesneriaceae Myoporaceae	Digitalis Jacararida Acanthus Streptocarpus Myaparum
Plantagionales	Plantaginaceae	Plantago
Campanulales	Campanulaceae, (including Lobeliaceae) Compositae	Lobelia

Angiosperm (Monocotyledon)

Plants of this phylum have an embryo with one cotyledon. The leaves of many herbs are parallel veined. The stele has scattered, closed vascular bundles and flowers in general are trimerous.

Following are examples of few orders and families of pharmaceutical interest (Table 2.4).

This system of classification very useful for the study of evolutionary development, it does not reflect any therapeutical/chemical relationship thus of not much use to pharmacists/pharmacognosists. This system represent plants as a whole while pharmacist is concerned for the active part only hence it is not of much significance from the identification point of view as well as pharmacological screening.

This system actually is arrangement of plants for botanical or zoological studies, in which the plants are grouped in families on the base of their distinguishing characters. Examples, the cremocarp fruits drugs (caraway, cumin, fennel, anise, etc.) are considered along with other drugs of umbelliferae.

Plants having alternate leaves, bisexual flowers (pentamerous) cymose inflorescence and capsular or berries fruits (belladonna, hyocyamus, stramonium) are considered with solanaceae, the family have about 90 Genera and over 2000 species that is a large group of plants.

Drugs obtained from the plants having square stem, opposite leaves with glandular hairs containing aromatic oils and bilabiate flowers (peppermint, spearmint, lavendula, thyme) are considered with Labiateae family. This family has about 200 Genera and 3300 species.

Table 2.4: Angiosperm (Monocotyledons)

Orders	Families	Drugs
Liliflorae	Liliaceae	Allium Spp.
	Agavaceae	Agave
	Amaryllidaceae	Leucojun Spp.
	Hypoxidaceae	Hypoxis Spp.
	Dioscoreaceae	Dioscorea Spp.
	Iridaceae	Crocus
Bromiliales	Bromeliaceae	Ananas Spp.
Graminales	Gramineae	Oryza Spp.
Principes	Palmae	Calamus Spp.
Cyperales	Cyperaceae	Cyperus Spp.
Microspermae	Orchidaceae	Vanilla Spp.

Animals are grouped as mammals, fish, insects, anthropods, etc.

PHARMACOLOGICAL CLASSIFICATION

Since ancient times medicinal plants are used for the treatment of illness and are evaluated on the basis of their therapeutic efficacy/potency for the convenience of physician and pharmacological screening they are grouped into classes having similar pharmacological action, irrespective of their morphology, phylogeny or chemical relationship, e.g. senna, ispaghula, cascara sagrada and castor oil are kept in group of laxative because of their action on intestines. Drugs having pharmacological action on cardiac muscles are grouped into one group: digitalis, strophanthus, scilla and arjuna in the category of cardiac tonic. To illustrate it further following are the example Classification of medicinal plants on the basis of their pharmacological action/properties:

Pharmacological properties	Medicinal plants
Anti-inflammatory	Aloe, turmeric, liquorice
Antiamoebic	kurchi
Anticancer	Colchicum, vinca, taxus, podophyllum
Antiasthmatic	Ephedra, lobellia
Anthelmintic	Male fern, quassia wood
Bitter tonic	Quassia, gentian, chirata, kalmegh, cinchona, picrorhiza
Carminative	Fennel, peppermint, coriander, ajowain, dill

Purgative/Laxative	Senna, ispaghula, agar, castor oil, *cascara sagrada*
Emetic	Ipecac
Cardiotonic	Digitalis, strophanthus, scilla, arjuna
Antispasmodic	Datura, belladonna, hyoscyamus
Antitussive	Codeine, liquorice
Bronchodilator	Vasaka, viola
Antidiabetic	Karela, jamun, aloe, fenugreek, kalmegh, garlic, gurmar
Antihypertensive	Rauwoalfia, garlic
Analgesic	Opium

Chemical Basis of Classification

In this system of classification plants are grouped together on the basis of chemical constituents responsible for therapeutical use as well as for their pharmaceutical additives, irrespective of their morphology.

Carbohydrates and Related Constituents Containing Drug/Plant

Chemical constituents	Drug/plants
Polysaccharides	
Starch	Corn, potato, rice, wheat
Gums and Mucilages	Acacia, tragacanth, karaya, Indian tragacanth
Mucilages	Plantago seed, linseed, cydonium seed (quince seeds)

Glycosides	
Anthraquinone	Aloe, rhubarb, senna
Saponin	Quillaia, glycyrrhiza, dioscorea
Cynogenic	Wild cherry bark
Cardiac	Digitalis, strophanthus, scilla
Bitter glycosides	Gentian, quassia, chiarata, kalmegh
Tannins	Nutmeg, hamamelis, amla, ashoka bark, acacia bark
Lipids	Fixed oils: olive, almond, cod-liver oil, shark liver-oil, mustard oil, coconut oil
Fats	Theobroma oil, lanolin, woolfat
Waxes	Bees wax, spermaceti
Resins	Colophony, benzoin, balsam, myrrh, storax, asafoetida, ginger, capsicum, podophyllum
Alkaloids	Aconite, cinchona, ephedra, ergot, datura, belladonna, hyoscyamus, henbane, ipecac, lobelia, nux vomica, opium, rauwolfia, stramonium, tobacco, taxus, withania

Merits: This is most commonly followed method of plants classification by official book as well as by textbooks dealing with natural products and by phytochemist.

Demerits: Plant drugs contain numbers of phytoconstituents of different groups leading to repetition in different groups. Thus, it is not of much use for pharmacist and physician.

CHEMOTAXONOMY

It is based on the existence of biochemical relationship between the similarities and differences of taxon. These characteristics are genetically controlled and advantages over morphological ones, as have definite structural and configurational chemical formula, it helps in understanding their biosynthesis, which is matter of fundamental systemic importance.

In chemotaxonomic study only those chemical constituents are taken in consideration which are uniformly present almost in all parts of the plant, examples:

Carbohydrates in Chemotaxonomy

Carbohydrates are universally present and widely spread in all plants and thus having little importance in chemotaxonomy, however, there are few rare sugars (6-deoxyhexose, 2,6-dideoxyhexoses, gentiobiose, gentianose, polyole, cyclitoles and polysaccharides) having taxonomic significance.

6-deoxyhexose: It occur as methyl esters are specific to drugs containing cardiotonic glycosides.

2,6-dideoxyhexoses are also often methylated and specific to cardiac glycosides (cardinolides) containing such sugars are particularly abundant in the family Apocynaceae and Asclepiadaceae.

Gentiobose and gentianose: These are characteristic of the rosaceae family and gentian genus family Gentianaceae respectively.

Polysaccharides

Inulin: It is characteristic of family Compositae.

Fructans: It is characteristic of Gramineae.

Glycosides in Chemotaxonomy

C-glycosides found in plants containing anthraquinone derivatives as example aloin in aloe (liliaceae) and cascarosides of cascara (Rhamnaceae).

S-glycosides: These glycosides on hydrolysis liberate isothiocyanate, found in Cruciferae.

Isothiocyanate: These compounds are characteristic of Cruciferae and related families Capparaceae, Moringaceae and Rosaceae.

Cynogenetic glycosides: About 100 plant species have ability to produce hydrocyanide (HCN) on enzymatic hydrolysis. This property is particularly common in Rosaceae, Passifloraceae, Leguminosae, Spindaceae and Gramineae family.

Glucosinolates as chemotaxonomic marker: It is useful taxonomic marker within Ibris and Arabis genera (Cruciferae) the compound occur abundantly in Cruciferae and related family Capperidaceae.

Phenolic Compounds

Flavone: On the basis of flavone present in the heartwood of Pinus genus subgenera Hapoxylon were differentiated from diploxylon which do not contain flavone in the heart wood.

Leuco-anthocyanins (colourless flavone): On the basis of leuco-anthocyanins all woody dicotyledons families can be differentiated from herbaceous families lacking leuco-anthocyanin.

In dicotyledons family from Casuarinaceae (magnoniales) to Ebenaceae (ebenales) are kept in one group while families from Aristolochiaceae to Compositae are in another group. Similarly in monocotyledons plants, all species of woody Palmae family contain leucoanthocyanins and such compounds are extremely rare in herbaceous Graminae and Orchidaceae.

Alkaloids in Chemotaxonomy

Alkaloids distribution in Angiosperm is uneven. The Dicotyledons order Salicales, Fagales, Cucurbitales and Aleales at present appear to be Alkaloids free.

Alkaloids are generally found in order Centrospermae (chenopodiaceae) Magnoliales (Ranunculaceae) Papaverales (Papaveraceae) Rosales (Leguminosae subfamily; Papilionaceae) Rutales (Rutaceae) Gentianales (Apocynaceae, Loganiaceae, Rubiaceae) Tubiflorae (Boraginaceae, Convolvulaceae (Solanaceae) and campanuales (Campanulaceae, subfamily Loboliodae, Compositae subfamily Senacioneae) in the dicotyledon and liliales and orchidales in monocotyledons.

Alkaloid type can be considered as a source of taxonomic evidence as chemical or biogenetic group of species as a particular taxon is the same. For instance Papaveraceae synthesise isoquinoline alkaloids those of the Fabaceae: (lupin alkaloids), Rubiaceae (Quinoline alkaloids) Apocyanaceae (indole alkaloids) and those of Solanaceae (Tropane derivatives).

Terpinoids and Steroids in Chemotaxonomy

The oxidised terpinoids derivatives are useful taxonomic markers as **cucurbitacins** are the characteristic of Cucurbitaceae family while **malicins, limonoids** and **quassins** are found in closely related Maliaceae, Rutaceae and Simarubaceae families.

Diterpinoids alkaloids of the aconitine type are characteristic of the related Aconitum and Delphinium genera of the Ranunculaceae, they also occur in Garryaceae, a family difficult to classify on the basis of morphological grounds.

Monoterpinoids composition of the Pinus genus (Pinaceae) has been useful in tracing hybridisation between species and migration of the genus while cultivators of the blue spruce (Picea pungens, family Pinaceae) have been identified from their monoterpinoid composition.

Iridoids

Iridoids are highly characteristic metabolites, which occur mainly in number of assumed phylogenetically related dicotyledonous families. The detection of iridoids in Callitrichaceae, part of Icacinaceae. Liquidambar, part of Loasaceae, Thaligonaceae and other often mono or oligotypic taxa had a considerable contribution to their appropriate classification.

Both Smith and Swain (1966) commented on the possible value of taxonomy of iridoids (Monoterpinoid cylopentanoid lactones), of these asperuloside is found in Rubiaceae and Scrophulariaceae and also in Buddlia and Garryaceae.

Essential oils in Chemotaxonomy

The bulk of essential oil bearing plants belongs to the seed plants. In **Thallophytes** true essential oils occur in some fungi (e.g. in the genus Lactarius) and in a number of *Chlorophyta, Rhodophyta* (Red Algae) and *Phaeophyta* (Brown Algae); in these plants essential oils are deposited in specialised cells (excretory hyphae or cells of idioblastic nature). In **Bryophyta** essential oil are restricted to Liverworts. In **Pteridophytes**, only rarely noticable amount of essential oils are produced. In **Spermatophytes** (seed plants) the essential oils ubiquitous in **Coniferopsida and Taxopsida** (Gymnosperms), which possess schizogenous cavities and canals. In

Coniferopsida the essential oils seems to be restricted to *Ginko biloba* (Lysigenous cavities). Chlamydospermae seems to be devoid of essential oils. In angiospermae (flowering plants) most of them having essential oils. These are classified in 62 orders (Engler's syllabus, Vol. 1964).

From the chemotaxonomical point, the bulk of well known constituents of essential oils occurs in many taxonomically unrelated taxa, e.g. **Eugenol, cis-asarone, thymol, limonene, sabinene, apinene carvone and linalool**. Such compounds are taxonomically useful only at the **generic level**. Other oil constituents can be termed **taxon specific** because they seem to occur in only a few species, e.g. **Sec-butyl-propenyldisulphide** (component of the oleoresin of a few species of *Ferula* (Umbilliferae) and **Nitrophenylethane** (Cinnamon-scented constituents of the essential oils of Aniba and Ocotea-taxa family Lauraceae).

On the basis of chemical constituents of essential oils, the medicinal plants can be classified into following groups.

   i. Rutaceae
  ii. Myrtaceae
 iii. Umbelliferae
 iv. Compositae

Rutaceae

Rutaceae family plants are chemically characterised by the synthesis and accumulation of essential oils, furanocoumarins, anthranilic acid derived alkaloids and limonoids. Prenylations of aromatic compounds is common in this family, e.g. of this tendency are furano and dimethylpyrano-coumarins and a number of essential oil constituents such as **Evodionol** (a phloracetophenone derived 2,2'-dimethylchromene. Similar tendencies are perceptible in Umbelliferae (coumarins) and Compositae (Precocene and 6-desmethoxy derivative).

Myrtaceae

Myrtaceae family consists of tannin-rich essential oil plants. Methylated, prenylated and (or) acetylated phloroglucinol derivatives occurs frequently in their essential oils; production

of this very characteristic type of acetogenesis (Torquatone, a phloroglucinol derivative; present in some species of *Eucalyptus*) represent a chemical trend of this family.

Umbelliferae

Umbelliferae family constitute the plants with furano and dimethylpyrano-coumarins and essential oils which tends to contain phthalides, e.g. **Ligustilide** (phthalide occurring in the essential oils of species of *Angelica, Cinidium, Conioselinum, Levisticum* and *meum*) (Umbelliferae) ferulol type monoterpenoids and acetylenic compounds like falcarinone. The latter link the family chemically with **Araliaceae, Pittosporaceae and Compositae**.

Compositae

Compositae plants are chemically characterised by synthesis and accumulations of many classes of natural compounds. In Asteroideae (= Tubiflorae) essential oils are common. They often contain acetylenic compounds, e.g. matricaria ester (an ester of a C-10 polyacetylenic carboxylic acid occurring in essential oils of many compositae plants) and tend to comprise complex derivative of thymol; in some genera and tribes, e.g. Nematicidal thymol derivatives occurring in several species of *Helenium* (Compositae). As indicated by many metabolic trends in the synthesis of series of essential oils, an evolution line from Rutales ® Umbelliferae (Umbelliferae and Araliaceae only) ® Asterales can be drawn.

Amines in Chemotaxonomy

The widespread of amines in plants limit the usefulness of amine in chemotaxonomy. In general plants with flowers synthesising volatile aliphatic amine are common amongst the **Caprifoliaceae, Cornaceae, Rosaceae and Araceae families, while the Papilionoideae and Labiatae** are almost devoid of such flowers.

The di and polyamines occurs widely but monoamine and 3-aminopropionitrile has been found only in three species of Lathyrus (Leguminosae), *L. odoratus, L. hirutus* and *L. roseus*.

Some of **heterocyclic amine**, such as nor-adrenaline, ephedrine and histamine have an erratic distribution while **mescaline** appears to be restricted to members of the **Cactaceae.**

SEROTAXONOMY

Classification of medicinal plants/drugs by means of **protein component** of the plants/drugs; this is based on the highly specific relationship between **antigen** and **antibody reaction.** In this method the specific properties of antisera produced by animals blood against plant proteins is used as character to assess plants relationship.

In this technique proteins of different plants of the taxa is extracted. Seeds of the plants are taken from the selected plant species, as the seeds are rich source of protein but they also contain oils and other constituents therefore the seeds should be made free from all these components before the extraction of protein by extraction with light petroleum ether (40°C).

Protein solution in concentration of 0.2% in Freund's complete adjuvant, injected subcutaneously to the test animals (rabbit or rats) to develop antibodies. Serum of the animals is collected and made to react with antigen of another plant *in vitro* in agrose gel by diffusion method or by cup plate method. (Immunodiffusion in Agarose Gel), the precipitation reaction indicate the similarity of antigens. Degree of precipitation determine the proportion of homology, hence the precipitation reaction is considered as polygenic marker and taxonomic character.

This method is quite useful in establishing a satisfactory and natural classification of plants families.

This method is used to develop species relationship within a genus and the arrangement of genera into tribes as well as to establish the possible boundaries of families within its neighbours. This system of classification is more convenient for practical study, especially when chemistry of the drug is not known, then this is quite useful, in identification of the adulterants.

Rives, Nelson and Biskeland and Moritz made significant contribution to the application of serology to systematic.

For examples, on the basis of Serotaxonomy system of plant classification, inclusion of Gentianaceae in Comiflorae could be made possible, because of homogeneity of iridoids producing plants. Lee and Fair brothers (1978) used serological technique to study the Rubiaceae and related families. Ansen (1968) reported the close serological relationship of Ranunculaceae and Hydrastis than Berbaridaceae and Hydrastis.

Chrispeel and Gartner on the basis of serological evidence supported the relation of *Phaseolus aureus* and *P. mungo* with genus Vignae.

FURTHER READING

1. Chemotaxonomy and Serotaxonomy Google Books. *https://books.google.com›Science›Life Sciences›Biochemistry*

2. Classification of crude drugs and serotaxonomy https://www.slideshare.net›Sudheer Kandibanda›classification-of-crude-

3. Cronquist A. 1981. An integrated system of classification of flowering plants. Columbia University Press, New York.

4. Evans WC. 2009. Trease and Evans Pharmacognosy, 16th ed., Elsevier; New York.

5. Hawkes JG. 1967. Chemotaxonomy and serotaxonomy: proceedings of a symposium held at the Botany Department, Birmingham University.

6. Kirikar KR, Basu B.D. 1933. Indian Medicinal Plants Vol. 1–4. Bio-Green Books.

7. Quality Control methods for herbal Material-WHO, Updated edition of quality control methods for medicinal plant materials, 1998. Through www.who.int

8. Serotaxonomy/Encyclopedia.com, Oxford University Press. URL: www.encyclopedia.com>science>serotaxonomy

9. Serotaxonomy: Definition, History and Roles/Plant Taxonomy. www.biologydiscussion.com›plant-taxonomy›serotaxonomy-definition

10. Stuessy T. 1990. Plant Taxonomy. Columbia, NY.

11. Sudheer Kandibanda. Classification Of Crude Drugs & Serotaxonomy, Slide Share, URL: https://www.slideshare.net/Sudheer Kandibanda/classification-of-crude-drugs-serotaxonomy

12. Takhtazan AL. Outline of the classification of flowering plants (Magnoliophya). Bot Rev. 1980;46(3):225–359.

13. Thorne RF. Phytochemistry and angiosperm phylogeny: a summary statement. In: Young DA, Seigler DS (eds) Phytochemistry and angiosperm phylogeny. Praeger, New York. 1981;233–95.

14. Tod F Stuessy. 1990. Plant Taxonomy: The Systematic Evaluation of Comparative Data. Columbia University Press.

15. Wallis J TE, Churchill A. 1960. Textbook of Pharmacognosy. 4th ed. Little, Brown and Co.

16. Wallis TE. Textbook of pharmacognosy. CBS Publishers and Distributors, New Delhi, 2005; 68–101.

17. Winston JE, Metzger KL. Trends in Taxonomy revealed by the published literature. Bio Science. 1998;48:121–8.

Quality Control of Drugs of Natural Origin

INTRODUCTION

As per WHO estimate about 80% population of developing countries relies on traditional medicines, mostly of plant origin for their primary healthcare needs. The widespread popularity towards the traditional medicine in Asia, Europe and USA has induced high growth and development worldwide. Hence quality specification of crude drugs in demands are being taken up by number of pharmacopoeias (British Pharmacopoeia, the European Pharmacopoeia the United States Pharmacopoeia, Indian Pharmacopoeia), the National formulary and other national publications. The quality specifications are usually characterised in monograph of crude drugs. A monograph usually comprises of:
• Name with biological and geographical source of origin of crude drug
• Morphological characters
• Identity comprising macro- and microscopic characters and chemical tests for the active components
  – Purity test
  – Quantitative determination
  – Biological evaluations
  – Storage conditions.

ADULTERATION OF DRUGS OF NATURAL ORIGIN

Adulteration in broad and legal sense is an addition of another substance, plant part or plant product to increase the bulk of material with the result, loss in quality of the raw material.

Types of adulteration:
1. Intentional
2. Accidental/un-intentional

Intentional adulteration: Deliberate admixture of inferior, spoiled, deteriorated drug and substitution with the intention to increase the profit margin.

Unintentional or accidental adulteration: It is usually attributed to ignorance, carelessness, engagement of unskilled labour, and by lack of storage facilities.

Intentional Adulteration

Addition of undesirable part of the drug, e.g. in male fern (roots and dead portions are included into the Rhizome and leaf bases) Tamarind (outer part of the pericarp of the fruits are not properly removed and preserved in sugar); Ginger (cork not-removed from the Rhizome); Quillaia (Rhytidome are also included with inner part of the bark.

Inferiority: Admixture the raw material having low concentration of chemical constituents, e.g.

Mixing the wildly cultivated drug with the cultivated one because of the morphological resemblance with authentic drug.

The inferior drugs may or may not have the therapeutic component, e.g. different species of senna leaflets, Arabian senna, (*Cassia angustifolia*); dog senna (*Cassia obovata*) and ranawara (Tamil) *Cassia auriculata*.

Glycyrrhiza glabra L. roots are being mixed with *Glycyrrhiza glandulifera* stolon and roots. Japanese ginger (*Zingiber mioga* Roscoe) and

Martinique ginger (*Z. zerumbet* Rose) with *Zingiber officinale* (medicinal ginger).

Powdered ginger is adulterated with rice powder, wheat flour and with ginger waste.

Adulteration (sophistication): Cheaper natural drug with genuine drugs.

It is deliberate mixing of inferior material with the genuine to increase the bulk, e.g. asafoetida (*Ferula asafoetida*) is adulterated with Gum arabic or wheat flour. Chirata (*Swertia chirata* with *Swertia paniculata*).

Substitution with a factitious material: Addition or replacement of the genuine drug with factitious mixture of similar composition, e.g. Lemon oil-replaced with citral (from the oil other than lemon oil) and terpene removed from the oil of lemon. Nutmeg-broken kernel, moulded with clay and shaped pieces of wood.

Substitution with entirely different drug: Supplying the drug with similar morphological characters but different chemically, e.g. palm oil with olive oil. Belladonna leaves are substituted with *Solanum nigrum* leaves.

Substitution with artificially manufactured substitute: Invert sugar having similar colour and taste with natural honey and the beeswax is substituted with yellow coloured paraffin wax.

Accidental spoilage: Crude drug stored at unhygienic house may gets spoiled by microbial, fungal or bacterial growth; with the result loss in therapeutic efficacy of the drug. Drug may get toxic to human being because of phytotoxin growth on the drug.

Adulteration by admixture of foreign materials: Sometime to increase the bulk of the drug materials; sand, stone pellets are mixed with resinous drug, gum acacia, gum tragacanth and lime stone in asafoetida, coal tar in opium.

Addition of synthetic material: Addition of citral to lemon oil; benzyl benzoate to balsam of Peru.

Many drugs are processed on large scale for the isolation of active principles and subsequently exhausted material are substituted for genuine drugs, e.g. clove, umbelliferous fruits and cardamom (volatile oils removed); Indian Hemp and Jalap (resins removed);

ginger (volatile oils and resins removed); Balsam of tolu (balsamic acid removed) and liquorice (glycyrrhizin and other water soluble matter removed), etc.

Addition of vegetative part of the plant: Addition of stem part into senna leaflet, buchu and digitalis leaves, blown up clove flower to clove bud.

Deterioration of Herbal Drugs

Crude drugs are prone to deterioration while stored in store house because of light, temperature, and humidity produce detrimental effects on the active principle of the drugs with the result loss in therapeutic potential. Above that the drugs may also get attacked by insects to eat out the nutrients.

Factors Affecting the Deterioration

Light: Photosensitive drugs are affected by light—should be kept away from light or the containers should be resistant to sunlight as amber coloured glass containers or the containers be wrapped in light resistant paper. The following is the list of drug which can be affected by light:

Worm seeds which on exposure to sunlight darkens and eventually becomes dark.

Santonin and Rhubarb powder. Its yellow colour gets deteriorated in sunlight and it changes to red colour.

Moisture or humidity: Drugs containing cardiac glycosides gets hydrolysed in the presence of moisture and temperature, e.g.

Digitalis leaves and Scilla scale leaves, it also contains hygroscopic mucilage which become sticky.

Temperature: When drugs exposed to high temperature and moisture the enzyme present in cell, gets coagulated and becomes inactive to protect the secondary notabilities, e.g. volatile oils containing, drugs, e.g. Labiatae family, rose petals and chamomile.

Adsorbent—Cotton fibre becomes non-absorbent on storing at high temperature which is because of fat contents which gets spread over the surface of fibre, thus make it non-absorbent.

Oxygen: Air also effects the crude drugs as it causes oxidation of the drugs, e.g. volatile oils.

The oxidation process alters the odour of the oil, viscosity and its therapeutic potency. The main constituents of the essential oil on combining with atmospheric oxygen causes negative chemical change (oxide and peroxide are often formed), e.g. limonene-2-hydroxide formed from limonene, which is slightly toxic. Rancidification of the fixed oil due to peroxidation thus, loss in vitamin, e.g. cod liver oil.

Mould attack: The crude drugs are also being attacked with same type of mould as those are found in food product, the commonly found moulds are species of *Rhizopus*, *Mucor*, *Penicillium* and *Eurotium*. Their presence identified by their characteristic smell because of oxidation. Conversion of alcohol to aldehyde or ketone and aldehyde to carboxylic acid.

Esterification: Glycosylation, acetylation, condensation, etc. with the result new chemical changes take place which otherwise not present in the normal components of the drugs.

Insects and other pest attack: Most of the drugs, even stored well are liable to attack by insect pests (especially beetles), who remained hidden in the drug but at the certain stage (larvae) of development they appear on the surface of the stored drug through small circular holes and fine powdered material appear at the bottom of container. The drugs which are commonly infested are ginger, belladonna leaves and roots, nutmeg, coriander, stramonium and dandelion.

The insects eat both carbohydrates and protein components of the drug.

Following are the most commonly reported insect found in drugs: *Stegobium paniceum* (Drug-room beetle or Biscuit weevil) *Ptinus fur* and *Ptinus tectus*, *Lasioderma serricorne* (cigar-beetle), *Lyctus brunneus* (powder-post beetle), *Niptus hololeucus* (The Golden spider beetle) *Calandra granaria* and *Calandra oryzae* (Grain weevils).

In addition to the beetles mentioned above Mites may also attack drugs like Ergot, Cantharides and crushed linseed by tearing up tissues with their mandibles. Commonly founded mites are *Tyroglyphus longior*, *Aleurobius farina* and *Glycyphagus spinipes*.

A damp atmosphere is favourable to the development of fungi and drugs may become covered with *mould*. The commonest fungi found are species of *Penicillium* (Blue mould), *Eurolium* (Green mould) and *Mucor*. Certain beetles, e.g. *Cryptophagus acutangulus Gyil*, feed exclusively on the fungi developed on the bales of drugs (liquorice) store in damp warehouse.

DRUGS EVALUATION

It is the process of analysing the drugs for its identity, purity, quality and detection of type of adulterants by comparing the parameter with the reference sample.

The following are parameters to be checked:

   i. Organoleptic properties

  ii. Morphological characters

 iii. Microscopic characters

 iv. Physical

  v. Chemicals

 vi. Biological evaluations.

ORGANOLEPTIC PROPERTIES (EVALUATION)

Organoleptic: Involving the use of sense organs as taste, colour, odour and feel of drugs/substance/food. These characters are useful, often in a supplementary way in evaluation of drugs, especially applicable to drugs containing volatile oils or pungent-constituents, e.g. capsicum and to the detection of the effect of inadequate drying of drugs.

Colour: The drugs of the aerial part of the plants—leaves, leaflets, stems and branches are always green in colour. The intensity of the colour also indicates the quality of the sample.

Underground part of plant is always non-green (free from chlorophyll). Flowering part (petals) always are coloured orange, pink, violet, etc.

For proper examination, untreated samples are examined under defused sunlight or artificial light having same wavelength as that of daylight. Colour parameter helps to segregate the parts of the plant drugs.

Odour: Odour can be examined by slow and repeated inhalation. In the case of innocuous odour even the small portion of the plant sample is sufficient, e.g. asafoetida.

In case of weak smelling drug, the sample is lightly crushed either in hand or by applying light pressure and putting it on boiling water in watch glass or Petri dish followed by inhalation.

The odour parameters: These are rancid, fruity, aromatic, musky and mouldy. The quality or adulteration can be characterised by weak, distinct and strong odour.

Rancid odour indicates spoilage of fixed oil containing drugs.

Taste: Before proceeding to taste of the unknown sample, one has to be sure about its non-poisonous properties, otherwise it can be fatal. This parameter is useful to evaluate the drugs having characteristic taste, e.g. bitter (cinchona, chirata, etc.) sweet (honey, stevia).

Sour taste—Tamarindus, Salty—*Cassia tora*, Bitter—*Andrographis paniculata*, Pungent—*Elettaria cardamomum*, Astringent—*Saraca ashoka*.

Feel or Texture

This parameter is helpful in evaluation of the surface characters like smooth, rough, hairy and gritty. This can be achieved by rubbing the sample between thumb and forefingers. Bending the sample gives information regarding the softness or brittleness. Then check the freshly fractured surface whether it is fibrours or smooth, rough, granular, etc., e.g. *Centella asiatica* smooth surface.

Spongy: Cork oak (*Quercus robur*)

Soft-silky: *Eschscholzia californica* (California poppy), *Aegle marmelos* (leaves beneath).

Furry plant: *Artemisia* spp.

Texture is anything with an irregular surface. This is because of fine hairs, scales, thorns and lumps or any other protuberance.

Rough stem plant: Spinach and sunflower.

Morphological Evaluation

For morphological evaluation, the crude drugs are classified into leaves, stem, flowers, fruit seeds, bark, wood and roots. The adulterant shows marked difference in morphology from the authentic material.

Leaves: Leaves are flattened outgrowth of stem. They are of two types—simple and compound leaf. **Simple leaves** have bud in their axil while no bud in the axil of **compound leaves**. The whole leaf is divided into many segments which arise on a common rachis known as leaflets.

Leaves are of different size, shape, apex, margin, base and venations; are the parameters used for the identification/evaluation of leafy crude drugs.

Shape of lamina: The flat part of the leaf, which is green in colour, is known as lamina which always have different shape and venation, which are characteristic point for identification (Fig. 3.1).

Shape: The common structure of lamina has the following description—circular, oblong, cordate, ovate, obovate, oval, linear and lanceolate.

Apex of leaf: The outer end of leaf lamina that is opposite the petiole. It varies from plant to plant and is useful in identification and evaluation. Term used to describe the apex are acute, acuminate, obtuse and tunicate (Fig. 3.2).

Base of leaf: Lower end of leaf lamina which may be symmetrical, asymmetrical, cordate and decurrent (Fig. 3.3).

Margin of leaf: Margin of the leaf lamina may be entire, serrate (sharp edge), dentate, crenate and sinulate (Fig. 3.4).

Venation: The pattern in arrangement of veins in the blade or lamina of a leaf is called venation. There are three types of venation: Reticulate, pinnate and parallel venation. Most of the monocot plant leaf shows parallel venation (Fig. 3.5).

Compound leaf: When attachment of leaf to stem is examined, it can be determined if leaf is attached directly to stem, leaf is simple (pinnate or palmate). In compound leaf it is paripinnate or imparipinnate (Fig. 3.6).

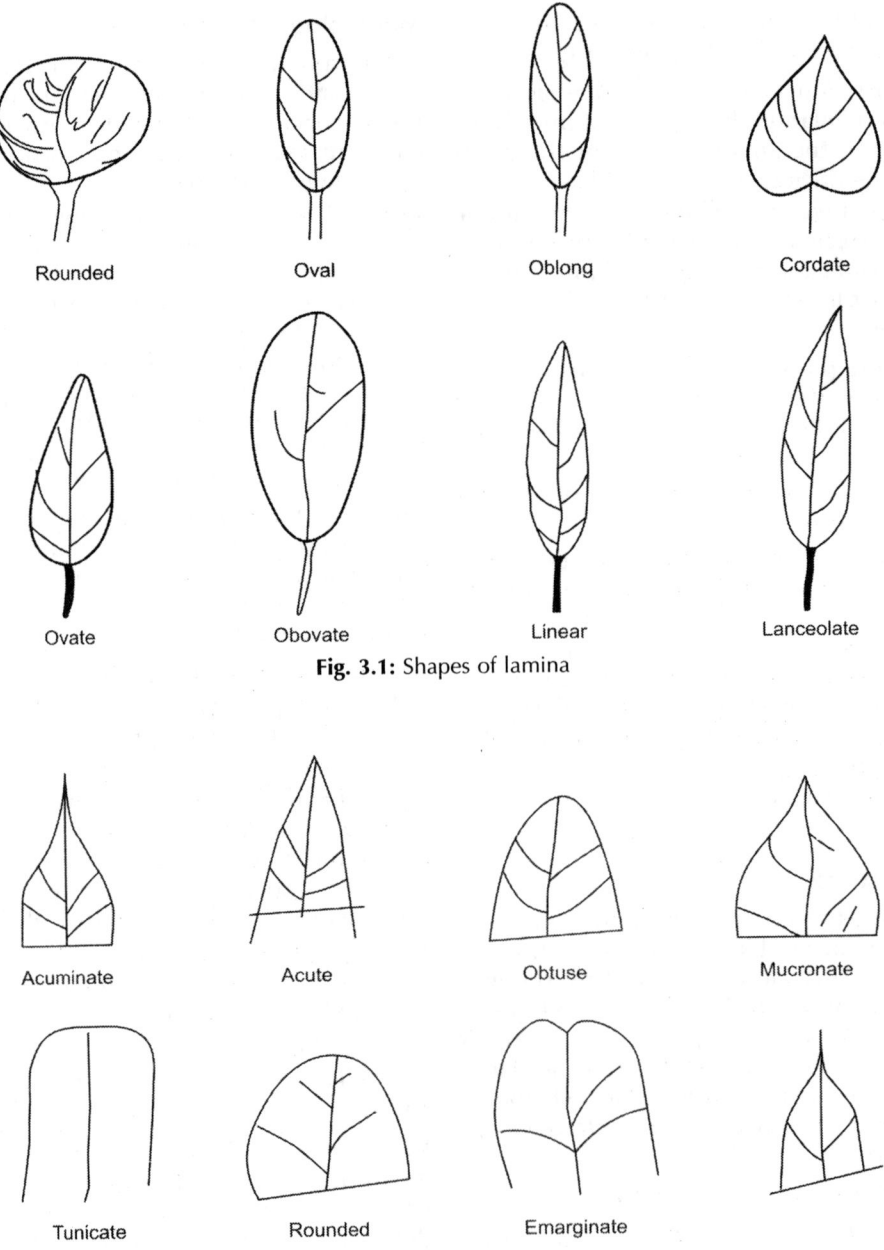

Fig. 3.1: Shapes of lamina

Rounded Oval Oblong Cordate

Ovate Obovate Linear Lanceolate

Acuminate Acute Obtuse Mucronate

Tunicate Rounded Emarginate

Fig. 3.2: Apex

Parallel, Pinnate and Reticulate (Fig. 3.5)

Parallel venations: The secondary veins run paralled to each other of a central primary vein, e.g. Banana leaf venation.

Pinnately: Veined leaves have a single primary vein from which smaller veins branched off like the division of feather (Fig. 3.5).

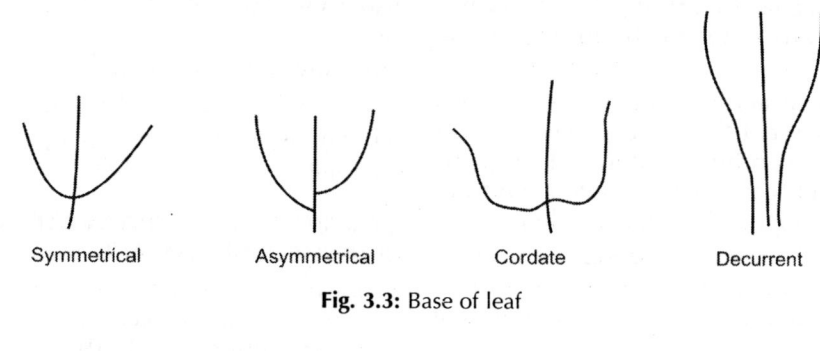

Symmetrical   Asymmetrical   Cordate   Decurrent

Fig. 3.3: Base of leaf

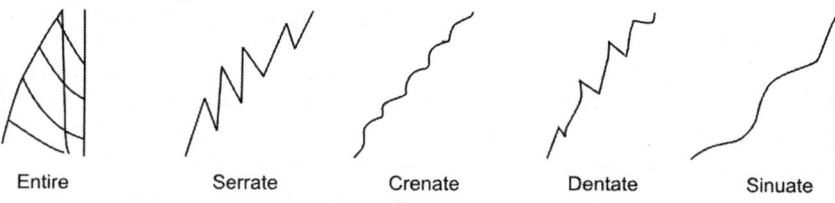

Entire   Serrate   Crenate   Dentate   Sinuate

Fig. 3.4: Margin of leaf

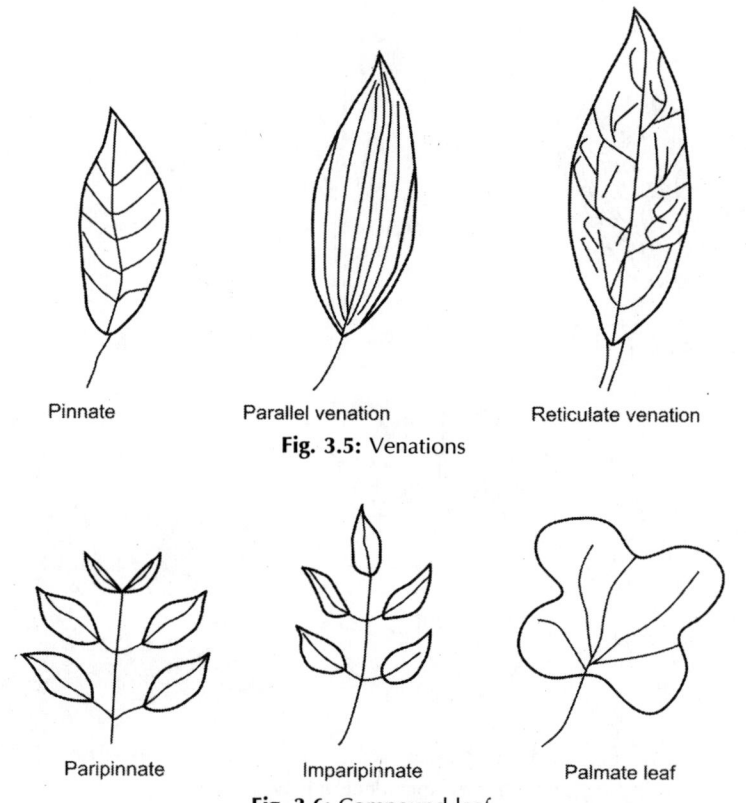

Pinnate   Parallel venation   Reticulate venation

Fig. 3.5: Venations

Paripinnate   Imparipinnate   Palmate leaf

Fig. 3.6: Compound leaf

Reticulate: Veins are arranged in a net-like pattern on both sides of the midrib. Dicot plants.

Description of aerial stem: The stem is an aerial axis of plant that bears leaves, flowers and fruits. It conducts water and minerals from root and food from the site of synthesis to part of the plant where it is needed.

Herb sample stem can be described in terms of shape, colour, dimension, upright or creeping, smooth or ridged, hairs are present or absent.

Arrangement and Position of Leaves on Stem

The terminologies used to describe the arrangement is as follows:

Cauline: Leaves arising from the stem.

Radical: Leaves starting from the crown of the stem.

Adnation: Part of leaves remain fused with stem.

Opposite and decussate: It is cauline but arises in pairs, alternately at right angles to the stem.

Alternate: The leaves arise from stem in alternate manner (Fig. 3.7).

MORPHOLOGICAL CHARACTERS OF UNDERGROUND ORGANS

Crude drugs from underground organ consist of root structure and stem structure as storage organ including true **bulbs, corms, tubers,** enlarged hypocotyls and **rhizomes**. Rhizome looks to be similar to root but has internal structure arrangement similar to a stem, e.g. gentian and rhubarb. These drugs are commonly classified as root but actually both of them consist of rhizomes.

Rhizomes have scale leaves with axillary buds on the surface and have adventitious roots or

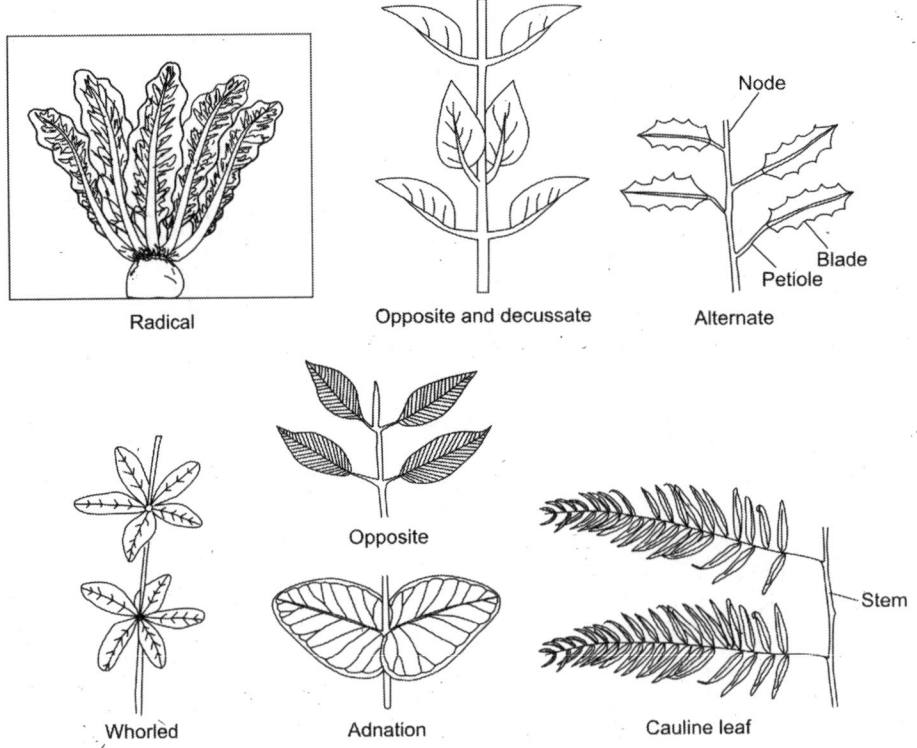

Radical   Opposite and decussate   Alternate

Node

Blade
Petiole

Opposite

Whorled   Adnation   Cauline leaf

Stem

Fig. 3.7: Arrangement of leaves on stem

scars, whereas roots do not have scale leaves and buds. They have main tap root and the lateral root—no nodes/internodes (Fig. 3.8a).

Underground organs are characterised by the absence of chlorophyll. They are often swollen, hence they are cut into small pieces and dried for storage and transportation.

Underground organs are of following size and shape—straight, conical, cylindrical, tortuous and fusiform (Fig. 3.8b).

Morphological Evaluation of Bark

Bark is the outer protective layer of woody plants, roots and shrubs. It refers to all tissues outside the vascular cambium.

A young bark is composed of:
1. **Epidermis:** Closely packed cuticle, parenchymatous cell with occasional stomata.
2. **Primary cortex:** It is usually made up of chlorophyll-containing collenchyma and parenchyma tissue.

Endodermis: Innermost of cortex, closely packed parenchyma often containing starch.

Pericycle: Composed of parenchyma and fibre tissue. Sometimes pericyclic fibres are in groups opposite to patches of phloem.

Phloem: Composed of parenchyma, sieve tube and companion cell separated by radially arranged medullary rays (Fig. 3.9a).

In **old bark** secondary growth appears because of activation of cork cambium or **phellogen** with the result **primary bark** is tangentially stretched, and outer layer compressed and torn out or divided by radial walls and the parenchymatous cells of the cortex—becomes thickened and converted into sclerenchymatous cells. Inner side cambium produces secondary phloem consisting of alternating zone of sieve elements and phloem fibres. Pericyle layer also ruptured and even in few barks it disappears as sclerenchyma.

In the epidermis and primary cotex, cork cambium or phellogen may arise, which on outer side produce cork and in inner side **secondary cortex** or **phelloderm** (chlorophyll containing suberized cell). All these three layers are known as **periderm** (Fig. 3.9b).

The primary cortex will lie on the outer side of cork and will gradually thrown off, the stomata will be replaced with **lenticells** for the gaseous exchange.

The barks are flat when removed freshly but on drying its curvature increases except in the case of large pieces of trunk bark, if subjected to pressure are flat. The terminology used to

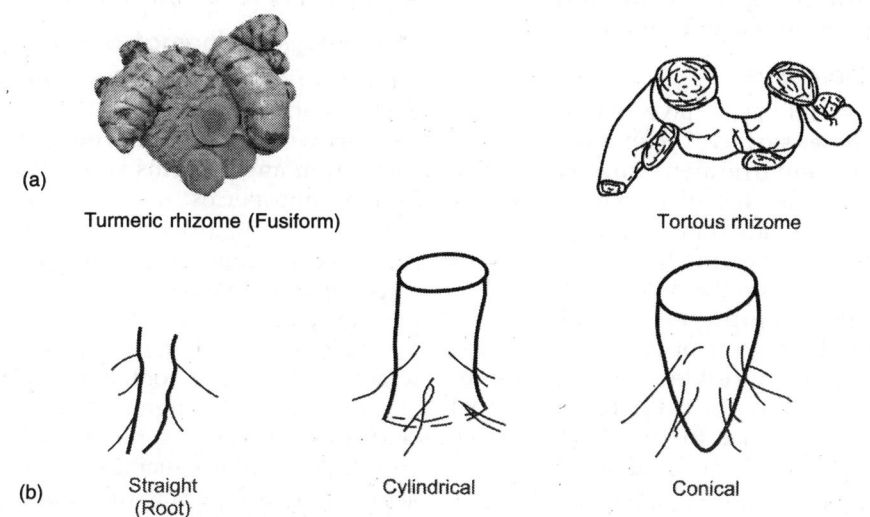

(a) Turmeric rhizome (Fusiform)

Tortous rhizome

(b) Straight (Root) — Cylindrical — Conical

Fig. 3.8a and b: Shape of underground drugs

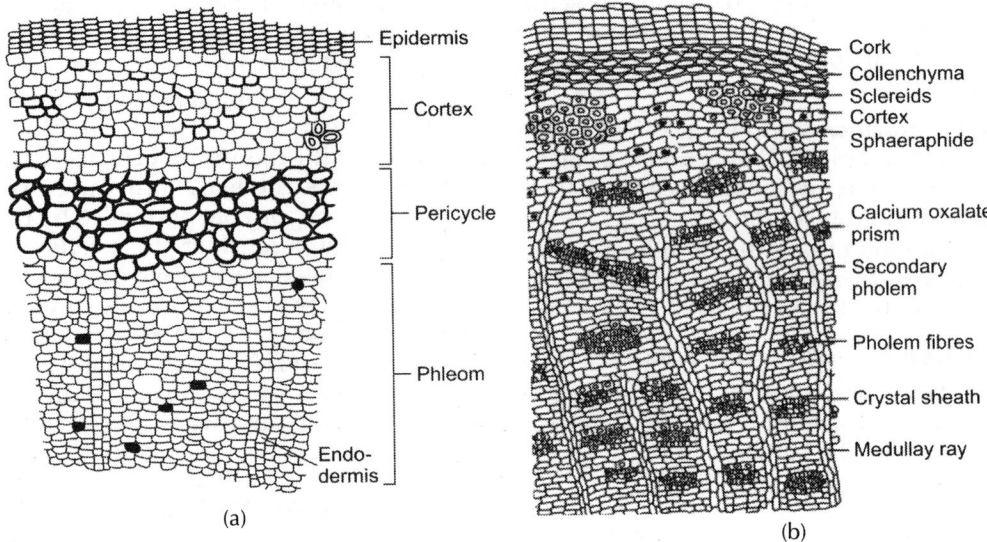

Fig. 3.9: Microscopic structure of bark; (a) young bark; (b) old bark

describe the curvature shown in (Fig. 3.10). These curvatures are characteristic of official barks.

For pharmacognostical evaluation the bark may be described under following headings:

i. **Origin:** Trunk bark or root bark.

ii. **Size and nature of curvature:** According to the extent of curvature every bark develops its specific shape.

Quill, double quill, compound quill, channelled, recurved and **curved** (Fig. 3.10a).

Surface Characters

The commercial barks have two surfaces—**outer and inner surface.** Depending upon the surrounding environment **epiphytes** may grow on the surface of a plant in forest. Hence, when trunk barks are removed and prepared, there is presence of epiphytes like **lichens** and **moss** may appear on the outer surface.

Other than epiphytes on old barks **rhytidome** (dead layer of cork cells) is seen which looks like wrinkles. Some barks are scraped at the time of preparation to give smooth surface. Hence, to describe the surface characters of bark, terms used are:

Outer surface: The presence of lichens, mosses, lenticells, cracks/furrows, colour before and after scraping.

Inner surface: Colour, striations.

Fracture: Outer surface generally have short but inner surface fracture depends upon the extent of secondary growth, i.e. **fibrous, splintery** or **granular.**

Transverse surface: Freshly broken (fractured) bark on staining with phloroglucinol and hydrochloric acid shows lignified elements (sclereids and vessels), medullary ray and cork.

Morphological Characters of Wood

Wood is a porous and fibrous structural tissue of stems and roots of tree. It is of two types, i.e. **hardwoods** and **softwoods.** Hardwood come from angiosperms and softwood come from gymnosperms.

Wood made up of secondary tissues produced by cambium on inner side. These consist of fibres, vessel elements, tracheids and parenchyma. All the tissues are generally lignified but exceptions are there as in case of wood of belladonna root, non-lignified tissue are predominant to lignified one. This can be confirmed by staining the cut surface of the wood, with phloroglucinol and hydrochloric acid. Medullary rays: width and height of the ray are characteristic in wood of quassia and rhubarb.

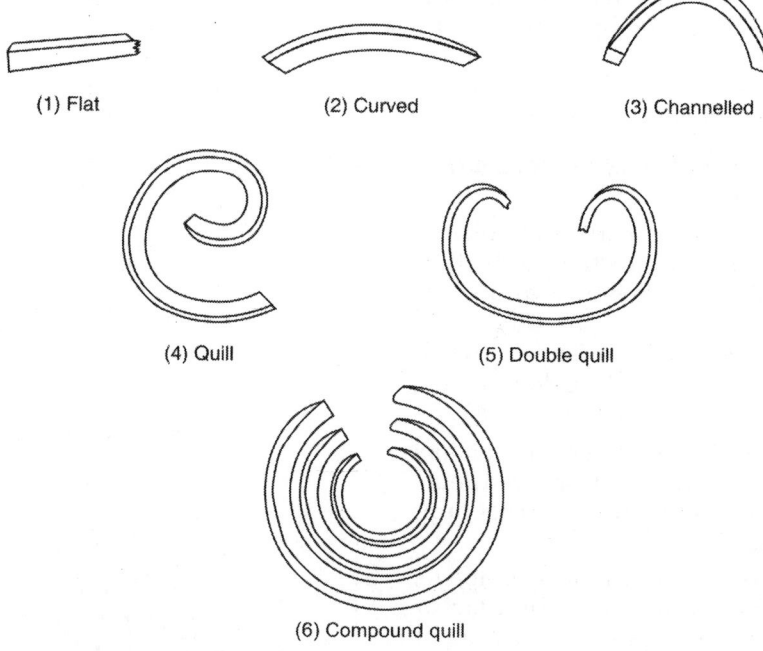

(1) Flat (2) Curved (3) Channelled

(4) Quill (5) Double quill

(6) Compound quill

Fig. 3.10a: Curvature of bark

The wood block has two regions:
1. Heart wood
2. Sap wood.

Heart wood: It is the central region which is coloured because of the deposit of waste products such as resins, tannins and colouring matter in the wood of old tree.

Sap wood: It is the outer wood still retains its normal appearance and functions. Each year tree forms new cells arranged in concentric rings known as annual rings or annual growth rings. In some tropical species these rings are not well marked because of the seasonal interruptions in growth, hence false annual rings are formed.

Annual ring shows amount of wood produced during one growing season. It appears as darker ring in transverse section. These rings are formed due to activity of **extrastelar cambium** or **intrastelar cambium** or both (Fig. 3.10b).

Wood grains which describe the alignment, texture and appearance of wood fibres are also characteristic of plants.

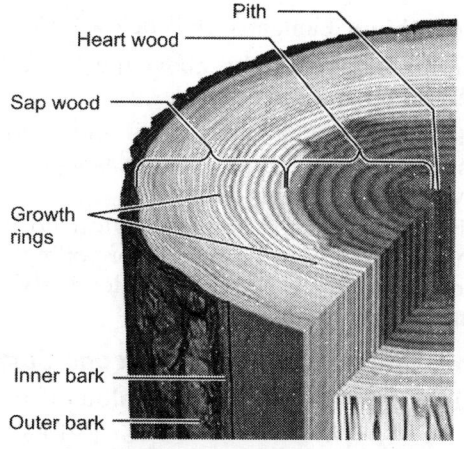

Fig. 3.10b: Internal structure of wood

Grains of wood are indicator of the arrangement of annual rings and medullary rays.

Wood can be identified under the following headings:

Size and colour: Colour depends upon the ration of heart wood and sap wood.

Surface: To see the arrangement of lignified tissue, wood fibres or wood parenchyma in transverse section.

Longitudinal section/surface to measure the length and width of medullary rays.

Morphological Evaluation of Herbal Drugs Containing Flowers

Flowers are reproductive part of the plants. They are useful as drug for the production of essential oils for cosmetics and food nutrients.

Flower drugs include true flowers (rose), flower buds (clove) and inflorescence (*Chrysanthemum indicum, Coptis chinensis*).

Morphology of flower: Each flower has four sets of organs inserted on preduncle (i) Calyx, (ii) Corolla, (iii) Androecium, (iv) Gynoecium.

Types of flowers: Complete or incomplete, unisexual or hermaphrodite, regular or zygomorphic, hypogynous, perigynous or epigynous.

Receptacle of flower:

Hypanthium: Elongated stalk below the calyx.

Gynophore: When calyx above the ovary, the stalk is known as gynophore.

Calyx: Generally green in colour and leaf-like in structure. Individually known as sepal. The calyx encloses flower bud.

Petals which are usually coloured and conspicuous and attract insects for pollination. Their structure is like leaf, collectively the petals make up the corolla.

Terms Used to Explain the Calyx and Corolla

Calyx: Polysepals or gamosepalous (free or fused sepals), caducous (e.g. poppy) or persistent (e.g. belladonna). Perianth (calyx) having colour of petals (Fig. 3.11).

Corolla: Polypetalous (free petals), gamo-petalous (petal fused) and special character if any, like venation or oil glands (Fig. 3.12).

Androecium: The next to Corolla to form floral apex are the stamens (male organ). Number varies from one to many depending on the species (Fig. 3.13).

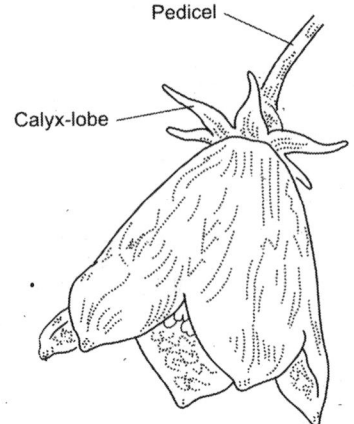

Fig. 3.11: Calyx

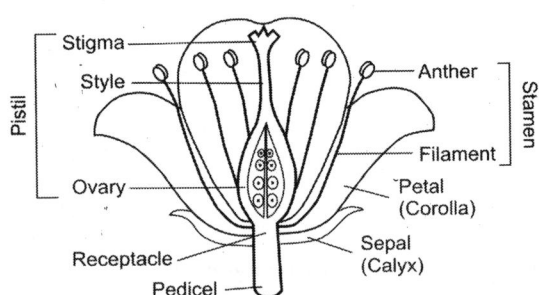

Fig. 3.12: LS of flower

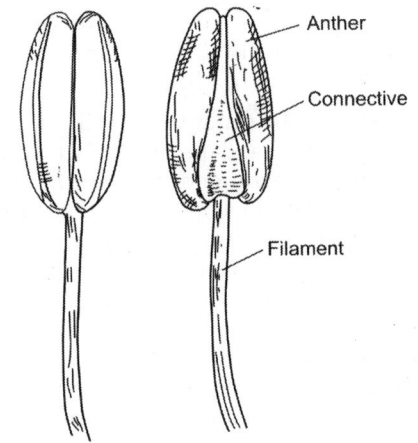

Fig. 3.13: Androecium

Each stamen has three parts—filament, anther and connective. Anthers bear four chambers for the storage of pollen grains.

Terms Used for Stamen

Monadelphous or diadelphous (free or fused) at the base).

Monadelphous: Stamens united by their filaments, so as to form one group.

Diadelphous: United into two sets by filaments.

Didynamous or tetradynamous [stamen 2 + 2 and 4 + 2 (long and short)]

Epipetalous, etc. (on the petals)

Dehiscence of anther splitting of pollen at maturity generally released from the anther through a longitudinal slitlike opening.

Gynoecium: The upper and inner most part of the flower, usually the last floral part to mature are the carpels (gynoecium or pistils) female organ (Fig. 3.14).

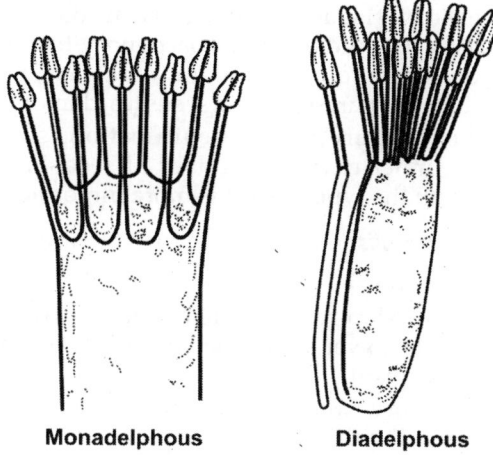

Monadelphous   **Diadelphous**

Fig. 3.15: Stamens arrangement

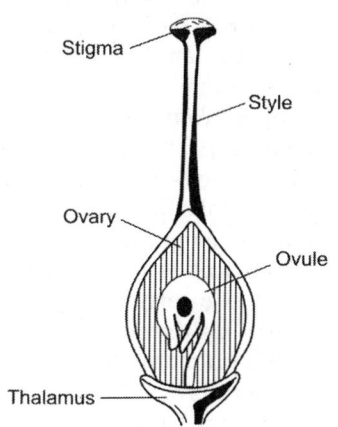

Fig. 3.14: Gynoecium

The carpels consist of hollow expanded base or ovary (matured ovary form fruits), stigma (flat and sticky surface to receive pollen grains), style (slender stalk to connect stigma and ovary) (Fig. 3.15).

Terminology Used

Apocarpus or syncarpus—free carpels or joined carpels

Superior or inferior.

Size and shape of stigma, style and ovary.

Transverse section of the ovary to find number of loculi and placentation (parietal, axile, free central).

Ovules: Egg-like bodies present in locule of the ovary. Each ovule encloses a large oval cell known as the embryo sac. Pollen grains after being deposited on stigma form long tube, which travel down through stigma and style enter one of the ovules in the ovary to form zygote on fusion with nucleus of egg.

Terminology

Orthotropous ovule: Straight ovule with the micropyle at the apex.

Campylotropous ovule: A curved ovule with the micropyle almost touching the funicle.

Anatropous ovule: Completely inverted ovule, turned back at 180° on its stalk.

Syncarpous ovary—Carpels are fused by their style or stigmas but possess distinct ovaries, e.g. Apocynaceae.

Superior ovary (Hypogynous): Superior ovaries are those that are present above the flower stalk (on the receptacle), e.g. Wild geranium (*Geranium maculatum*), tomato, chilli.

Inferior ovary: Ovary embedded within the receptacle. Term used is epigynous, e.g. Gourd (Cucurbitaceae), orchids.

Seeds: Matured ovules form seeds.

Fruits: Fruit is reproductive structure of an angiosperm which develops from ovary and accessory tissue, which surrounds and protects the seeds. In pharmacognosy fruit is used as a whole (capsicum, caraway and fennel) or its part separated seeds (cardamom).

For the purpose of identification, size, shape, inner cavities, number of seeds and above all the type of fruit is more important.

Types of fruits

A. Simple fruits

Fruits develop from a single matured ovary in a single flower, i.e. formed from gynoecium with one pistil.

Accessory fruits having some other flower part fused with ovary, e.g. Hip.

B. Aggregate fruits

These fruits are formed from number of matured ovaries of a single flower over the surface of a single receptacle. The individual ovaries are called fruit, i.e. formed from more than one pistil.

Etaerio of berry, e.g. raspberry or may be etaerio of achenes (traveller's joy).

Note: Generally fruits are formed by fertilisation. This process initiates complex changes in the ovules of ovary leading to formation of seeds and fruits respectively but there are exceptions where fruit can form without fertilisation (parthenocarpy) and such fruits are seedless. On maturity, ovary walls thicken and become differentiated into three distinct layers. These three layers together form pericarp which surround the seeds.

Following are the three layers of pericarp:

Exocarp: Outermost layer (epidermis)

Mesocarp: Middle one

Endocarp: The inner most one which varies from species to species.

Classification of Simple Fruits

1. **Fleshy fruit:** Pericarp becomes fleshy on maturity. Seeds set free after decomposition of the pulp.
   a. **Berry:** Fruits are made from one or more carpels with one seed or many seeds. Pericarp fleshy, e.g. orange lemon, colocynth.

Pepo: A fleshy several-seeded fruit that has developed from one flower having single ovary divided into several carpels, e.g. melon, cucumber.

Hesperidium: Specialised berry with leathery rind and many seeds, e.g. orange and other fruits of family Rutaceae.

   b. **Drupe** (stone) developed from single carpel. Endocarp is hard (woody), encloses one seed (almond).
   c. **Pome:** An accessory fruit, developed from many carpels. Pericarp is fleshy. Inner portion of pericarp papery or cartilaginous forming a case, e.g. apple, pear.

2. **Simple dry fruits (indehiscent):** Pericarp dry but does not open at maturity.
   a. **Achene:** One seed, attached at one point to the fruit, e.g. the fruits of Compositae family buck wheat.
   b. **Nut:** Hard one seeded like achene but developed from compound ovary and hard pericarp throughout, e.g. dock fruit.
   c. **Samara:** One or two seeded fruit with pericarp looks like wings.
   d. **Caryopsis or grain:** One seeded fruit in which seed is fused at all points to the fruit, e.g. cereals.

3. **Simple dry dehiscent fruit:** The fruits which open on maturity.
   a. **Folicle:** Fruits develop from one carpel, which open from one inner suture (ventral), e.g. Calotropis.

   Legume or pod: It is many seeded developed from both the sutures ventrally and dorsally, e.g. Senna pod.

   Capsules: It is dry many chambered fruit from polycarpellary pistil, which dehisce by means of number of parts, e.g. Datura, cotton.

   Siliqua: It is many seeded fruit developed from superior bicarpellary pistil which open from the base upward, but seeds remain attached with the false septum, e.g. mustard (Cruciferae fruit).

4. **Schizocarpic fruits, i.e. cremocarp fruits:** These fruits develop from inferior

bicarpellary pistil. After ripening they split into two mericarps but remain attached to an axis, e.g. coriander fruits of Umbelliferae family.

Multiple fruits: Whole inflorescence develops into a single fruit.
a. **Sorosis** in collective/multiple fruits developed from a spadix inflorescence with fleshy axis, e.g. pineapple jack fruit.
b. **Syconus:** It develops from the special inflorescence with fleshy hollow receptacle, e.g. mulberry; pineapple.

MICROSCOPIC EVALUATIONS

Microscopic examination of stained section of the drug (whole or powdered) is aimed to: study the internal arrangement of cells/tissue; their shape, size and the chemical composition of the cell walls and the cell contents.

Microscopical examination of epidermal trichomes and calcium oxalate crystals is very much important; especially to specimens in broken or powdered conditions, e.g. solanaceous leaves.

It is of two types:
i. Qualitative
ii. Quantitative microscopy (*see* page 65).

Qualitative Microscopic Evaluation

I. Clearing

For the microscopic evaluation of herbal drug (leaves) are to be cleared from chlorophyll by heating the sample drug with chloral hydrate in aqueous solution (5 : 2). It will remove the colouring matter and also will remove the common cell contents.

II. Staining

To differentiate the lignified and non-lignified tissues, cleared sample is treated with phloroglucinol (1% solution in alcohol) and hydrochloric acid. It will stain the lignified tissues from pink to red.

Hydrochloric acid (dilute) is strong clearing agent. It will also dissolve many cell contents as well as calcium oxalate, hence for the study of cell contents, drug sample should not be treated with hydrochloric acid.

Microscopic Evaluation for Leafy Drugs

Powder drug: The basic general characters which can be observed in the slide of unknown powder sample are epidermal cell, stomata, trichomes and small size vascular vessels (lamina), oil glands, palisade cells, cell contents (calcium oxalate crystals) patches of pericyclic fibre.

Fresh sample: Transverse section (TS) of the sample drug is prepared from the midrib region containing small portion of lamina. After clearing, stained with phloroglucinol and hydrochloric acid, mount under compound microscope in 50% glycerine/water solution.

TS of fresh leave has following general characters. It has two parts—lamina and midrib.

Lamina portion: Epidermis—single layer of parenchyma with number of stomata and trichomes on epidermal cells are very often covered by cuticle.

Palisade: Next to epidermal cells there is layer of palisade cells discontinued in the midrib region. The palisade tissue may be one sided, i.e. may be on the upper surface only (e.g. Duboisia) or in some drug on both the surfaces (upper and lower), e.g. Indian Cassia (*Cassia angustifolia*).

Mesophyll: Next to palisade is mesophyll which is always parenchymatous cells but it may also sometimes have collenchyma or sclerenchyma. Mesophyll region may be full of chloroplast or mucilageous contents. Very rarely oil secreting cells (Rutaceac family). Narrow vascular elements are also present.

Midrib region is characterised with vascular bundles generally collateral and open in the centre. Above and below of midrib region collenchyma and sometimes sclerenchyma is also present. Vascular bundles are enclosed in endodermis which may sometimes have starch grains in the form of sheath (e.g. Solanaceae).

Development of pericycle (parenchymatous) is variable in some plants. Sclerenchyma fibres may also be present in pericycle (Fig. 3.16a).

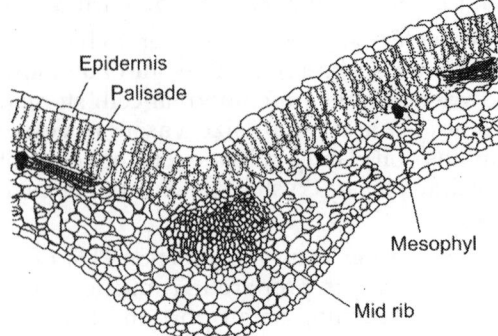

Fig. 3.16a: Microscopic structure of leaf

Characteristics Identifying Structure

Type of stomata

- Trichomes
- Type of vascular bundles
- Venations
- Palisade cells on one surface or both
- Cells contents.

Microscopic Identification of Stem Drugs

A young stem has the following basic anatomical structures:

Epidermis, cortex, medullary rays, pith and vascular system (dictyostele) (Fig. 3.16b).

Epidermis: It is outermost layer consisting of single layer of compactly arranged parenchyma cell having occasionally stomata.

Cortex: The cortex is generally parenchymatous cell in young stem. Upper layer of the cortex just below the epidermis is collenchyamous cell known as **hypodermis.** **Endodermis** is fully developed in the case of underground stem (resemble root) has well developed endodermis having casparian strip (suberised cell wall).

Pericycle: In the beginning may be parenchymatous cells or may have the patches of fibre just opposite the phloem bundles.

Vascular systems: The vascular bundles in young stem are in the form of dictyostele and are collateral open but in some families they are bicollateral (Cucurbitaceae, Solanaceae) in which xylem is differentiated into **protoxylem** and **metaxylem** (centrifugally). The protoxylem is endarch. Phloem is differentiated centripetally exarch protophloem. In bicollateral bundles the intrafascicular cambium is present between the xylem and outer phloem group.

Secondary growth: As the plant grows old secondary growth takes place by the tangential division in the intrafascicular cambium (VB) with the formation of complete ring of cambium. As the process of secondary growth proceeds, the dictyostele is converted into a solid stele continuous layer of xylem vessel and phloem and thus cambium cylinder is completed. The secondary growth in vascular

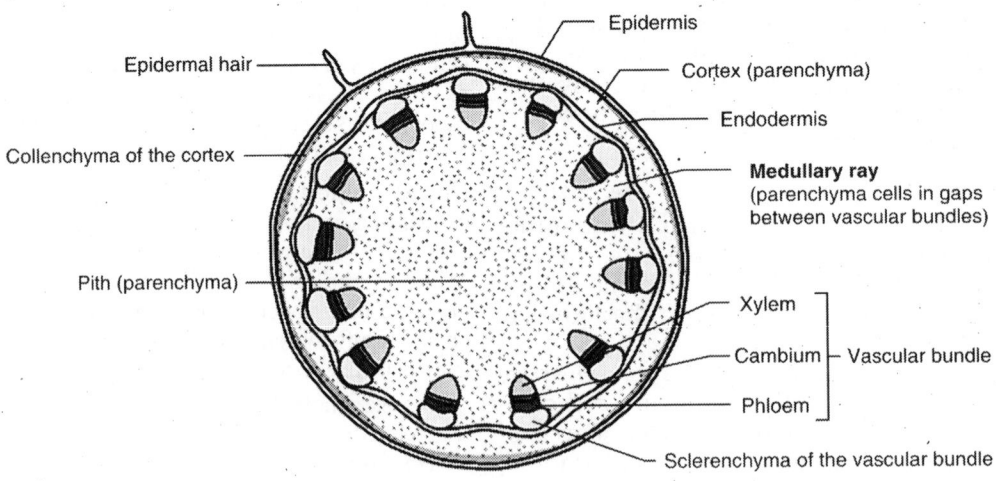

Fig. 3.16b: Internal structure of stem

stele is accompanied with the increase in diameter as well as increase in the outer tissue with the result secondary growth in the primary cortex and epidermis with the formation of **phellogen** in epidermis, cortex or pericycle and give rise externally to cork and internally **phelloderm**.

The **powdered stem** sample can be identified by the presence of cork, vascular tissue (lignified) abundant parenchyma, starch grain, calcium oxalate and other cell contents variable, from species to species.

The number, size and shape of the structural elements are the characteristic point for identification of the adulterants.

Microscopy of Bark

Bark

In transverse section of the bark, layers of cork tissue are tangentially elongated and arranged in radial rows. **Phellogen** and **phelloderm** may be present. In surface view, cork cells are polygonal in shape.

The cortex region generally shows one or two layers of collenchyma followed by parenchyma cells. Secretion cells, sclereids of pericycle fibre, occur scattered in cortex. Medullary rays are present. Phloem region have sieve tube, companion cell, phloem parenchyma.

Xylem tissue usually absent. If present then in small number in inner surface of the bark (Fig. 3.9a and b).

Cell contents: Suberin, tannins, calcium oxalate crystals and starch grains may be present.

Powdered Bark Sample

Pericyclic fibre, sclerides calcium oxalate, parenchyma with starch grains and secretory tissue. Xylem vessels are absent. Chemical test positive for tannins.

Microscopy Examination of Wood

Dry wood softened by keeping in boiling water for 1 to 2 hours or by keeping in mixture of alcohol, water and glycerin in proportion of 1 : 1 : 3.

Transverse section and longitudinal thin section to be prepared and stained by rinsing with 1% solution of safranin for 1–3 minutes. After the removal of extra safranin by rinsing with water are mounted in aqueous glycerine (1 : 1) and examined under high power microscope.

Wood from living trees can be sectioned without boiling in water.

Heart wood is often not stained with safranin.

Microscopy

Wood is highly lignified fibrous tissue (xylem) differentiated inside the cambium of a stem towards its centre. Bordered pits occur on radial side of the fibrous vessel (tracheids) (Fig. 3.16b).

Identifying Characteristics

Dicotyledons wood: Wood with vessels—size of pore, distribution patterns of the large and small vessel. Vessels are not uniformly distributed throughout the wood. Vessel width is the identification of early part of growth.

Medullary rays—length and width. Parenchyma cells containing chemical substance.

Coniferous wood: It is the wood without vessels with tracheids only having resin canals.

PHYSICAL AND CHEMICAL EVALUATION OF CRUDE DRUGS

Physical Methods of Evaluation

1. Solubility
2. Extractive value
3. Moisture contents
4. Ash value
5. Specific gravity
6. Melting point for solid unorganised drug
7. Boiling point for liquid drugs
8. Optical rotation
9. Refractive index for liquids
10. Determination of volatile oil contents.

Solubility: Amount of solid substance (solute) dissolved in a unit volume of suitable solvent to give a clear solution; under specific conditions (temperature and pressure). It is expressed as moles of a solute per 100 g of solvent (aqueous or organic).

On the basis of solubility, the solid can be hydrophilic (aqueous soluble), e.g. alkaloidal salts, glycosides and tannins, etc. or can be lipophilic (soluble in organic solvent), e.g. lipid, fixed oils, etc.

BP Solubilities Terms

Very soluble: 1 gm of drug substance dissolves in less than 1 ml of solvent:

Freely soluble:	From 1 to 10 parts of solvent
Soluble:	From 10 to 30 parts
Sparingly soluble:	From 30 to 100 parts
Slightly soluble:	From 100 to 1000 parts
Very slightly soluble:	From 1000 to 10,000 parts

Practically insoluble: More than 10,000 parts, e.g. urea is very soluble in highly polar solvent (water) less soluble in fairly polar solvent (methanol) and practically insoluble in non-polar solvent such as benzene. Hence, it is hydrophilic substance.

Caffeine at room temperature 2 g/100 ml, freely soluble but in boiling water 6 g/100 ml.

Colophony: Light petroleum.

Castor oil: Light petroleum (half to the volume of castor oil).

Extractive value: It is the percentage (%) of drug components soluble in solvent (aqueous/ organic). These constituents or substances are known as extractive. Regardless whether these are single component or mixture. It is considered as chief constituents of the drug.

Determination of extractive value of crude drugs is useful for their evaluation, especially when the constituents of drugs cannot be measured or estimated by other available methods. It gives the idea of the nature of chemical constituents.

Water soluble extractive value: Coarsely powdered drug (10 g) to be macerated with 100 ml of water in a closed vessel for 24 hours, with frequent shaking for first six hours and allowed to stand for 18 hours, filtered, volume make up to 100 ml. Then 25 ml of the filtrate

evaporated to dryness and dried at 105° to constant weight. Percentage of water extractive to be calculated with reference to the air dried sample, e.g. Aloe, gentian root, senna leaves and ginger.

Water soluble extractive value, e.g.

Aloe	25% w/w
Ginger	>10% w/w
Senna leaflet	>30% w/w
Liquorice	>20% w/w

Alcohol soluble extractive value: Air dried coarsely powder drugs (10 g) macerated with 100 ml of 90% alcohol in closed flask for 24 hours, shaking frequently during first six hours. Then allowed to stand for 18 hours. Filtered, rinsed, make up the volume to 100 ml. 25 ml of the filtrate evaporated to dryness in tared flat bottom shallow dish. Dried at 105° and weighed. Percentage alcohol soluble is calculated with reference to air dried drug/ sample or by soxhlet apparatus extraction technique is used.

Example of alcohol soluble extractive:

Aloe	>10% w/w
Benzoin	
i. Sumatra	>75% w/w
ii. Siam	>90% w/w
Ginger	>4.5% w/w
Asafoetida	60% ethanol extractive

Volatile oil contents: Weighed amount (5 g) of fresh leafy drug is distilled with water (Clevenger apparatus) and distillate, collected in a graduated tube. The aqueous portion separates automatically back into the distillation flask. The volatile oil collected in the side graduated tube is measured (Fig. 3.17).

If the volatile oil has density higher or near to water difficult to separate from aqueous phase. The solvent with a low mass density (xylem) added to the measuring tube, the dissolved oil will float on the top of aqueous phase and measured. Calculation to be done with respect to weight of drug sample.

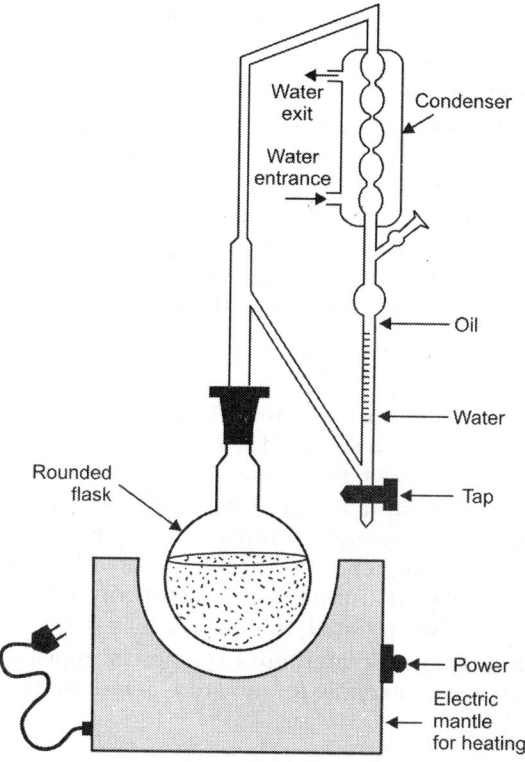

Fig. 3.17: Clevenger apparatus

Minimum limit for the percentage of volatile oil present in particular drug is given in pharmacopoeias IP, BP, BPC.

Moisture contents determination: It helps to reduce the error in the estimation of the actual weight of the drug.

Low moisture contents within the prescribed limit help in their stability against degradation of the drug in warehouses (check enzymatic and hydrolytic reaction, microbial contamination).

Moisture contents determination can be done by following methods as per WHO guidelines.

1. By heating a drug at 105°C in oven to constant weight.
2. *Gravimetric:* Loss on drying.
3. *Volumetric:* Azotropic toluene distillation method.
4. *Instrumental:* GC, NMR, etc. (BP and USP).

Loss on drying: 2–5 g of the test sample is placed in tared weighing bottle or china dish and heated in oven over diphosphorus pentoxide at room temperature or within specified temperature range in oven at 100 to 105°C.

This method is applicable to those drugs which contain little or no volatile oils, as the small amount of volatile oils can also contribute to loss in weight, e.g. digitalis, starch, aloes and fibres, etc.).

For materials having volatile contents like balsams, etc. drying is done in desiccator after spreading the drug in thin layer on glass plates over phosphorus pentoxide or in vacuum desiccator over an absorbent, at a specified temperature.

Toluence distillation method (separation and measurement of water):

The drug sample (5–10 g) to be analysed is distilled with suitable water saturated immiscible solvents (toluene, xylene and carbon tetrachloride) in an apparatus devised by Dean and Stark (Fig. 3.18). The water present in the sample is co-distilled with the immiscible solvent and collected in the graduated tube as a separate layer that can be measured and percentage is calculated with reference to weight of drug sample.

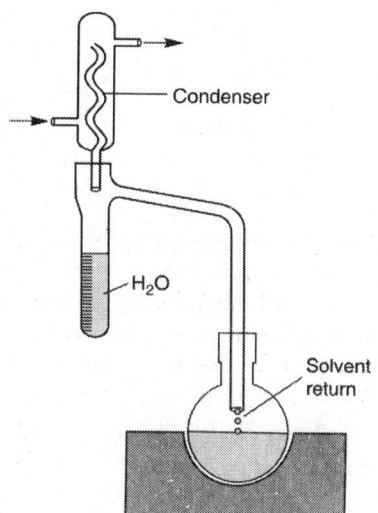

Fig. 3.18: Dean and Stark apparatus (water moisture apparatus)

Gas chromatography method: In this method drug sample to be tested is extracted with anhydrous or dry methanol, the aliquot submitted to chromatography on a column of either 10% carbowax on Fluoropak 80 or Porapak (polymer suitable for GLC). The water separated is measured readily from the resulting chromatogram.

Chemical methods (Karl Fischer method): It is very common procedure for water determination in pharmaceuticals, foods, chemicals and petrochemicals as well as in drug samples, even for the expensive drugs such as dry extracts of alkaloids containing drugs and fixed oils (castor oil, olive, arachis and sesame oil for parenteral use). It is mentioned in BP.

Method: The crude drug sample (digitalis) is extracted with anhydrous solvent (dioxane) till exhaustion of water and aliquot used for titration.

Reagent: Iodine, sulphur dioxide and pyridine in dry methanol. This reagent on titration with sample containing water, brown colour of the reagent disappears. At the end point (no water traces available) the brown colour persists. The basic reaction is the reduction of iodine by sulphur dioxide in the presence of water.

$$SO_2 + I_2 + H_2O + 3 \text{ Pyridine} \longrightarrow 2 \text{ (Pyridine·N^{±}HI)} + \text{Pyridine·N·SO}_2\text{—O}$$

Pyridine

Pyridine sulphur trioxide

Reaction is completed by the removal of sulphur trioxide as pyridine sulphur trioxide.

Pyridine sulphur trioxide in turn reacts with methanol to form pyridine salt of methyl suphate. In the absence of methanol the

Pyridine sulphur trioxide $+ CH_3OH \longrightarrow$ Pyridine salt of methyl sulphate

Pyridine sulphur trioxide (SO_2—O)

Pyridine salt of methyl sulphate (H, SO_4CH_3)

pyridine suphur trioxide reacts with another molecule of water.

Precautions

1. This test is water sensitive hence it should be performed under an atmosphere of dry nitrogen.
2. The reagent is prone to self-oxidation should be standardised immediately before or after use by using standard water solution in methanol.

Not: Nowadays karl fischer reagents are available which are less toxic than pyridine.

Other chemical methods: Treating the sample with carbides, nitrides and hydrides. Gas evolved measured by gas chromatography.

Spectroscopic method: Water absorbs energy at various wavelengths throughout the electromagnetic spectrum, this could be used as base of quantitative determination in spectroscopy analysis (NMR).

Electrometric method: Commercial moisture meter is available for moisture determination.

Ash Values

Ash is solid residue of mineral substances left-over the incineration of vegetable drugs derived from the cell wall and cell contents. **Chemically**, it is phosphate, carbonates and silicates of sodium, potassium, magnesium, calcium, etc. These are present in definite amount in a particular drug, hence its quantitative values of particular drug helpful in quality evaluation.

This can be used to determine foreign inorganic matter present as adulteration, as in the case of ginger a minimum percentage of water soluble ash is determined to detect the exhausted drug present as adulterant.

In case of hyoscyamus, being sticky trichomes attract the grit unavoidably, hence higher acid insoluble ash value is allowed (12%).

Types of ash: Total ash, acid insoluble ash, and water soluble ash.

A quantitative method for the determination of the yield of the ash is given in the pharmacopoeia for most of the official drugs, to evaluate the proportion of extraneous mineral matter. Included at the time of collection or during processing.

EP and BP use sulphated ash which is more consistent, and the drug is treated with dilute sulphuric acid before ignition thus all oxides and carbonates are converted into sulphate and ignition is done at higher temperature 600 ± 50°C.

Total ash value: To determine total solid residue that remains after ignition at low temperature (450°C) but carbon must be removed completely at low temperature as at higher temperature, alkali chloride will be volatilised. In the case carbon still remains at moderate temperature then, water soluble ash may be separated and the residue again ignited (BP) or as per USP ash may be treated with alcohol and then ignited.

Classification

Physiological ash: Derived from plant tissues.

Non-physiological ash: Residue left after the ignition of extraneous matter (sand and soil) total ash consist of carbonate, phosphate, silicate and silica.

Acid insoluble ash: Total ash treated with dilute hydrochloric acid, filtered, the residue leftover is the acid insoluble ash which is mainly of silica, e.g. senna, clove, tragacanth, liquorice and valerian, etc. are contaminated with earthy material. Senna leaf powder should have low acid insoluble ash (2.5%) while hyoscyamus 12%.

Water soluble ash: In the case of determination of total ash values, the carbon must be removed at a low temperature (450°C), without producing flames. If carbon still remains at moderate temperature then ash is treated with water (water-soluble ash) and separated and the residue again ignited as described in pharmacopoeia.

Method: Total ash is boiled with distilled water (25 ml) for 5 minutes, filtered on ashless filter paper, rinsed with hot water, ignited the residue to constant weight. The weight of water-insoluble subtracted from the total ash. The percentage is calculated with respect to the air dried drug.

	T. Ash %	Acid insoluble
Tinospora cordifolia	7.5	1.16
Cannabis	15.0	5.0
Ginger	6.0	1.7
Asafoetida	6.0	Water soluble

Optical Rotation

It is the property of certain liquid drugs to rotate an incident plane of polarised light to specific angle to the plane of incident light is known as optical rotation.

It is of two types: dextrorotatory, those rotate the light to clockwise direction (+) the symbol used is 'd' and levorotatory when the rotation of the incident light is anticlockwise (–) symbol 'l'.

The measurement of optical rotation is done using a polarimeter, the general equation used in polarimeter

$$|a|_\lambda^t = \frac{100a}{lc}$$

a is the specific rotation, t is time λ is wavelength, l is path length in decimeter, c is the concentration of the solute in g per 100 ml.

The BP uses the D-line of sodium ($\lambda = 589.3$ mm), a layer 1 dm thick and a temperature of 20°C.

Many volatile oils contain optically active components, their property of rotation and magnitude of rotation is a useful criterion of purity, hence employed for purpose of evaluation of adulterant, example, caraway oil +74° to +80°, lemon oil +57° to +65°, cinnamon oil 0° to –2°, citronella oil (Java) –5° to +2°, citronella oil (Ceylon) –9° to –18°, peppermint oil –16° to –30°; spearmint –45° to –60°.

Optical rotation observation conditions, i.e. temperature and wavelength for a particular drug are given in monograph of pharmacopoeias IP, BP, BPC and Herbal drug pharmacopoeia.

For essential oils the optical rotation requirement is expressed in terms of observed rotation, a measured under conditions defined in monograph of pharmacopoeias.

Refractive Index or Index of Refraction

It is the bending of a ray of light when passing from one medium to another. It may be measured as the ratio between the velocity of light in air and velocity in the medium of substance under test $\eta = c/v$, i.e. the sine of angle of incidence divided by the sine of angle of refraction. It varies with the temperature and the pharmacopoeial determinations are made at 20°C.

The most convenient instrument used for the measurement of refractive index is **Abbe refractometer** in which angle measured is critical angle for the total reflection between glass of high refractive index and sample to be examined (Fig. 3.19).

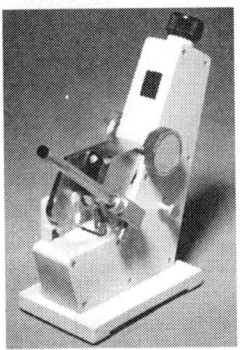

Fig. 3.19: Abbe refractometer

Measurement of refractive index is useful for the quality evaluation of volatile oils and fixed oils. Reference values are available in EP, BP, BPC and other pharmacopoeias, e.g. oils of cassia 1.61, oil of cinnamon 1.573–1.595 and cinnamon leaf oil has refractive index 1.53 thus making possible to differentiate the oils.

Lemon oil is 1.474–1.476 and that for terpeneless lemon oil 1.482–1.485.

Specific Gravity

It is the ratio of mass of a substance to the mass (density) of reference substance for the same given volume.

The reference substance for liquid is water at its densest at 4°C or 39.2°F, for gases it is air at room temperature (20°C or 68°F). Pressure is nearly always 1 atm (101.325 kPa).

The specific gravity can be expressed as follow:

$$SG\ true = \frac{P\ sample}{P_{H_2O}}$$

where P_{sample} is the density of the sample and P_{H_2O} is the density of water.

$$SG\ apparent = \frac{W_A\ sample}{W_A\ H_2O}$$

where W_A sample represents weight of the sample measured in air and W_A H_2O the weight of water measured in air.

Specific gravity can be measured by number of ways but most commonly used method is by the use of specific gravity bottles known as pycnometer, e.g.

Fluid	SG
Water	1
Ethanol	0.78
Urine	1.003 to 1.035
Blood	1.060
Linseed oil	0.932 at 24°C
Linolenic acid	0.902 at 25°C
Acetic acid	1.049
Glycerin 100%	1.2631 at 20°C 1.26170 at 25°C

Melting point: It is the temperature at which solid/semi-solid crude drug (animal/plant) gets liquefied. The crude drugs contain number of chemical constituents hence their melting points are not sharp. Therefore, always mentioned in range, whereas, the melting point of isolated pure compound is always sharp. Melting point is also one of the criteria to identify quality of the drugs.

Standard range of melting point of number of drugs is given in pharmacopoeias for comparison, e.g.

Hard paraffin	50–57°C
Hydrous wool fat	34–40°C
Cocoa butter	30–33°C
Caffeine	235–237°C
Piperine	130°C
Nicotine	79°C
Chloral hydrate	57.5°C

Boiling point: Normal boiling is the temperature at which the vapour pressure is equal to the standard sea level atmospheric pressure (760 mm). At sea level water boils at 100°C. Or it is defined as the point at which liquid can change its state from a liquid to a gas throughout the volume of liquid. It varies with atmospheric pressure.

It is the criteria of purity for liquid drugs. This can be compared with the standard boiling point given in pharmacopoeias.

Nicotine 247°C

Chloral hydrate 97.8°C–98°C.

Swelling index: BP define as volume in millilitre (ml) occupied by 1 g of drug, including any adhering mucilage after it has been swollen in water for 4 hours.

Number of herbal drugs have their specific therapeutic activity because of their swelling property especially gums and other drugs having constituents like mucilage, pectin or hemicellulose. Its determination is based on the addition of water or swelling agent as specified in pharmacopoeia in a measure cylinder with stopper for specified period of time.

1 g of drug treated with 1 ml of (96%) alcohol and 25 ml of water in a graduated cylinder shaken every 10 minutes for 1 hour and allow to stand, as specified, standard given in pharmacopoeia; for mucilaginous drugs, e.g.

Agar ≮ 10, Fenugreek ≮ 6, ispaghula husk ≮ 40, ispaghula seed ≮ 9, linseed ≮ 4, and psyllium ≮ 10.

Ispagol: Occupies volume not less than 10 ml.

Foaming index: The foaming ability of an aqueous decoction of plant material and their extracts are measured in terms of a foaming index.

Method: Prepare the decoction with 1 g of plant material as per WHO guideline. Put the decoction into 10 stoppered test tubes (height 16 cm and diameter 16 mm) in successive portions of 1 ml, 2 ml, 3 ml, etc. up to 10 ml and adjust the volume in each tube up to 10 ml, with water. Stoppered the tubes and shake them lengthwise for 15 seconds (two times per second). Allow to stand for 15 minutes

and measure the height of the foam, the results are observed as follows:

- If the height of foam in every tube is less than 1 cm the foaming index is less than 100.
- If height of foam is 1 cm in any tube. The volume of material decoction (α) in this tube is used to determine the index. If this tube is in the series of first or second then intermediate dilution of material decoction is prepared to get precise result.
- If the height in more than 1 cm in every tube the foaming index is over 1000. In this case repeat the process using new series of material decoction to obtain the result.

Calculation

$$\frac{1000}{\alpha}$$

where 'α' is the volume in ml of decoction used to prepare the dilution in tube where the height is 1 cm observed.

CHEMICAL METHODS OF EVALUATION

Chemical evaluation of crude drug means, the evaluation of the drug based on chemical analysis, as its potency and efficacy depends on the contents of phytochemical constituents present in the drug, e.g. alkaloids, glycosides, tannins, flavonoids, terpenoids, steroids, essential oils, etc. Estimation of the chemical contents by chemical method is known as chemical evaluation. This can be achieved by:

1. Qualitative estimation/determination
2. Quantitative estimation of chemical constituents.

The chemical methods of evaluation consist of:

a. Isolation, purification and identification the active chemical constituents by their **chemical tests**, e.g. alkaloids in opium, rauwolfia, cinchona and belladonna, etc. glycosides in digitalis, senna, cascara and strophanthus, etc. tannins in acacia and catechu, etc. (qualitative estimation).

b. **Chemical constants**, like acid value, iodine value, saponification value and acetyl value for the evaluation of fixed oils and fats.

c. Quantitative analysis of the active constituents.

General Methods of Extraction of Chemical Constituents from Plant Material

Extraction is the process of isolation of the chemical constituents from the plant material in soluble form. Before extraction the plant material should be properly authenticated. The extraction methods to be adopted depend on the nature of the plant material and the chemical constituents present in plant material. As all the chemical constituents are not soluble in the same solvent, e.g. fixed oils, essential oils, alkaloids (base), and steroids are soluble in organic solvents (petroleum ether, chloroform and solvent ether, etc.); alkaloidal salts, glycosides, flavonoids, phenolic compounds, etc. are soluble in polar solvents (alcohols and water).

Methods used for extraction are **maceration** (repeated), **decoction** and **percolation** (cold and hot) and continuous hot soxhlet extraction.

For essential oils special methods for the volatile oils extractions: are steam distillation and enfleurage process are used.

Ultrasound may enhance the extraction in some plant materials.

Dried plant material is usually powdered before extraction, whereas the fresh plant material is crushed and homogenised or macerated with solvent such as alcohol which is solvent with the extensive extraction power for almost all natural substances (low molecular weight) like alkaloids, saponins and flavonoids. Alcohol mixed with water induces swelling of the plant-particles and increase the porosity of cell walls, which helps in diffusion of cell contents into the surrounding solvent. In general, ratio of alcohol/water for bark, roots, woody parts and seeds is about 7 : 3 or 8 : 2. For leaves or aerial parts the ratio is usually 1 : 1 in order to avoid the extraction of chlorophyll. (Drug/solvent ratio is 1 : 5 or 1 : 10 in maceration)

Water immiscible solvents are widely used for the extraction of essential oils, fixed oils and steroids (light petroleum), for alkaloids base and quinones (ether and chloroform), for the extraction of organic bases (alkaloid) usually basification of the plant material is required, whereas for the extraction of aromatic acids and phenols, acidification is required.

Qualitative Chemical Tests (See detail in Chapter 7)

Qualitative chemical evaluation: Chemical tests are performed with specific chemical reagents to detect the type of chemical constituents, e.g. alkaloids, carbohydrates glycosides, flavonoids, tannins, saponins, steroids, terpenoids, fixed oils lipids, proteins, amino acids, essential oils, resins to detect the adulteration.

Quantitative chemical analysis: For the estimation of total quantity of phytoconstituents, to evaluate the quality of the drug.

Qualitative chemical test: Plants are subjected to preliminary phytochemical screening for the detection of class of phytoconstituents.

Chemical tests of identifications with the plant extract are as follow:

Tests for Alkaloids

Acidified solution of most of the alkaloids give precipitate with: **Mayer's reagent** (potassium mercuric iodide solution)—creamy coloured precipitate.

Wagner's reagent: (Solution of iodine in potassium iodide)—reddish brown precipitate.

Dragendorff's reagent: (solution of potassium bismuth iodide)—reddish brown precipitate.

Hager's reagent (a saturated solution of picric acid)—yellow colour precipitate.

Test for Carbohydrates (See detail page 146)

Molisch's test: All carbohydrates give purple colour with molisch reagent (α-naphthol in conc. sulphuric acid).

Reduction of Fehling's solution: All reducing sugars (monosaccharide and many disaccharide like lactose, maltose, cellobiose and gentiobiose) give brick red precipitate on boiling with Fehling soltution. Non-reducing carbohydrates (some disaccharides like sucrose and trehalose and polysaccharides), will reduce Fehling solution, after boiling with hydrochloric acid (hydrolysis) and followed by neutralisation (hydrolysis of non-reducing before testing with Fehling solution).

Tests for Glycosides
Cardiac Glycoside
Raymond's test: To identify the active methylene group.

To the solution of drug (50% ethyl/alcohol) add 0.1 ml of 1% solution of m-dinitrobenzene in ethanol. To this solution add 2–3 drops of 20% sodium hydroxide. Violet colour appear.
Legal's test: Deep blue colour with sodium nitroprusside in alkaline solution.

Killer-Killiani test: Blue colour appear—the presence of deoxy sugar.

Xanthydrol test: Red colour confirm the presence of deoxy sugar.

Baljet test: Yellow to orange colour with sodium picrate reagent on fresh TS of leaf.

Kedde test: Development of blue colour with 3,5-dinitrobenzoic acid and aqueous potash, for the confirmation of cardinolide group.

Saponin Glycosides
Foam test: Persistent foam produced

Haemolytic test: Haemolysis of RBC

Anthraquinone glycosides: Borntrager's test—in alkaline aqueous solution (KOH), red colour more or less purple colour develop.

Test for Lipids
Concentrated sulphuric acid test: Blue-red to cherry colour developed on treating the chloroform solution of lipids with concentrated sulphuric acid.

Libermann Burchard's test: A red to bluish green colour will develop on the treatment of chloroform solution of lipid with concentrated sulphuric acid in the presence of few drops of acetic anhydride.

Tests for Tannins
Gelatin test: About 0.5–1% solution of tannins gives precipitate with 1% solution of gelatin (10% sodium chloride).

Phenazone test: All tannins give bulky precipitate with 2% solution of phenazone in the presence of sodium acid phosphate.

Goldbeater's skin test: Brown or black colour develop on the hydrochloric acid (2%) treated goldbeater skin, in the presence of ferrous sulphate (1%) solution.

Matchstick test: A matchstick wood dipped in tannins extract, on treatment with concentrated hydrochloric acid, develop pink or red colour on exposure to heat.

Test for Proteins
Biuret test: Alkaline solution of protein gives purplish to violet colour with 5% solution of copper sulphate.

Physicochemical Constants Tests for Fixed Oils and Fats
Acid value: It is the number of milligram's of potassium hydroxide required to neutralise the free fatty acid in 1 g of the fixed oil.

It is a measure of free fatty acid present, which usually should be between 1 and 6 for each oil or fat.
Saponification value: It is the number of milligram's of potassium hydroxide required to neutralise the free fatty acids and to saponify the glycerides present in 1 g of fixed oil or fat.

This value is useful for detecting the adulterations of mineral oils with fixed oils, e.g. liquid paraffin, which do not saponify (being esters are absent), hence it proportionately reduce the saponification values of the fixed oils or fats.

Iodine value: The number of gram of iodine absorbed by 100 g of the fixed oil or fat under defined conditions.

It is the measure of the proportion and characters of the glycerides of unsaturated acids. The values of acids of **acetic series** will have low iodine values, while those of the linoleic and **linolenic series** will have high values, e.g. Linseed oil has not less than 175 and olive oil has 79 to 88; arachis oil and almond oil have 85 to 100, and 95 to 100 respectively while that of coconut oil 8 to 19.

Ester value: Number of milligrams of potassium hydroxide required to neutralise the complete hydrolysis of the 1 g substance.

BIOLOGICAL EVALUATIONS

Biological evaluations or biological assay are performed in living animal, isolated living organs or tissues or in microorganisms (bacteria, fungi, etc.). This method of drug evaluation is based on the pharmacological potential of the drug, which is directly affected by the concentration of active phytochemicals present in the drug. Hence, it is supplement to physical and chemical evaluation. It is also essential in the case of drug quantity being not sufficient enough to carry out all the tests for chemical evaluation.

Following are the properties analysed for the biological evaluation:

1. Anti-inflammatory properties.
2. Antipyretic activity—rabbit or guinea pig.
3. Anti-diabetic—rabbit or guinea pig.
4. Analgesic activity.
5. Anti-ulcer activity.
6. Anthelminitic activity—an earthworm.
7. Cardiac activity—frog and pigeon.
8. Antimicrobial—bacteria, fungi.
9. Anti-cancer
10. Anti-lithiatic.

Anti-inflammatory Activity

The chemicals used as anti-inflammatory drugs suffer from the disadvantage of side effects and high cost of treatment. Alternative to these drugs are natural products, derived from medicinal plants, e.g. curcumin, resveratol, boswellic acid, betulinic acid, ursolic acid and oleanolic acid, colchicine, capsaicin, quercetin and epigallocatechin-3-gallate (EGCG).

What is inflammation

It is a physical condition of the body or part of the body, becomes reddened, swollen, hot followed by pain and subsequently edema in response to injury or infection.

There are three stages of inflammation:

   i. Acute: Swelling stage.
   ii. Subacute: Regenerative stage.
   iii. Chronic: Scar tissue maturation and constant for number of days depending on immunity of the person and intensity of the infection or disease.

Mechanism: The inflammation occurs in response to injury caused by bacteria, trauma, toxin, heat or chemicals. The damaged cells release chemicals including histamine, bradykinin and prostaglandins. These chemicals cause leakage of fluid from vessel to tissues causing swelling.

This inflammation can be cured by the use of natural or synthetic drugs known as anti-inflammatory agents.

The anti-inflammatory drugs (non-steroidal) alleviate pain by counteracting the cyclo-oxygenase (cox) enzyme, which synthesises prostaglandins creating inflammation, e.g. aspirin, ibuprofen and naproxen.

All these drugs have side effects. Hence, there is need to screen some natural plants.

Screening the anti-inflammatory drugs: There are various *in vitro* and *in vivo* models available for the evaluation of anti-inflammatory potential but the most common screening model is carrageenan induced paw oedema in rats; cotton pellet induced granuloma. Acetic acid induced vascular permeability, histamine induced paw oedema in rats.

Subacute model: Formalin induced paw oedema.

Chronic model: Cotton-pellet induced granuloma in rats.

For evaluating the most effective and widely used method among all the above-mentioned models, the **carrageenan** induced paw oedema model is commonly used.

What is carrageenan?

It is a mixture of polysaccharides composed of sulphated galactose units, derived from Irish sea moss, *Chondrous crispus*.

Carrageenan Induced paw Oedema

It is biphasic event. The initial phase is the release of histamine and serotonin. The second phase is oedema due to release of prostaglandins, protease and lysosome.

The **first phase** starts immediately after the subcutaneous injection of carrageenan and remains for two hours.

The **second phase** begins at the end of first phase and remains for three to five hours duration.

Procedure: Healthy animals (rats) weighing 150–250 g to be selected and divide them into three groups each having six animals. Starve them overnight with water *ad libitum*. Next day record weight individually. The control group to be given vehicle 10 ml/kg orally while other group receives test drug and standard drug respectively. The left paw marked with ink at the level of lateral malleolus; basal paw volume is measured by means of plethysmographically by volume displacement method using plethysmometer by immersing the paw till the level of lateral malleolus. The animals are given drug treatment. One hour after dosing the rats, inject carrageenan 0.1 ml (1% solution in normal saline) into sub-plantar side of the left hand paw. The paw volume is measured again at one hour intervals for five hours after the challenge with injection.

The increase in paw volume is measured as percentage compared with the basal volume reading. The difference of average volume between treated, control and standard drug calculated for each interval and evaluated statistically. The percent inhibition calculated as per the following equation:

% oedema inhibition $[1 - (V_t/V_c)] \times 100$

V_t and V_c are oedema volume in the drug treated and control group respectively.

$$\text{Oedema rate (E)\%} = \frac{V_t}{V_c} \times 100$$

$$\text{Inhibition rate (I)\%} = \frac{\Sigma_c - \Sigma_t}{\Sigma_c} \times 100$$

where V_t is the oedema volume of drug treated animal. V_c is oedema volume of control group whereas Σ_c is the oedema rate of control group and Σ_e oedema rate of treated group per hour.

Cotton Pellet Granuloma

Procedure: In this method healthy Wister albino rats of either sex weighing 150–200 g to be selected and keep them in polypropylene cages at an ambient temp. $(25 \pm 2°C)$ with relative humidity 55–65°C.

The animal to be divided in groups (each having six animals) as per the requirement of the experiments. One group as control, second as standard and others—two as test drugs (lower and higher dose). The animals administered with test drug, vehicle (10 ml/kg b. wt.), and standard drug. After thirty minutes of administration anaesthetise the animal with diethyl ether or thiopen sodium 40 mg/kg; I.P.) followed by implantation of sterile cotton pellet weighing (20 mg). The animals are treated for 7 days subcutaneously or orally, then the animals are to be sacrificed. Remove the pellets and dry to constant weight. The net dry weight, i.e. after subtracting the weight of cotton pellet is determined.

Evaluation: The average weight of the pellet of control group as well as of the test group is calculated. The percent change of granuloma weight relative to vehicle control group is determined.

Analgesics and Antipyretics

Analgesics are the drugs which relieve the pain. The most common analgesics in USA are ibuprofen and aspirin. Both are non-steroidal and anti-inflammatory.

Antipyretics are substances which reduce the raised body temperature, e.g. acetaminophen (Paracetamol). Traditional use of higher plants as antipyretics are commonly referred to as febrifuge.

What is pain: It is somatic sensation and acute discomfort because of some physical hurt or disorder or emotional distress.

It is of two types: Acute and chronic pain

Acute pain: Fast and sharp followed by aching pain. It is of short duration.

Chronic pain: Pain that lasts longer, constant or intermittent and generally harder to treat than acute pain.

Following are models for the evaluation of analgesic activity of drugs.

Hot plate method, tail immersion test, formalin-induced pain.

Eddy's hot plate method used to assess the thermal pain, chemical pain through writhing method and for mechanical pain through tail clip method.

Procedure

Selection of the animals: Healthy animals of either sex (rats or mice) weighing 150–200 g (rats), 20–30 g mice. Acclimatize them to the laboratory conditions for at least one hour before testing.

Grouping: Divide the animals (rat/mice) into three groups (each group containing six animals), i.e. control, test and standard.

Drug administration: Administer the drug to test group orally and the control group the vehicle (10 ml/kg b. wt.) and the standard analgesic drug.

Experiment: One hour after the drug administration or as per the pharmacological action of the drug in reference monograph.

Eddy's hot plate: Place the animal on hot plate, having electrically heated surface, maintained at 55°C temperature.

Observation: Jumping, withdrawal of paws and licking of paws are to be counted. Time period, i.e. when animals start showing the response to be recorded by stop watch after 0, 30, 60, 90, 120 minutes.

Evaluation: The values to be compared with standard drug and the control groups.

Writhing method: In this model acetic acid 0.06% to be used as irritant to produce constrictions. Administer intraperitoneally, the irritant to drug treated animals and start noting the characteristic stretching behaviour. A series of constrictions occur which travel along the abdominal wall. Sometimes there are turning movements of the body along with the extensions of hindlimbs. The animals are transferred into glass chamber to record the number of writhes in fifteen minutes time.

Evaluation: The percentage of inhibition are calculated as follows:

% of inhibition = Average number of writhes in control/test group

$$= \frac{\text{Writhes in test group}}{\text{Writhes in control group}}$$

The time period with highest percentage of inhibition considered to be peak time.

Tail clip method (Haffner's method): At the root of tail of the animal (mice) place the Haffner's clip followed by the application of noxious stimulus, observe the reaction of mice in response to noxious stimulus as biting the clip or tail at the point of clip. This response to be recorded by a stopwatch after 15, 30 and 60 minutes.

Haffner's tail method: The method was described by Haffner as early as 1929 who observed the raised tail in mice tested with morphine or similar opioid drug.

Procedure: An artery clip is applied to the root of the tail of mice and the reaction time is noted. Male mice (18–25 g) are used.

Control group: Consists of 10 mice. Test drug is administered subcutaneously or orally (depending upon the nature of drug) to fasted animals. Drug is administered 15, 30 or 60 minutes prior to testing. The artery clip is applied to the root of tail (approximately 1 cm from the body) to induce pain. The animal quickly responds to this noxious stimuli by biting the clip or tail near the location of clip.

The time between stimulation onset and response is measured by a stopwatch in 1/10 sec. intervals.

Evaluation: A cut-off time is determined by taking average reaction time plus 3 times the standard deviation of combined latencies of the control mice at all time period. Any reaction time of test animals which is greater than the cut-off time is called **positive response** indicative of analgesic activity. The length and time, until response indicates, the period of greatest activity after dosing. An ED_{50} value is calculated at the peak time of activity. ED_{50} value found by the method were

1.5 mg/kg subcutaneously (SC) for morphine and 7.5 mg/kg for codeine SC.

Yanagisawa et al (1984) described a tail pinch method *in vitro* for testing anti-nociceptive drug consisting of an isolated spinal cord, spinal nerve root and the functionally connected tail of newborn rats. Change in electric potential in the ventral root is induced by noxious pressure on the tail. In addition, response after electric stimulation of the dorsal root were recorded.

Evaluation of Drug for Antipyretic Activity

To evaluate this property of drug, fever is induced in rabbits or rats by injection of lipopolysaccharide or Brewer's yeast. As subcutaneous injection of Brewer's suspension is known to produce fever in rats, a decrease in temperature can be achieved by the administration of compound having antipyretic activity.

Procedure: Wistar rats of either sex weighing about 150 g are selected. Divide into three groups (each having 6 animals), i.e. control, test and standard groups. Body temperature is to be recorded by the insertion of thermocouple to a depth of 2 cm into the rectum. The animals are fevered by the subcutaneous injection of 10 ml/kg of Brewer's yeast suspension (15% in 0.9% w/v saline). The site of injection is massaged in order to spread the suspension beneath the skin.

Animals are to be kept in room having ambient temperature, i.e. at 22 to 24°C. Immediately after the Brewer's yeast administration, food is withdrawn and after 18 hours of injection body temperature of animal is recorded. The measurement of temperature repeated after 30 minutes. The animals having rectum temperature more than 38°C are taken as test animal. Drug under investigation at different doses administered orally or SC and rectal temperature is recorded at 30, 60, 120 and 180 minutes, post-dosing of drug, standard as well as of control group.

Evaluation: The difference between the actual value and the starting for each time interval is recorded. The maximum reduction in temperature in comparison to control is calculated. The results are compared with reading of standard drug, i.e. aminophenazone 100 mg/kg b.wt. or paracetamol.

Antidiabetic Acitivity

To evaluate antidiabetic potential of the drug from natural source or compound, diabetes is induced in animals by the use of alloxan or streptozotocin in several species such as dog, rabbits rats or mice.

Alloxan-induced diabetes: Diabetes can be induced in rabbits weighing 2.0 to 3.5 kg by infusion of 150 mg/kg alloxan via ear vein. Rats of Wistar or Sprague Dawley strain weighing 150–200 g are injected subcutaneously (SC) with 100–175 mg/kg alloxan.

Male Beagle dogs weighing 15–20 kg are injected intravenously with 60 mg/kg alloxan. Subsequently, the animals are givan daily 1000 ml 5% w/v glucose solution along with 10 IU regular insulin for one week and canned food *ad libitum*. Thereafter a single daily dose of 28 IU insulin adminsistered subculaneously (SC).

Modification of the method

Neonatal: New diabetes model induced by neonatal alloxan treated rats (Kodoma et al, 1993). Male Sprague Dawley rats 2, 4, or 6 days of age are injected intraperitoneally with 200 mg/kg of alloxan monohydrate after 16 hours fast. But rats of 6 days are most suitable for the neonatal diabetes model.

In most species a triphasic time course occurs. An initial rise of glucose followed by a decrease, subsequently followed by sustained increase.

Streptozotocin-induced diabetes

Rakietin et al (1963) reported the diabetogenic activity of the streptozotocin (antibiotic) because of its cytotoxicity to beta cells of pancreas.

Procedure: Male Wistar rats weighing 150–200 g fed with standard feed are injected with streptozotocin 60 mg/kg IV or 50–60 mg/kg body weight intraperitoneally to overnight fasted animals to induce diabetes. As in alloxan three phases of blood glucose changes take place, initially blood glucose is increased, reaching to 150–200 mg%, after 6–8 hours time serum insulin values are increased up to 4 times, resulting in hypoglycaemia (need glucose administration) followed by persistent hyperglycaemia (depending on dose). Steady stage reaches after 10–14 days.

Administration of streptozotocin

Streptozotocin: It should be freshly prepared (50 mg/kg body weight) in 0.1 M citrate buffer (pH 4.5) to overnight fasted rats followed by 20% w/v glucose solution *ad libitum* for 24 hours to prevent streptozotocin induced hypoglycaemia. After one week time, blood glucose is analysed and animals having glucose level more than 200 mg/dl are to be selected as diabetic animals for the evaluation study.

Preparation of diabetic animal by alloxan monohydrate

Rabbits: Rabbits weighing 2.2 to 3.5 kg are selected. Alloxan monohydrate (150 mg/kg) freshly prepared in distilled water (5% w/v) is injected IV through marginal ear vein of the rabbit. Precaution to be taken that injection is given slowly to avoid sudden death of the animal. In the case of rats and mice alloxan monohydrate 150 mg/kg body weight is dissolved in distilled water and administered intraperitoneally.

Grouping of animals: Diabetic animals (rabbit/rats) are randomly divided into four to five groups of six animals each. Number of groups depends upon the dose of testing compound or plant extract. The control group (Group 1) administered vehicle (10 ml/kg body weight) 1% aqueous solution of carboxymethyl cellulose orally. Group 2 administered with standard (reference) antidiabetic drug suspended in 1% w/v aqueous solution of carboxymethyl cellulose. Group 3 and 4 administered with lower and higher dose of plant extract suspended in vehicle and administered orally using stainless steel cannula (feeding needle) attached to plastic syringe of 10 ml capacity.

Collection of blood: Blood samples 0.2 ml are collected (ear vein in the case of rabbit and retro-orbital plexus under mild anaesthesia in rats) before the drug/vehicle administration and one, three, five and twenty-four hours after the plant extract, compound and standard drug administration for the study of blood glucose level.

Drug administration: Normal diabetic animals are kept overnight fasted but water *ad libitum*. Blood samples are withdrawn before the administration of vehicle (control) and drug/plant extract are to be suspended in vehicle (1% w/v CMC) 10 ml/kg body weight.

Evaluation: Average blood glucose levels of test groups are compared with the control diabetic group as well as with the average blood glucose level of standard drug treated animals.

Oral glucose tolerance test (OGTT) or glucose-induced hyperglycaemia: Normal healthy animals (rabbits/rats) are divided into four to five groups, six animals in each depending upon doses of plant extract. Animals are kept overnight (18 hours) fasted but water *ad libitum*. Their fasting blood glucose level (FBS) are measured, before the administration of the test drug/plant extract at different doses to separate groups and vehicle to control group. One hour after the drug administration blood sample withdrawn for blood glucose level, followed by glucose (1 g/kg b. wt.) administered orally to drug treated and vehicle treated animals. Thereafter, blood sugar is determined at half an hour intervals for three hours. Glucose tolerance curve is plotted and peak rise in blood sugar level after glucose load is compared with vehicle control group as well as with standard drug treated animals. Time taken for clearance of glucose from the body (fasting level) is also measured and compared with control group.

The last sample to be withdrawn at 5th hour to measure the blood sugar level to see hypoglycaemic effect, if any.

Evaluation of Anti-ulcer Activity

Peptic ulcer and gastric hyperacidity are very common problems and one of the major gastrointestinal disorders. For the evaluation of plant product or plant extract for anti-ulcer activity, ulcer is induced in animals by the administration of 100% ethanol at a dose of 5 ml/kg body weight; or aspirin at the dose of 2000 mg/kg body weight; or indomethacin at the dose of 5 mg/kg and by pyloric ligation or by cold restraint stress induced ulcer methods.

Procedure: Pylorus ligation in rats.

Healthy female: Wistar rats weighing 150–170 g are selected, grouped into 10 animals in each group. The animals fasted for 48 hours having access to water *ad libitum* during fasting. Animals should be kept separately in cage with raised bottom of wide wire mesh to avoid cannibalism and coprophagy. Under anaesthesia, midline abdominal incision is made, pylorus is ligated with precaution of any traction or any damage of blood supply to pylorus region. The abdominal wall is sutured. The test compound (plant extract, standard drug and vehicle) is administered orally by gavage or by subcutaneous injection based on the nature of the drug under investigation.

The animals are placed for 19 hours in plastic cylinder with inner diameter 45 mm being closed on both ends by wire mesh followed by sacrifice of the animals under anaesthesia. Stomach is opened, ligated around oesophagus near the diaphragm. Remove the stomach and collect the gastric fluid in centrifuge tubes. The stomach is opened along the greater curvature and pinned on a cork board plate and examined for ulceration. The number of ulcers are noted and the severity recorded with the following score.

0   = No ulcer
1   = Superficial ulcer/spot colouration
1.5 = Haemorrhagic streak
2   = Deep ulcer
3   = Perforation

Measure gastric volume after centrifugation. Acidity determined by titration.

Evaluation: Ulcer index (U_i) is calculated as follows:

$$U_i = U_N + U_s + U_p \times 10^{-1}$$

U_N = Average number of ulcers/each animal

U_S = Average severity score
U_p = Percentage of animal with ulcers

Percentage inhibition

$$\% \text{ inhibition} = \frac{U_l \text{ control} - U_l \text{ treated}}{U_l \text{ under control}}$$

Ethanol-induced ulcer: Ethanol is reproducible method to produce gastric lesion in experimental animals (Robert et al, 1979).

In this model, animal (male Wistar rats) weighing 250–300 g are used, grouping is done as per the experiment design. The animals are deprived from food for 18 hours but water *ad libitum*. During that period they are kept segregated in raised wire mesh cages to prevent coprophagy. The rats are treated with test drug and vehicles respectively half an hour prior to administration of absolute alcohol (1 ml) to drug treated or (3 ml/kg b. wt.) to vehicle controlled animals one hour after the alcohol administration. Animals are sacrificed after anaesthetisation, incised along the greater curvature, gently rinsed under tap water and stretched by pinning on a cork board and evaluated for ulcer grade as per the formula given.

Indomethacin-Induced Ulcer Method

Indomethacin-induced gastric lesions in man and in experimental animals, by inhibition of gastric cyclo-oxygenase.

Procedure: Animals used are the Wistar rats weighing 150–200 g and group of 8–10 animals each. Test drug is given orally by dissolving in 0.1% TWEEN 80 solution 10 minutes prior to oral administration of indomethacin 20 mg/kg (4 mg/ml dissolved in 0.1% TWEEN 80 solution). Six hours later animals are sacrificed after anaesthesia. The stomach is removed and totally ligated and stored overnight after injecting the formol saline (2% v/v) solution. Next day open the stomach along the greater curvature and washed with warm water and examined with magnified lens. Lengths of the longest lesions are measured in millimetre.

Evaluation: Inhibition of the lesion production is expressed as percentage value.

Ulcer can also be induced with aspirin 200 mg/kg body weight in Wistar rats.

Evaluation of Hypolipidemic Activity

Hyperlipoproteinemia is the condition when there is increased concentration of cholesterol and triglyceride-carrying lipoprotein.

Lipoproteins are further divided into six major classes: Chylomicron, chylomicron remnants, VLDL (very low density lipoprotein), HDL (high density lipoprotein) and IDL (intermediate density lipoprotein). HDL promotes the removal of cholesterol from the peripheral cells and facilitates its delivery back to liver. Hence, higher level of HDL is better for good healthy heart and helps in the protection from arteriosclerosis.

Procedure of evaluation: Healthy animal (rabbits/Wistar rats). Rabbits weighing 2–3 kg and Wistar rats weighing 200–250 g are selected. Divide into groups of ten animals each (male). Animals (Wistar rats) kept overnight fasted but allowing water *ad libitum*. Their blood samples are withadrawn by retro-orbital plexus under mild anaesthesia before the administration of test drug or standard in various doses as per the experimental design. The test drug or standard were given orally by dissolving in vehicle 5 ml/kg body weight (PEG 400 or CMC 0.5% solution) followed by high fat diet. The control groups are given vehicle only. The treatment is continued for a period of eight days. Body weight of each animal is recorded at the beginning and at the end of experiment, i.e. on ninth day. At the end of treatment animals are kept overnight fasted with water *ad libitum*. Blood samples are withdrawn by retro-orbital puncture. Immediately thereafter the animals are sacrificed and liver removed, blotted free from blood and weighed and frozen in liquid nitrogen and stored at −25°C for lipid analysis.

Blood samples are centrifuged at 3000 rpm for 15 minutes and used for the estimation of total cholesterol by cholesterol oxidase and peroxidase method (CHOD/PAP) method, total glycerides (TG) by glycerine phosphate oxidase peroxidase (GPO/PAP) method, LDL_C, $VLDL_C$ (Friedewald's formula) and HDL_C level (PEG precipitation method), hepatic enzymes SGOT and SGPT by UV spectrometer.

Frozen liver samples are thawed and extracted with chloroform/methanol (2 : 1) in Teflon Potter Elvehjem homogeniser. Extract to be purified (Folch et al, 1957). Aliquot of the extract (solvent) are evaporated for the determination of cholesterol and triglyceride.

Evaluation: Average value of body weight, total cholesterol, triglycerides, HDL, VLDL, LDL, SGOT, and SGPT are compared with the average values of control group as well as the standard drug treated animals. Statistical difference between the control, standard drug treatment and test drug treatment are to be evaluated by means of two way ANOVA.

Triton-induced Hyperlipidemia

Triton $C_{14}H_{22}O(C_2H_4O)n$ (n = 9–10) a viscous colourless liquid, density 1.07 g/cm^3 is non-ionic surfactant having hydrophilic polyethylene oxide chain. Its systemic administration to mice or rats induce biphasic elevation of plasma cholesterol. Hence, it can be used to develop a hyperlipidemic model for the evaluation of plant extract for its hypolipidemic activity.

This model can be developed to study the antihyperlipidemic acitivity with the following mechanism:

1. Those plant drugs which interfere with the uptake of plasma lipid by the tissue as the triton increases the serum cholesterol level 2 to 3 times within 24 hours.

2. Plant drug interfering with cholesterol excretion, as the increased level of serum cholesterol decreases nearly to control levels within 48 hours.

Procedure: Keep healthy animals (male Sprague Dawley or Wistar rats 200–350 g fasted for eighteen hours, then next day record their weight and collect the blood sample withdrawn by retro-orbital puncture method, followed by administration of 20 mg/kg body weight triton injection intravenously. Test group of animals are subsequently administered with plant drug/test drug, control group vehicle only and reference group with standard drug. Blood samples are withdrawn after 6, 24 and 48 hours after triton injection for the estimation of total cholesterol from the blood serum.

To the another group of animals test drug and standard drug are administered 22 hours after the triton injection and blood samples are withdrawn after 6, 24 and 28 hours after the injection.

Evaluation: The results are compared with the average value of serum cholesterol of test group with control and the standard drug and statistical difference calculated by using Student's t-test.

Fructose-induced Hypertriglyceridemia

Rats with diet having higher cone. of fructose and rich protein diet develop hypertri-glyceridemia. Hence, higher concentration of fructose is used to develop hypertriglyceridemia model.

Procedure: Male Sprague Dawley rats weighing 200–250 g are selected and divided into groups of 10 animal in each group. Number depends upon number of doses of test drug, control and group for standard drug (clofibrate 100 mg/kg b. wt.). Their weights are taken and recorded. Blood samples withdrawn by retro-orbital puncture, analyse for serum triglyceride level. Then the animals are fed over a period of one week a diet enriched in protein and reduced carbohydrate contents. After one week time the animals are treated for three days with test drug, standard drug (clofibrate 100 mg/kg body weight) and vehicle (PEG 400) by oral route. From 2nd to 3rd day water is withheld for a period of 24 hours. Immediately after animal are provided with 20% fructose solution *ad libitum* for a period of 20 hours. At this time (i.e. 20 hours after the last dose of drug administration) blood samples withdrawn under mild anaesthesia, centrifuged to separate the serum and analysed for total cholesterol and triglyceride contents of the sample.

Average values of total glycerol of the treated group are compared with the control and standard groups using Student's t-test.

Evaluation of Hepatoprotective Activity

Liver is vital organ in the body. It plays an important role in drug elimination and detoxification. Liver diseases are characterised by fibrosis, cirrhosis and hepatocellular carcinoma and are associated with high morbidity and mortality.

The hepatotoxicity can be produced by alcohol and chemicals. Paracetamol-induced toxicity in animals is one of the most common experimental models to evaluate the hepatoprotective activity. At therapeutic dose it is considered safe for liver. However, when it is given at overdoses, it is leading cause of damage to liver, kidney and other organs in both humans and animals.

Acetaminophen/paracetamol

Experimental model: To induce liver injury in mice/rats, the chemical can be paracetamol, thioacetamide, azoxymethane and carbon tetrachloride. Synergistic effect of two drugs at lower doses are best alternative, e.g. paracetamol 500 mg/kg body weight and azoxymethane 200 mg/kg body weight.

Procedure: Healthy animals mice/Wistar rats of either sex are to be selected, divided into different groups six in each (control, test drug and standard). Animals are administered orally with test drug, standard drug (silymarin 50 mg/kg body weight), and vehicle to the control group for 14 days. Liver toxicity to be produced by administering paracetamol 500 mg/kg body weight alone or paracetamol 250 mg/kg and azithromycin 200 mg/kg together for seven days from 7 to 14 day. On the 14 day after test dose administration, the animals are subjected to biochemical investigation.

Blood samples are withdrawn by retro-orbital puncture under mild anaesthesia. The animals are sacrified by bleeding. The livers are carefully collected, dissected, removed and rinse with ice cold isotonic saline and then kept on ice, separated and weighed. Prepare 10% (w/v) tissue homogenate in 0.1 M phosphate buffer (pH 7.4), centrifuge at 10,000 × g for 15 minutes and aliquot of suspension separated and used for tissue biochemical estimation. Remaining part of livers are stored in 10% formalin for histopathological investigation.

Blood serum separated from the blood sample is investigated for serum glutamate oxaloacetate transaminase (SGOT), serum glutamate pyruvate transaminase (SGPT), alkaline phosphate (ALP) and total bilirubin using commercial enzymatic biochemical diagnostic kits as per the instructions of the manufactures.

Estimation of Tissue Biochemical Parameter

Tissue suspension used for the estimation of total lipid peroxidation by measuring malondialdehyde (MDA), reduced glutamine level, catalase and protein level.

Evaluation: The average results of the estimations are compared with the average results of control groups as well as that of standard drug treated group.

Statistical analysis is to be done by using Turkey's multiple comparison analysis.

Carbon Tetrachloride-induced Hepatotoxicity

To induce hepatotoxicity with carbon tetra-chloride (CCl_4). Administration of single dose (1 ml/kg b. wt) of CCl_4 to rats produces centrilobular necrosis and fatty changes within 24 hours. It reaches at maximum level within administration of three doses. Thereafter, it falls whereas at the dose of 2 ml/kg body weight sub-cutaneously for 2 days in rats have significant increase in serum SGPT and SGOT levels.

Evaluation of Anti-epileptic Activity

The evaluation of plant drug for anit-epileptic activity. Maximum electroshock seizure (MES) model and pentylenetetrazole (PTZ) induced convulsions model are commonly used.

Maximum electroshock seizure (MES) model. The generalised tonic-clonic seizures in rats are induced by applying current (150 mA, 0.2 second) through corneal electrodes using electroconvulsiometer. The antiepileptic activities are assessed by observing the extent of tonic hindlimb extension (THE), extension/flexion (E/F) ratio.

Pentylene tetrazole (PTZ) induced convulsions: Absence seizures are induced by a single dose administration of PTZ (50 mg/kg I.P.) to the rats which are placed in individual plexiglass cages (50 × 50 × 40 cm), to observe the behaviour by camera, connected to computer. PTZ is administered intraperitoneally once one hour after the last dose of plant extract on 7th day. The observation to be measured are first myoclonic jerk, onset of jerks, number of jerks, latency to clonus forelimb tonus with hindlimb clonus and duration of clonic convulsions. Changes in the time duration and absence or presence of different phases were taken as the measures of effectiveness of different doses of plant extract and the standard drug.

Procedures MES model: Male Wistar rats (200–250 g) are divided into number of groups (as per approved experiment design) each having six animals each (vehicle control, standard drug control and test drug low and high dose). The animals are treated with vehicle, test drug lower and higher dose for one week, by dissolving in 10% aqueous TWEEN 80. Standard drugs phenytoin 25 mg/kg b. wt. and diazepam 2 mg/kg b. wt. once on 7th day intraperitoneally 45 minutes before the induction of seizures and electric current is given.

Observation

Assessment of locomotor activity: Locomotor activity is an index of wakefullness of mental ability and assessed to study the sedative effect of the plant extracts/drug. The observation of each animal is to be done over a period of 5 minutes in a square (30 cm) closed arena equipped with light sensitive photocells and value expressed as counts per 5 minute. The beam in actophotometer cut by the animal is taken as a measure of movements. The apparatus to be placed in darkened, sound attenuated and ventilated testing room.

Assessment of rotarod test: Rats able to remain on the rotating rod with speed of 10 rpm for 5 minutes or more are to be selected and divided into different groups (n = 6). The animals are placed on the rotarod after 30 minutes of drug administration and latency to fall from the rotarod is noticed.

Evaluation of Cardiac Activity

Note: As per CPCSEA order the use of frog is prohibited. Hence, suitable animal model for cardiac activity is either Wistar rats or guinea pigs.

Aortic banding rat model: Banding of the ascending arota in rodents is the most commonly used method for the induction of hypertension as well as cardiac hypertrophy within several weeks. Angiotensin enzyme inhibitors even at subantihypertensive doses inhibit the cardiac hypertrophy. This method is leading method for assessing, subclinical left ventricular (LV) systolic abnormalities.

Partial aortic constriction by aortic banding leads to rapid increase in cardiac load and, therefore, cardiac hypertrophy. Under anaesthesia, ascending aorta is exposed by left thoracotomy which is constricted to about 30% of the original cross either with silver clip or by cannula No. 1 (0.9 × 40 mm) or with a weak hemoclip. Thus, heart weight is increased by 47% in 28 days banding.

Procedure: Ref. Vogel.

Male Sprague Dawley rats weighing 250–280 g are selected and divided into groups (n = 6) (control, standard and test drug) and their weights are recorded. Animals are kept fasted for twelve hours before surgery but water is allowed *ad libitum under anaesthesia* (IP injection of 200 mg/kg b.w. hexobarbital). Shave the abdomen followed by cleaning with disinfectant and by cut parallel to the linea alba, taking care to avoid any injury to the lung while making incision between the ribs. The aorta is made free from connective tissue above the left renal artery and underlaid with silk thread. Followed by placing the cannula No. 1 (0.9 × 40 mm) longitudinally to the aorta

and both aorta and cannula are tied, or you can place a small sized titanium clip around the ascending aorta with the help of an applicator whereby constricting the aorta lumen as per the diameter of cannula. The intestines removed during surgery are placed back with the application of 5 mg rolitetracycline (antibiotic). In sham operated controls no banding is performed. The skin is closed by clipping.

Animals are treated once daily with designed dose of testing drug and with standard antihypertension drug (as a reference). At the end of the experiment after six week treatment, blood pressure is measured under anaesthesia via indwelling catheters in the left carotid artery.

Heart is removed, rinsed in saline until free of blood and gently blotted to dryness. Total cardiac mass is determined by weighing on sensitive electronic balance (0.1 mg sensitivity). The atria and all adjacent tissue are trimmed off and weight of left ventricle including the septum as well as remaining cardiac tissue representing the right ventricle are weighed separately and calculated the weight per 100 gm body weight.

Evaluation: Total cardiac mass and weight of left ventricle and right ventricle of treated rats are compared with operated, control and sham-operated, control and with standard drug treated and analysed statistically.

Mineral Corticoid Hypertension Model

Salt retention is characteristic of human hypertension and can be achieved in unnephrectomised rats by mineral corticoid administration by weekly subcutaneous injection of deoxycorticosterone acetate (DOCA) and salt loading with 1% sodium chloride (NaCl) in drinking water will produce a major increase in blood pressure with increase in cardiac and renal weight. Hypertension develops more quickly and becomes more severe in male than female. DOCA salt have no signs of congestive heart failure at 6 weeks.

This model is in use for hypertension research or angiotensin-independent model.

Procedure: Healthy animal Sprague Dawlay rats weighing 175–225 g are selected. The animals are placed in well-maintained, under standard laboratory conditions, provided with normal feed. One day prior to the experiment animals are divided in groups each containing six animals (control, standard drug and the plant under investigation) as per the experimental design.

Hypertension is induced by DOCA salt (20 mg/kg SC) administration, two times in week for four weeks. The change in blood pressure to be recorded at the end of every week by the cuff method. When blood pressure reaches > 140 mm Hg, each group is given drug treatment for seven days in 5th week. The control group (normal control and hypertension control) is given vehicle only.

At the end of 5th week again blood pressure is recorded to evaluate the change in blood pressure.

Results are calculated as mean + standard error of the mean and compared with control group as well as drug treated and standard drug treated animals to evaluate the plant drug/extract for its cardiac activity.

Evaluation of cardiac glycosides activity: As the cardiac glycosides were standardised in units of an international standard and were adopted by many pharmacopoeias have nowadays of historical interest only. The frog and pigeon methods were suitable for this standardisation.

Frog method: Frog method was adopted by the US pharmacopoeia. It is one hour test.

Frog weighing 20–30 g are selected and record their weight, one hour before the analyses are placed in wire cages with a water depth of 1 cm. The dose of digitalis calculated in such a way that it should be 0.015 ml per g of body weight. Injection is made into ventral lymph sac. One hour later the animals are pithed, heart removed and examined. Systolic arrest of the ventricle and widely dilated atrium indicates the typical result.

International units are made from the percentage of dead animals in the test group versus those in the group receiving international standard.

Pigeon method: In this model adult pigeons weighing 300–400 g are injected with a solution of the cardiac glycoside into the suitable wing vein in the axillary region, vomiting occurring within 15 minutes is regarded as positive result, as intravenous injection of cardiac glycosides have an emetic action.

Procedure: Two doses of test solution and standard drug are injected. The percentage of vomiting pigeon registered.

Evaluation: It is done by comparing the results.

Test on isolated tissue and organs

Isolated cardiac papillary muscle or left atrium tissue have been chosen to study the decrease of performance after prolonged electrical stimulation and potential of restoration of force under the influence of cardiac glycosides.

Source of papillary muscle: Cats (2.5–3 kg), Wistar rats, spontaneous hypertensive rats, human papillary muscle strips from patient with moderate heart failure and compared the effect with papillary muscle strips from patient with severe heart failure.

This model is useful for the evaluation of cardiac glycosides.

Procedure: The animals are anaesthetised with ether. Heart is removed by opening the thorax followed by removal of papillary muscle from the right ventricle. The muscle strip fixed in organic bath containing oxygenated Ringer's solution at 36°C: One end of the muscle is tied to a tissue holder and other one a strain guage. The muscle is stimulated electrically with 5–6 V, 2 msec duration and a rate of 30/min. Contractions are recorded on a polygraph. After one hour the muscle begins to fail and force of contraction decreases to a fraction of control. At this point the cardiac glycoside solution/extract/drug is added to the bath. Record the contraction force to level approaching the control.

Standard drug is 300 mg/ml ouabain.

Evaluation: Increase of contractile force is calculated as per the percentage of extract or dose of the drug compared to standard drug.

Dose curve response can also be estabilished using various concentrations of the plant extract.

Evaluation of Diuretic Activity

Diuretics are the drugs capable of increasing the rate of urine flow and sodium excretion and are used to adjust the volume and composition of body fluids in variety of clinical situations including hypertension, heart failure, renal failure, nephrotic syndrome and cirrhosis. These drugs act on kidney and are able to increase the volume of urine excretion.

Diuretic Activity in Rats (Lipschitz et al Test)

Procedure: Wistar or Sprague Dawley rats weighing 150–200 g of either sex are used. The animals are kept in laboratory, maintained as per the norms prescribed by CPCSEA committee for one week to acclamatise.

This method is used for testing diuretic activity based on water and sodium excretion in test animals and compared to rats treated with high dose of urea. The Lipchitz value is the quotient between excretion by the test animals and excretion by urea control.

Procedure: In this method (Wistar rats 100–200 g), three animals per group are placed in metabolic cages provided with a wire mesh bottom and a funnel to collect the urine. Stainless steel strainer/sieve is placed in the funnel to retain the faeces and urine. Animals are fed with standard diet and water *ad libitum*. Eighteen hours before the experiment, food and water are withdrawn. Three animals are placed in one metabolic cage. For screening three animals are used for one dose of test compound. Test compounds are given at a dose of 50 mg/kg in 5.0 ml water/kg body weight. Two groups of three animals receive only 1 g/kg urea. Additionally, 5 ml of 0.9% sodium chloride solution per 100 g body weight are also given by gavage.

Urine excretion is recorded after 5 and 24 hours. The sodium contents of the urine is analysed by flame photometry. Test compounds are again tested with lower dose.

Evaluation: Urine volume excreted per 100 g body weight is calculated for each group.

Results are expressed as the 'Lipschitz value', i.e. the ratio T/U in which 'T' is the response of test compound and 'U' is of urea treatment. Indices of 1.0 or more are regarded as positive effect with potent diuretics. 'Lipschitz value' of 2.0 or more can be found.

Calculating the index for 24 hours excretion period as well as five hours indicates the duration of diuretic effect. Similar to urine volume quotient can be calculated for sodium excretion.

Dose response curves can be established using various doses.

Loop diuretics are characterised by steep dose-response curve.

Saluretic drugs like hydrochlorthiazide show Lipschitz value around 1.8, whereas loop diuretics (or high ceiling diuretics) like furosemide, bumetanide or piretanide reach value 4.0 and more.

Antimicrobial Activity Screening

Because of increase in multidrug microbial resistance, danger leads to treatment failure associated with multidrug resistant bacteria and it has become a global concern in public health.

Plants and other natural sources can provide a wide range of complex and structurally diversed compounds.

Therefore, the natural products as therapeutic agents have become increasingly popular.

To study their antibacterial activity, various methods used are agar disc diffusion, agar well diffusion and agar/broth dilution and to evaluate the antifungal effects against the molds the poison food method is used.

Agar disc-diffusion method: Agar disc-diffusion method developed in 1940. It is actually used by clinical microbiology laboratories. With the advancement in plant product research, this method is also adopted for testing of herbal extracts. In this method, diameters of inhibition growth zones is measured, here filter paper discs (about 6 mm in diameter), containing the test compound at a desired concentration, are placed on the agar surface inoculated with a standardized inoculum of the test microorganism and incubate for 24 hr at 37°C. Antimicrobial agent form the filter paper discs diffuses into the agar and inhibits germination and growth of the test microorganism creating inhibition zones. It is not appropriate to determine the minimum inhibitory concentration (MIC).

Evaluation: The diameter of inhibition zones are measured and antibacterial activity is evaluated by comparing with the inhibition zone diameter of standard drug.

Agar well diffusion method: This method is widely used in the evaluation of antimicrobial activity of plant extracts and the compounds obtained from plants.

Agar well diffusion methods refer to the movements of molecules through matrix that is formed by the gelling of agar. The antibiotic is applied to a well that is cut into the agar.

Procedure: In this method agar plates are prepared and inoculated with a standardized inoculum of test microorganism by spreading a volume of the microbial inoculum over the entire agar surface. Then wells are made with a sterile cork borer or a cylinder having diameter of 6 to 8 mm. Then plant extract solutions of different dilutions are introduced into well (20 to 100 µl) volume. The agar plates are incubated under suitable conditions required for a particular microorganism. The antimicrobial agent diffuses into the agar medium and inhibits the growth of microbial strain.

Evaluation: Zone of inhibition are measured and results are compared with standard.

Curve obtained from the zone of inhibition of different dilutions of the standard drug. The serial dilutions yielded concentrations of 20, 15, 10 and 5 mg/ml for the pure compounds are to be prepared. Similarly different dilutions of the plant extracts are also prepared.

Agar/broth Dilution Methods

Dilution methods are the most suitable to determine the minimum inhibitory concentration (MIC), that, inhibit the visible growth of bacteria under investigation. It is usually expressed in µg/ml or mg/L.

This method is useful both for the determination of susceptibility of bacteria to drugs and to evaluate the activity of new antibacterial agents.

Procedure: According to the European Committee on Antimicrobial Susceptibility Testing (EUCAST), the total extract dissolved in 10% dimethyl sulfoxide(DMSO) and diluted to higher concentration, then a serial ½ dilution of the extract is prepared directly in a micro titer plate containing broth (micro dilution) minimum volume 2 ml or with smaller volume using 96–well micro titration plate (micro dilution). Then each well is inoculated with standard microbial suspension. After well-mixing, the micro titer plate is incubated under suitable condition depending upon the test microorganism.

Positive control is also prepared with the standard drug. Under the similar conditions.

MIC to be considered the lowest concentration of the plant extract that inhibits the bacterial growth.

The lower the MIC, the higher the activity.

Procedure for essential oils: The essential oils are volatile, insoluble in water, viscous and complex substances thus, the methods mentioned above are not suitable for the testing of antibacterial activity of oils. Therefore only broth dilution method, using 0.02% tween 80 to emulsify the oil has been recommended most reliable and correct method.

Anti-fungal Activity

Poisoned food method: Plant extract to be tested is incorporated into the molten agar (different conc. of the plant extract) and mixed well. Poured the incorporated media onto Petri dishes. After overnight pre-incubation the plates/Petri dishes are inoculated with mycelia disc (2 to 5 mm) which is deposited into the centre of the plate. Then incubate under the desired suitable conditions. The diameter of the fungal growth are measured in control and test plates.

Evaluation:

$$\text{Anti-fungal acitivity (\%)} = \frac{(DC - DS)}{DC} \times 100$$

DC = Diameter of growth in control

DS = Diameter of growth in test solution

Disk-diffusion and broth or agar diffusion methods. Other methods are used for testing antifungal activities.

QUANTITATIVE MICROSCOPY

LYCOPODIUM SPORE METHOD

Lycopodium spore method used in quantitative microscopy for the evaluation of powdered drug, particularly those which have one of the following characters:

1. Well-defined particles which can be counted, e.g. pollen grains or starch grains.
2. Single layered tissue or cells, the area of which can be traced at a definite magnification and the actual area calculated.
3. Characteristic particle of uniform thickness, the length of which can be measured at definite magnification and actual length calculated.

Lycopodium spores are obtained from spore of Clubmoss particularly of *Lycopodium clavatum* Linn (Family Lycopodiaceae) grown in Polland, E. Europe, India, Pakistan (Himalaya) and North America. These spore are of light-yellow in colour, uniform in size (about 25 mm), three sided pyramid shape with convex base; the surface is covered with polygonal shaped reticulation. They can float on water without being wetted.

One mg of lycopodium spore contains an average of 94,000 spore, these facts make it possible to use them for the evaluation of powdered drugs like pyrethrum, clove, ginger, nutmeg, etc. and measure the length of trichomes (e.g. nux vomica trichomes) and to measuse the area (e.g. Senna and linseed).

Procedure: Definite proportion of powder and lycopodium (1 : 1 or 2 : 1) are mixed and suspended in olive oil or castor oil or in mucilage tragacanth (1.25 g tragacanth, 2 ml alcohol 90% and water to 100 ml) one drop suspension is placed on microscope slide and spread with glass rod and after applying the cover slip, keep the slide to settle the fluid.

The lycopodium spores are counted in each of the field (25 different fields) in which the numbers or area of the particles in the powder are determined.

Lycopodium spore method: For determination of percentage purity of powdered drug calculation to be done by using the formula

$$\frac{N \times W \times 94000}{S \times M \times P} \times 100$$

where

N = Number of characteristic structure in 25 field

W = Weight in mg of lycopodium spore taken

S = Number of lycopodium spore in 25 fields

M = Weight in mg of sample

P = It is constant, e.g. in the case of ginger P = 286000.

Note: For further detail refer to BP 1973.

Leaf constants

Leaf constaints such as stomatal number, stomatal index, vein islet number and veinlet termination are used for identification, quality determination and evaluation of leafy drugs.

Stomatal number

The average number of stomata mm^2 of epidermis is termed stomatal number. It is to be counted for both the surfaces (upper and lower) and ratio of values for both the surfaces is the diagnostic importance, to distinguish between the allied species, e.g. Datura innoxia and other species of Datura.

Examples

Atropa belladonna	(U)	17–25	(L)	77.5–176
Occimum sanctum	(U)	66–75	(L)	165–245
Datura metel	(U)	147–160	(L)	200–209

It may vary for the leaves of same plant grown in different environment or under different climatic conditions.

Stomatal number also varies considerably with the age of the leaf hence this leaf constant is not of much distinguishable factor for the evaluation of leaves.

Stomatal index: It is the percentage proportion of the ultimate divisions of the epidermis of a leaf, which have been converted into stomata is termed stomatal index.

$$\text{Stomatal index} = \frac{S \times 100}{E + S} \times 100$$

where

S = Number of stomata per unit area

E = Number of ordinary epidermal cells in the same unit area.

Stomatal index is highly constant for a given species. It can be examined either from the powdered leafy drug or an entire leaf sample.

For the determination of stomatal number to calculate the index, compound microscope with a 4 mm objective and an eyepiece containing 5 mm square micrometre disc is required.

Selection of sample: Mature leaf to be selected and cut 5 mm piece from middle portion between the margin and midrib region of the lamina and peeled off.

Cleaning: Boil with chloral hydrate in a test tube in a water bath and place the sample (peeled epidermis) on the slide with the help of brush along with chloral hydrate and mount the slide after covering with cover slip and examine under microscope. OR

Prepare the imprint of the epidermis: Smear the hot slide with little gelatin (50%), place a fresh leaf and slightly press the leaf, invert the slide and cool till gel is solidify, then remove the leaf, it will leave imprint of the stomata and epidermal cell. Trace them out on the paper with the help of camera lucida. At least not less than 400 cell should be counted, for the calculation of stomatal index values.

Tracing: Draw square about 8–10 cm square on paper, placed the prepared slide on the stage of microscope, focus the epidermal cell first under lower (10 × 10) magnification followed by high power (10 × 40) magnification then replace the eyepiece with camera lucida and trace the epidermal cells.

Example

	Stomatal index	
Species	*Upper surface*	*Lower surface*
Datura inermis	18.1 to 18.3 to 18.7	24.5 to 24.9 to 25.3
Datura metal	12.7 to 17.4 to 19.4	21.2 to 22.3 to 23.9
Datura stramonium	16.4 to 18.1 to 20.4	24.1 to 24.9 to 26.3
Datura tatula	15.6 to 20.2 to 22.3	28.3 to 29.8 to 31.0
Atropa belladonna	2.3–9 to 10.5	20.2 to 21.7 to 23.0
Atropa accuminata	1.7–4.8 to 12.2	16.2–77.5 to 18.3

Vein islet number: It is the number of vein-islets per sq. mm (mm^2) of leaf, calculated from four contiguous square millimetres, in the central part of the lamina (midway between the midrib and margin, of the leaf. **"Vein islet":** It is the minute area of photosynthesis tissue encircled by the ultimate division of conducting strands.

Veinlet termination number: The number of veinlet termination per mm^2 of leaf surface, midway between midrib of the leaf and its margin. It is the ultimate free termination of veinlet or a branch of a veinlet (Fig. 3.20).

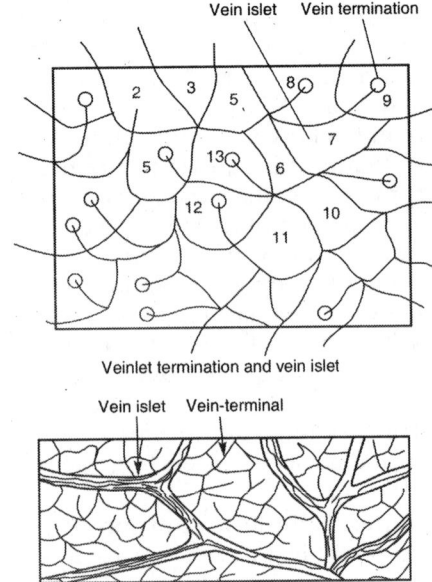

Fig. 3.20: Veinlet termination and vein islet

Vein islet			Vein termination number
Species	Range	Average	
Cassia senna	15–29.5	26	32.7–40.2
Cassia angustifolia	19.5–22.5	21	25.9–32.8
Digitalis purpurea	2–5.5	3.5	2.5–4.2
Digitalis lanata	2–3.5	2.7	
Digitalis lutea	1–1.5	1.2	
Digitalis thapsi	8.5–16	12.2	
Erythroxylum cocoa	8–12	11	16.8–21.0
Erythroxylum truxillense	15–26	20	23.1–32.3

Palisade ratio: It is defined as the average number of palisade cells beneath each epidermal cell is termed palisade ratio (Fig. 3.21).

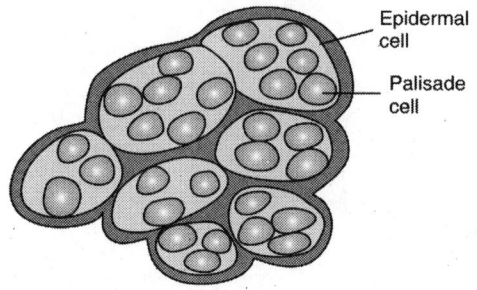

Epidermal cell

Palisade cell

Fig. 3.21: Palisade cell. Total: 7 epidermal cells. Palisade cell: 3 + 6 + 6 + 4 + 3 + 3 + 3 = 28. Average: 28/7 = 4

Procedure: For the determination of palisade cells, fine powder or fresh leaf can be taken as sample in the case of leaf (about 2 mm square or powder, are cleared by boiling) with chloral hydrate solution and mounted & examined with 4 mm objective. For tracing the object, camera lucida is required.

Example: Palisade ratio:

Atropa belladonna	6–11
Datura tatula	4–7
Datura atramonium	4–7
Cassia angurtse	5.1–7.5
Digitalis purpurea	3.7–4.2

Trichomes

Trichomes are unicellular and multicellular appendages of the epidermis. They are mainly of two types, i.e. Non-glandular and glandular:

1. **Non-glandular trichomes**
   a. Simple unicellular or multicellular
   b. Multicellular are of the following types:
      Stellated, e.g. *Styrax officinalis*
      Branched, e.g. *Verbascum* spp.
   c. T. Shaped–Stalk is one cell, with horizontally oriented terminal cell. *Artemisia annua.*
2. **Glandular trichomes:** The glands are involved in the secretion of various substances, e.g. salt solution, sugar solution (nector) lipids and gums (polysaccharide) (Fig. 3.22a and b).

Salt Secreting

1. Bladder like hairs consisting of large secretory cell on the top of a narrow stalk (Fig. 3.23).
2. Multicellular glands consisting of several secretory cell and basal collecting cell (Fig. 3.24).

Nectar secreting glands are found in corolla but not in leaf.

Mucilage secreting glands-arise from the leaf base of *Rumex* and *Rheum* (Fig. 3.25).

Example: *Rumex maximus*

Glands of carnivorus plant:
These gland are modified leaf and they prey insects and other small animals (Fig. 3.26) **example *Limonium latifolium.***

Stomata
These are intercellular spaces each of which is limited by two specialised cells (guard cells) hence stomata is opening between the two guard cells in the epidermis of leaf for gaseous exchange (Fig. 3.27).

Morphologically, four main types of stomata are distinguished in the dicotyledons. On the basis of arrangement of epidermal cells surrounding the guard cells. (a) Anomocytic, (b) Anisocytic, (c) Paracytic, (d) Diacytic, and (e) Actinocytic.

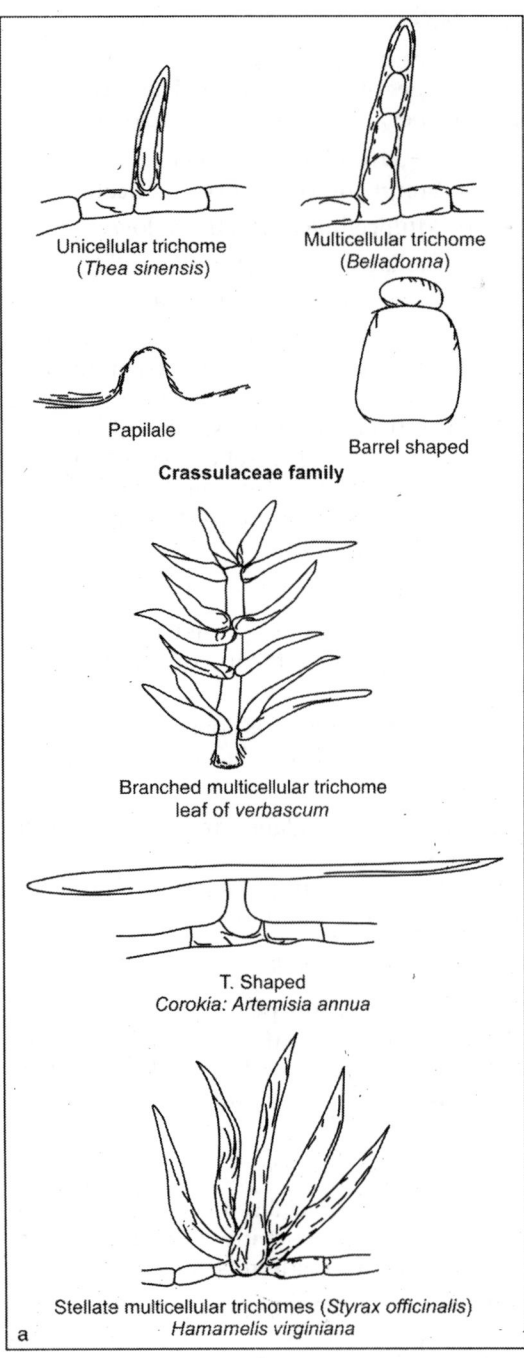

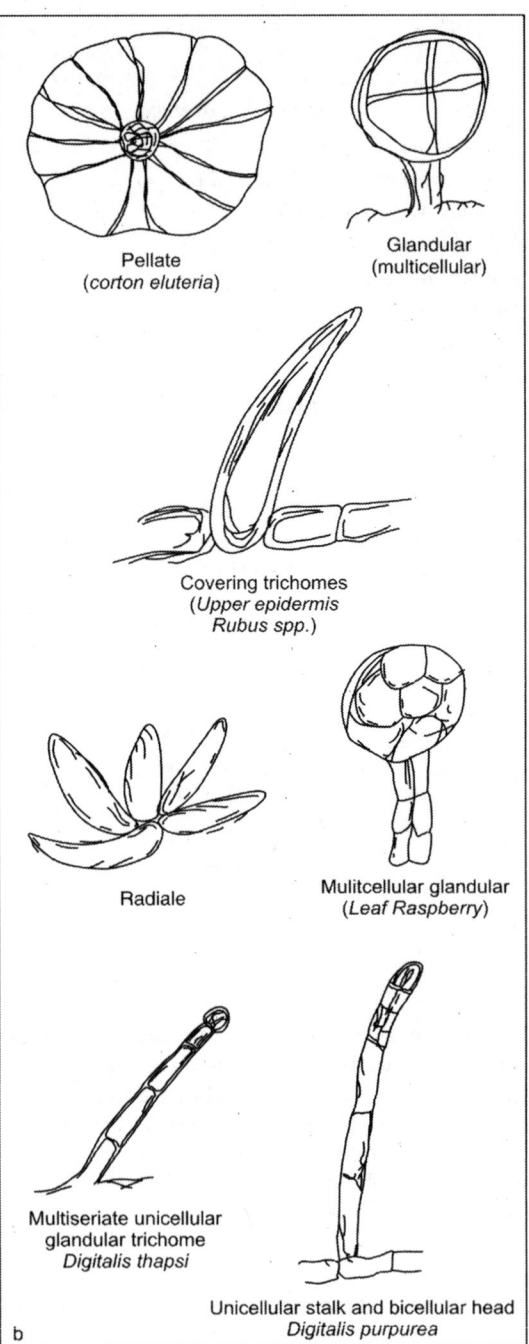

Fig. 3.22a and b: Trichomes

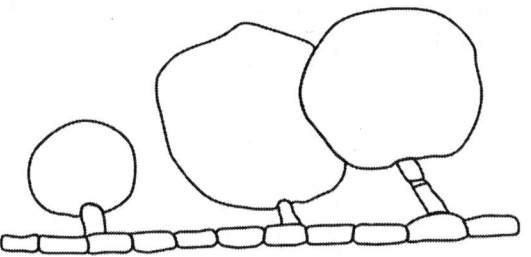

Fig. 3.23: Bladder like *vesiculate hairs of Atriplex protulacoides*

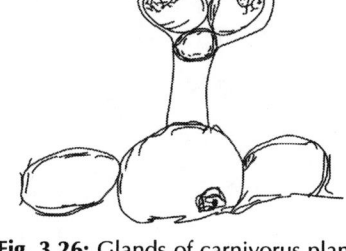

Fig. 3.26: Glands of carnivorus plants

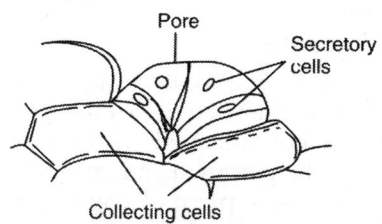

TS of leaf of *Tamarix*

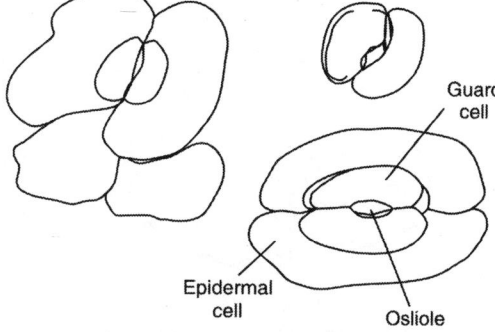

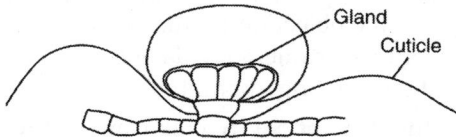

Fig. 3.24: Nectar secreting gland leaf of *Thymus capitatus*

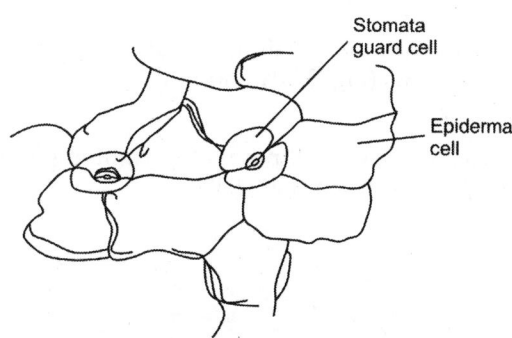

Fig. 3.27: Stomata

A. **Ranunculaceous (Anomocytic)** arrangement is, where stoma is surrounded by unmodified epidermal cells of varying size, e.g. digiltalis (lower epidermis) (Fig. 3.28).

B. **Anisocytic (Crueiferous)**
Stoma is surrounded by three or four subsidiary cells one of which is markedly smaller than the others (Fig. 3.29).

   Eample: *Hyoscyamus nigar,* (Lower epidermis)

C. **Paracytic (Rubiaceous).**

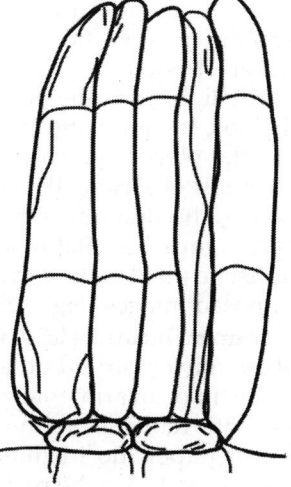

Fig. 3.25: Mucilage secreting gland *(Rumex maximus)*

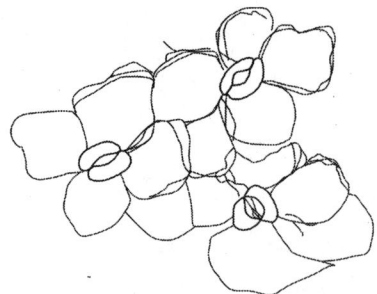

Fig. 3.28: Anomocytic

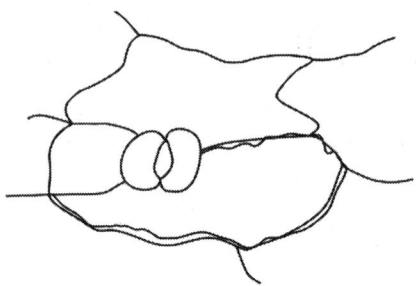

Fig. 3.29: Anisocytic stomata

Two subsidiary cells are parallel to the pore at long-axis (Fig. 3.30a and b).

Diacytic

Two subsidiary cell parallel to right angle to the pore of stoma (Fig. 3.30c).

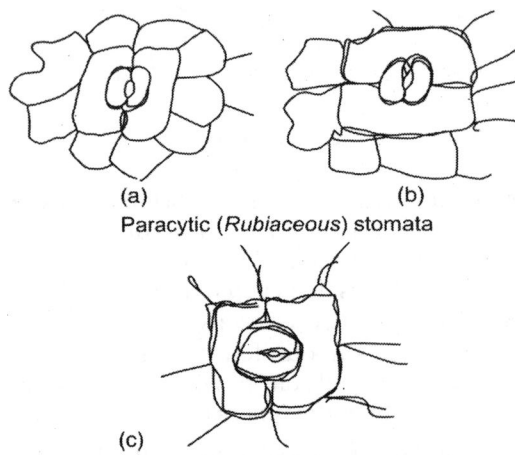

(a)   (b)

Paracytic (*Rubiaceous*) stomata

(c)

Diacytic (*Caryophyllaceous*) stomata

Fig. 3.30: Paracytic and diacytic stomata

Actinocytic: Stomata is surrounded by a circle of radiating cells, but this type is very uncommon (Fig. 3.31).

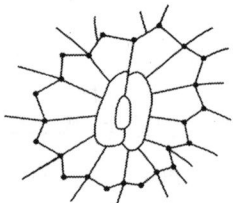

Fig. 3.31: Actinocytic stomata

Camera Lucida

Camera lucida is an optical device, invented in 1807 by William Hyde Wollaston (British Scientist), when attached with a compound microscope, help drawing microscopic images of the object on a piece of paper; preferably black paper and white pencil to draw image of the object. At present two types of apparatus have been designed to draw/trace a magnified image of the object under the microscope.

i. Swift ives camera lucida and

ii. Abbe drawing apparatus.

In the case of **Swift ives camera lucida:** consisting of attachment ring, the prism and the mirror. The attachment ring fit over the eyepiece, by attaching it with the body tube of the microscope, the prism just rest over the eyepiece, when light from the object passes direct to the observer's eye through an opening in the silvered surface of the prism, simultaneously light from the drawing paper and pencil look through the mirror super imposed on the object, which may thus be traced. Here while observing the object under the microscope, the illumination of both the object and paper must be suitably adjusted and the paper must be tilted at the correct angle to get superimposed images (Fig. 3.32).

In **Abbe's camera lucida** instead of adjustable prism, a plane mirror carried on a side arms attached at the tip of an arm, rotates to set at a angle of 45° with reference to the prism and plane piece of paper, no inclined board is required (Fig. 3.33), to see the paper too, so it appear that object if on the paper.

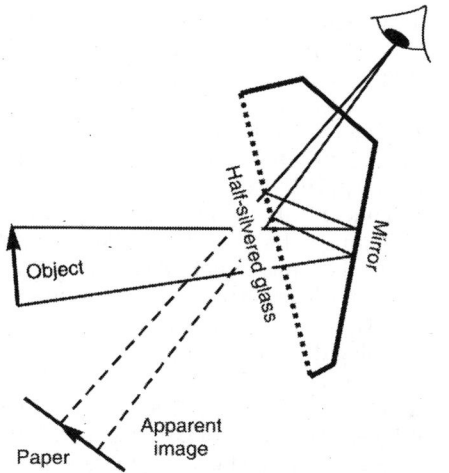

Fig. 3.32: Diagramatic representation of camera lucida

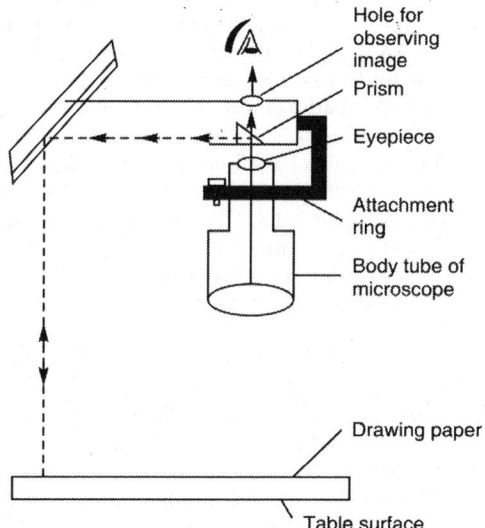

Fig. 3.33: Abbe's camera lucida

A camera lucida reflect a subject, so that it appears to be on your paper piece enabling you to simply trace it.

Appratus for making microscopic measurements and drawing object to scale with camera lucida

i. Stage micrometer.

ii. Eyepiece micrometer.

To make measurement or scale drawings, the calibrated divisions of a stage micrometer

are first traced on paper and then, using the same objective, eyepiece and length of draw tube, the object to be recorded is traced.

Stage micrometer: It is a glass slide 7.6 × 2.5 cm (3 × 1 inch) with a scale engraved on it. The scale is usually 1 to 1.1 mm long and is divided into 0.1 and 0.01 parts of a millimeter (Fig. 3.34).

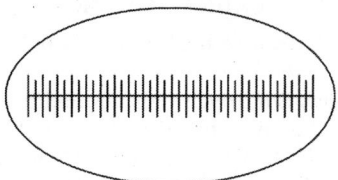

Fig. 3.34: Stage micrometer

Eyepiece micrometer: It is linear scale having 0–10 divisions. One eyepiece division is determined for every optical combination, as different combination of eyepiece and objective give different magnification and field of view.

When 4 mm objective is used, in the Fig. 3.35 above it is seen 7 line of stage micrometer coincide with 0 of the eyepiece, the 10 of the stage micrometer conincide with 7.7 of the eyepiece. As distance between 7 and 10 on stage micrometer is 0.3 mm. The 77 of small eyepiece division equal to 0.3 mm or

Focal length of objective	Initial magnification power	Approx. magnification (field of view in brackets) with eyepiece	
		×6	×10
16 mm (2/3 inch)	10	62 (20 mm)	119 (1.1 mm)
4 mm (1/6 inch)	45	285 (0.50 mm)	490 (.25 mm)

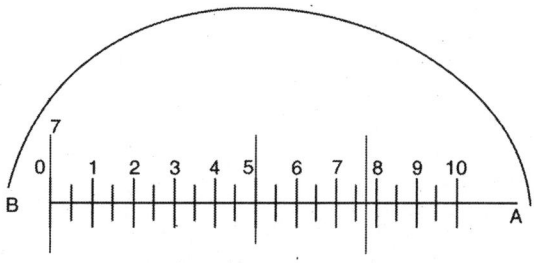

Fig. 3.35: Eyepiece micrometer

300 µm. Therfore 1 eyepiece division will be equal to 3.9 µm.

Thus, how the area under one division of eyepiece is calculated and used for measurement of the microscopic object traced on the paper with camera lucida.

FURTHER READING

1. Adv. Pharm. Technol. Res., US (3), July-Sept. 2-14, p. 129–33.

2. Ankush Sundriyal, Krishna Beddy V, Bijjem, Kalia AN. Antiepileptic potential of *Anisomeles indica* (linn) kuntze aerial parts in pentylene-tetrazole induced experimental convulsion in Wistar rats. Indian Journal of Experimental Biology, Sept. 2013;(51):715–20.

3. Bockman CS, Jeffries WB, Pettinger WA, Abel PW. Enhanced release of endothelium derived relaxing factor in mineralocorticoid hypertension, 1992; 20:304–13. [Pub. med.]

4. Cattell M, Gold H. Influence of digitalis glycoside on the force of contraction of mammalian cardiac muscle. J. Pharmacal Exp. Ther. 1938;62:116–25.

5. Evans WC. 2009. Trease and Evans Pharmacognosy, 16th ed., Elsevier; New York.

6. Fahn A. Plant Anatomy fourth Edition (1990) Aditya Book (P) Lid. New Delhi.

7. Flashade KO, Omoregie EH, Ochogu AP. Standardization of Herbal Medicines. Int. J. Biodivers Conservation. 2012;4(3):101–12.

8. General guidelines for methodologies on research and evaluation of traditional medicine. 2002. World Health Organization, Geneva.

9. Gerhard Vogel H, Wolfgang H Vogel. Drug discovery and evaluation. Springer publication, 1997;418–9.

10. Hem Singh, Asish Prakash, Kalia AN, Abu Bakar, Abdul Majeed. Synergistic hepatoprotective potential of ethanolic extract of *Solanum xanthocarpum* and *Juniperus communis* against paracetamol and azithromycin induced liver injury. Indian Journal of Complementary Medicine. 2015;1–7.

11. Ishpinder Singh, Tajinder Singh, Krishna Raddy V, Bijjim, Kalia AN. (2014). Anticonvulsant potential of Aniso and PTZ (50 mg/kg I.P.) was given on 7th day to induce generalized seizures.

12. Kan ST, Keddie JR, Andrew D. A method for screening diuretic agent in the rat. J. Pharmcol Meth. 1984;11:67–75.

13. Lipschitz WL, Hadidian Z, Kerpcsar A. Bioassay of diuretics. J. Pharmacol Exp. Ther.,1949;79:97–110.

14. Mounyr Balouiri, Moulay Sadiki, Saad Koraichi Ibnsouda. Methods for *in vitro* evaluating anti-microbial activity. A Review Journal of Pharmaceutical Analysis. 2016;(6):71–9.

15. Neeraj Chawdhary, Krishna Reddy V, Bijjem, Kalia AN. Anti-epileptie potential of flavonoids from the leaves of *Anisomeles indica* (Linn) kuntze aerial malabarica. Journal of Ethnopharmacology. 2011;35:236–42.

16. Quality control methods for medicinal plant materials, 1998. World Health Organization, Geneva.

17. Rifai N, Bachorik PS, Albers JJ. Lipid, lipoproteins and alipoproteins. In: Textbook of Clinical Chemistry, 3rd edition, edited by C.A. Burtis and B.R. Ashwood (W.B. Saunders Company, Philadelphia. 1979:809.

18. Swati Manik, Vinod Gautam, Kalia AN. Indian Journal of Experimental Biology. 2013;(51): 702–8.

19. Denslon TC. A Textbook of Pharmacognosy. 5th Edition London, 1951:631.

20. Wallis J, TE &. Churchill A. 1960. Textbook of Pharmacognosy. 4th ed. Little, Brown and Co.

21. Wallis TE. Textbook of pharmacognosy. CBS Publishers and Distributors, New Delhi, 2005.

Unit
II

Cultivation and Conservation of Medicinal Plants

4. Cultivation of Medicinal Plants

4

Cultivation of Medicinal Plants

HISTORY

Medicinal plants have been one of the important sources of medicines and are associated with health of mankind from the time immemorial. Archaeological discoveries of 60,000 years old Neanderthal burial ground in Iraque, reveal the use of several plants like marsh mallow (*Althaea officinalis*), yarrow (*Achillea millefolium*) and groundsel (*Senecio vulgaris*) that still figure in folk medicines. The medicinal plants always remained the local heritage with global importance. Herbs have always been remained major source of medicines in Asia and have made a good contribution in the development of ancient Indian **Meteria Medica**, one of the earliest treatise on Indian medicines. The **Charak Samhita** (1000 BC) has about 340 drugs of vegetable origin; most of them are being obtained from wild source to meet the demand of medicines for the ailment of human suffering. It is estimated that around 70,000 plant species have been used at one time or another for medicinal purposes. In ayurveda more than 2000 plant species are considered to have medicinal value, while Chinese pharmacopoeia have list of about 5,700 traditional medicines, most of them are of plant origin. Mexican Indian are reported to have used peyote cactus (*Lophophora williamsii*) for its hallucinogenic property. Ancient Egypt also gave the world one of the first medical text, the **Ebers Papyrus** named after the German Egyptologist George Ebers, believed to be written in 16th century BC containing about 700 drugs including aloe,

wormwood, peppermint, henbane, myrrh, hemp, castor oil and mandragora used for the preparation of wines, infusions, pills and poultice, etc.

The Chinese herbs have been used for centuries.

The oldest known list of medicinal plants is Shen Nung's Pem Ts'ao or Shennong Ben Cao Coo Jing (C.3000 BC), having record for 365 species of different parts of plants, animals and minerals. The record of the ancient literature reveals about the use of 13,000 medicines and over 100,000 medicinal recipe in China. The most common drugs were cinnamon, ginger, rhubarb, nutmeg and cubeb.

In 400 BC a Greek named **Hippocrates**, known as father of modern medicine has written a text including list of 300–400 healing medicinal plants.

Aristotle prepared catalogue having record of properties of various medicinal plants named **Aristotle's pupil Theophrastus** (3000 BC) a botanist whose treatise **Inquiry into plants**. He described the characteristics of herbs including cassia, mentha, belladonna, squill and several others. He was the person who could change the properties of some of these plants through cultivation (mutant varieties).

Dioscoroides (64–120 AD) has produced a list of several thousand plants in **De Materia Medica** having detailed identification characters, collection, adulteration and therapeutic uses of medicinal plants.

The medicinal plants provides the starting material for the isolation and synthesising the conventional drugs, in spite of the tremendous development in the field of allopathy during the development of 20th century, plants still remain one of the major source of drugs in the modern as well as in traditional system of medicines, throughout the world. It is estimated that in the primary health care, over 80% of world population still depends upon plants based medications (2002), as the medicinal plants play an important role in the lives of rural population, particularly in remote area of developing countries with a few health facilities.

The wild cultivation have been traditional source of medicinal plants and herbs. The position cannot be sustained much further because of over unauthorised collection of the herbs from the forest, and on the other hand, steadily shrinking of area under forest because of growing pressure of population and development of roads in remote area, has resulted in deforestation and loss of natural plant source.

In number of plants, the roots or the entire plants are being used in traditional medicines resulting to destructive collection, leads to extinction of medicinal plants. This has resulted in unscientific and over exploitation of medicinal plants in the forest. The Ministry of Environment and Forest has already banned harvesting, endangered species of medicinal plants from their natural habitat. Whereas medicinal plants are being utilised in the preparation of traditional medicines and modern drugs. Hence, there is increasing trends worldwide of using natural products in the form of pharmaceuticals, herbal food supplements, toiletries and cosmetics in the international market. Therefore trade in medicinal plants, globally, is expanding; it will reach to $ 5 trillion by 2050, while presently, it is about $ 62 billion. India's position in global market is just 0.5% although India is rich source for varieties of aromatic and medicinal plants. The agroclimatics conditions and rainfall favouring this biodiversity. As the demand for medicinal plants is rapidly increasing, therefore, organised cultivation of medicinal plants are urgently required for meeting the demand. Harvesting, drying and storage of medicinal plants must ensure the purity and safety against microbial contamination and quality deterioration to compete global market.

PROCESSING, STORAGE, COLLECTION OF DRUGS FROM NATURAL ORIGIN

Collection of drugs from natural (wild source) origin require very careful planning, to ensure the selection of part of the plant to be collected and processed at right time in peak conditions, followed by fast processing, to retain their active constituents. Wild source is actually source which provide free and natural source of herbal medicines, for the collection of drugs to the satisfaction of traditional process. Moreover, the active constituents are in high concentration, in comparison to classical cultivation, being grown in natural habitat.

FACTORS AFFECTING THE QUALITY OF DRUGS

Identification: It is an important factor, while collecting the drug from wild field, as many plants look similar, hence proper flower flora of the particular area along with the photo of flowering plants require to be carried, otherwise poisoning can result from misidentification. In many cases different parts of the same plant have quite different action and uses, hence be sure that the correct plant part has been collected. Plant should be healthy, free from disease, and insect damage; otherwise it will lead to disease or decay the dried plant material. Plant should be complete, otherwise will be problem of identification for the dried material.

Harvesting time: Picking of the plant and plant parts should be done at the right time of maturity, ensuring for the highest concentration of the active constituents, unless otherwise, it is mentioned for a particular plant species. **Leaves** are to be harvested during summer or spring month, **flowers** to be collected as they bloom, **fruits and berries** at the ripening time and the **roots** at the time of autumn when the maximum vitality of the plant is beneath the ground. Care should be taken that underground organ must be free from soil, by shaking the drug before, during and after drying, which is sufficient in the case of sandy soil. Whereas, when soil is clay or other heavy soil then washing becomes necessary as example in the case of valerian collected from wild soil is washed, before drying. In certain cases rootlets are cut-off; in large roots, like Columba roots and Inula rhizomes, to be sliced to facilitate drying. Some underground drugs are being peeled, e.g. rhubarb, ginger and marshmallow roots, etc. **Bark** of tree or shrubs to be taken after the rainy season by taking care of the survival of the plants (spring or autumn).

In general harvesting to be done in dry weather, preferably on sunny morning after the sunrise when the dew has disappeared, and care should be taken to exclude vegetable debris as for as possible.

Processing and Storage: In order to maintain the latent medicinal qualities of the drugs harvested, must be treated and modified in such a way that specific biological substances could be extracted, e.g. fermentation before drying.

Fermentation: In some plants enzymic transformation of the original phytoconstituents is required, these very plants needs to be placed in thick layers, sometimes covered and often exposed to raised temperature (30 to 40°C) and humidity, to accelerate the enzymic action, this process is known as **Fermentation**; the fermented product then dried to prevent the attack of mould and microorganisms. The fermentation process is used to make the drug free from bitter taste and sometimes unpleasant smell, e.g. vanilla, tea, and cocoa, etc. Sometimes it is required to hydrolyse the constituents, e.g. preparation of sapogenin, hecogenin (starting material for the synthesis of steroid hormones), by the fermentation of press juice of Agave (*Agave sisalana*).

Drying of Herbs

It is the process of reducing the water contents of fresh herb by 5 to 10%, to store the herb for longer period even up to three years. The fresh herb has a high water contents, leaves may contain 60 to 90% of water, roots and rhizomes 70 to 85% and wood 40 to 50% and often the seeds contain not more than 5 to 10%, therefore, the constituents of seeds do not have the same risk of degradation as those of the other plant parts.

Drugs containing the volatile oils are liable to lose their aroma if not dried or if the oil is not distilled from them immediately. The drying equipment or distillation stills should be installed as near as possible with the growing area.

The information on the moisture contents for particular plant material is available from pharmacopoeias or other authoritative monographs. Drying should take place as soon as possible after harvesting the plant material; if enzymic action is recommended in certain drugs like **Gentian root** or **Vanilla** pods, etc. then slow drying at moderate temperature is necessary, otherwise rapid removal of water from the material is required to prevent the degradation of the cell contents and it also prevent the external attack by the mould and other microbial infestation.

Methods of Drying

Drying is to be done at higher temperature, but the desired constituents are often sensitive to heat and hence care to be taken while selecting the method of drying the particular drug, it should be the balancing act between the quick drying and sensitivity to high temperature of the constituents.

As a general rule, leaves herbs and flowers may be dried at 20 to 40°C, barks and roots at 30 to 65°C and rapid drying is required for flowers and leaves to retain their colour, aromatic drugs to retain aroma, at a temperature suitable for the nature of drug.

Medicinal plants can be dried in a number of ways: in **open air** (shaded from direct sunlight); placed in thin layers on drying frames, wire-screened room or building: by direct sunlight, if appropriate: in drying ovens/rooms and solar dryers; by direct fire; lyophilisation; microwave or infrared devices. When possible temperature and humidity should be controlled to avoid damage to the active chemical constituents. The method and temperature used for drying may have considerable impact on the quality of the resulting medicinal plants.

The duration of drying process varies from a few hours to many weeks, and in the case of open air drying depends largely on the weather. In suitable climates open air drying may be suitable for drugs like: clove, colocynth, cardamom and cinnamon, but arrangement have to be made for keeping the drugs under the cover of shed or tarpaulins/canvas at night or even during the wet weather.

The plant materials are spread out in thin layers on drying frames and stirred or turned frequently, in order to secure adequate air circulation. The drying frames should be kept at sufficient height above the ground to achieve uniform drying of plant material.

Shade drying: Herbs should be dried in warm, shaded, well-ventilated areas. For drying in shed, small bundles of herbs are prepared and suspended from the roof, hanging them upside down, threaded on strings, or lay flat on screen, oven rack, placed on the counter or tinned wire netting to allow air to flow freely, through plants material while they are drying.

Papers spread on wooden framework are also used, especially for fruits from which seeds are to be collected.

Shade drying is preferred to maintain or minimum possible loss of colour of leaves and flowers; and low temperature should be employed in case of aromatic medicinal plants.

Artificial heat drying: Drying is rapid and efficient than open-air drying and is often necessary on rainy days or in regions where the humidity is high; tropical countries (e.g. South Africa and Honduras). Medicinal plants materials may be dried by means of ovens, stoves, rack dryer, belt dryer, other heating devices or with open fires.

The use of open fire should be avoided as much as possible, as the combustion residues may cause contamination. When open fire is used, the area must be well-ventilated.

Tunnel type dryers are most suitable for drying large crops, e.g. *Digitalis*; the material is spread out on shallow trays, which are placed on moving belt and passed into a tunnel having stream of warm air. As the rack move against the warm air, the plant material is exposed to dry air all times. The moist air is removed through vent at the back. Temperature, humidity and other conditions should be controlled by the physical nature of drug and the physical/chemical properties of active ingredients of the plants, under the process of drying, e.g. for thin material (leaves), temperature is kept at 20 to 40°C, and temperature raised to 60 to 70°C for hard drugs like roots, etc. girthy drugs are sliced into pieces for fast drying.

Over heating may lead to expensive loss of the volatile components and/or decomposition of chemical constituents. Even optimisation of the drying is a matter of practical experience, in case, of leaves and other delicate material is over-dried. They become very brittle and tend to break while transportation.

In dried plant material the enzymes are not destroyed but only rendered inactive due to the low water content. As soon as moisture is absorbed from the air, they become reactivated, hence dried drug must be protected from moisture during storage.

Lyophilisation

Lyophilisation is process of drying of pharmaceutical product. Which are thermolabile or unstable on storage in aqueous media for long-time. In this process, the water is freeze-dried and subsequent removal of ice by sublimation in vacuum and then by thermal desorption.

Characteristic of the freeze dry process are:

1. Minimisation of chemical decompositions (drying take place at low temperature).
2. Complete dissolution of dried product (resulting product has a very high surface area).
3. More compatibility with sterile operation (solution is sterile-filtered before filling vials).

4. Precise filling weight (fill weight control is more precise for liquid).

5. Absence of powder (particulate contamination is minimised).

Usefulness of lyophilisation or limitation of lyophilisation:

Lyophilisation or freeze drying is the method used for stabilisation of substances which are easily degradable:

• Microorganism
• Foods
• Biological products
• Pharmaceutical products.

Above that freeze drying technique is applicable in the production of:

• Injectable dosage forms
• For oral dosage forms, where fast dissolution rate is desired.

Process overview

The product is first frozen to low enough temperature to allow complete solidification of contents of each vial.

Then chamber is evacuated until the pressure is less than the vapour pressure of ice at the temperature of the product.

At this pressure heat is applied to the shelves to provide the energy required for sublimation of ice. Receding boundry in the vial indicate the drying process proceeds. This phase is called **primary drying**. When the ice disappear, additional drying time is required to remove water absorbed to or trapped by solid matrix stage is called **secondary phase**. When the product is dry, the vials are stoppered in place within the drier by the hydraulic compression of the shelf stack, pushing the stoppers to fully inserted led position.

This occurs under fully vacuum or by back-filling the chamber with inert gas.

The process is conventionally divided into three stages:

1. *Freezing*: Cooling the material until completely frozen.

2. *Primary drying*: Sublimation of ice from product reducing pressure in the chamber and providing heat to the product.

3. *Secondary drying*: Desorption of residual moisture from the product.

Process of freezing involves:

1. Dissolving the drug and excipients in a suitable solvent, generally water.

2. Sterilising the bulk solution by passing through bacteria retentive filter (0.2 microns).

3. Filling into individual sterile containers.

4. Freezing the solution by placing the open container on cooled shelves in a freeze drying chamber or prefreezing onto another chamber.

5. Applying vacuume to the chamber and heating the shelves in order to sublime the water from frozen state.

Characteristics

The characteristic of a freeze dried pharmaceutical dosage form include:

1. An intact cake occupying the same shape and size as the original frozen mass.

2. Sufficient strength to prevent cracking, powdering or collapse.

3. Uniform colour and consistency.

4. Sufficient dryness to maintain stability (< 2%).

5. Sufficient porosity and surface to permit a rapid reconstitution.

6. Freedom from contamination such as microorganism, pyrogens (5 endotoxins units/kg) and particulates (<50 particles of 10 mm per container and <5 particles of 25 mm per container), is an essential attribute.

These desired particulars can be achieved by proper formulation of the product and by employing optimum freeze drying cycles.

Development of Formulation

Formulation should be such, that it should complete the freezing process in the minimum possible time to produce stable and efficacious product, which:

- Contain low moisture content
- Undergo rapid reconstitution or redissolution
- Possess the desired appearance.

Composition

1. **Solvent:** Generally, water, organic solvent up to 20%, can be added to promote solubilisation, reduce the degradation rate of the drug and to reduce crystallisation of the drug in frozen state, e.g. ethanol, N-propanol and butanol, isopropanol, ethyl acetate and dimethyl carbonate.

2. **Bulk:** To increase the bulk to obtain the desired characteristic in the case of low dose product. Concentration of bulk should be between 5 and 15%.

   For example, mannitol, lactose, dextran, sorbitol, sucrose glycin, polyvinylpyrrolidone and sodium chloride, etc.

3. **Cryoprotectant agent:** To prevent damage during freezing, cryoprotectant (glycerol, ethylene glycol, propylene glycol and dimethyl sulfoxide (DMSO) albumin) may be added.

4. **Buffer agent:** Buffers like acetate citrate, phosphate and glulamate, etc. may be added to maintain pH for the stability of drug.

5. **Tonicity adjustment:** To prevent homolysis, or crenation of RBC in isotonic solution, e.g. NaCl 0.9% w/v or dextrose 5% w/v to maintain the cell tone.

6. **Antioxidant:** Sodium metabisulfite, sodium bisulfite tocopherol, butylhydroxyanisole and ascorbic acid to prevent the oxidation of the drug.

7. **Preservative,** e.g. benzalkonium and benzethonium chloride, benzyl alcohol, methyl and propylparaben or chlorobutanol to prevent contamination during the frequent use of multiple doses.

8. **Surfactants:** Polyoxyethylene sorbitan monooleate, and sorbitan monooleate are the example of surfactant used for the solubilisation of the drug.

Added substances

In case of potent drug to avoid adhesion of drug to the inner glass surface of the container silicon coating to be done.

Capacity of the container should not be filled more than one half or 1 to 2 cm in depth.

Circulating refrigerant: Such as Freon (CFC) cellosolve or trichloroethylene used for cooling the freezing shelf, on which containers are kept for freezing.

Storage of Crude Drugs

Fresh herbs: Refrigeration is required for the herbs to be used fresh in food, leaves (basil, mint, coriander, fennel, dill, rosemary and sage and flowers), edible flowers (e.g. calendula, broccoli, marigold, Maringa, chemmomile and lavender, etc.). These fresh herbs after washing with water and chlorine cut into small pieces, packed in small plastic containers in such a way, to protect their organoleptic characters. The package are then kept in refrigerator at low temperature (3–8°C), in the case of extension in storage period for 3–4 weeks, package to be done under vacuum before refrigeration.

Freezing: Fresh herbs like garlic, capsicum, and parsley, etc. to be stored for 1–2 year time require freezing at temperature below 0°C after packing in the plastic container.

Stability of air dried (10–12% moisture), herbal drug is limited, because of slow enzymic changes in the constituents, hence there is great differences in the stability of crude drugs, e.g. drugs such as Indian *hemp* and *sarsaparilla* deteriorate even when carefully stored; drugs containing glycosides and esters (*Digitalis*), are usually less stable than those containing alkaloids (*Cinchona*). The drugs like *Digitalis* and Indian hemp should never be allowed to become air dry or they lose considerable part of active constituents, they may be kept in sealed containers with a dehydrating agent (quicklime) at the bottom of container separated by perforated grid from the drug.

Drugs containing essential oils deteriorate more quickly through evaporation, oxidation and polymerisation of the substances, hence should be stored in sealed, well-filled containers in a cool, dark room; however, at the other hand tannins have unlimited stability.

The fixed oils particularly cod liver oil stored in a sealed container in which the air is replaced with inert gas.

In order to keep the crude drugs stored for longer period, it is advisable to store them in a dry condition, in carefully closed containers and away from light, because even it does not affect the constituents but causes the changes in the appearance of the drugs especially leafy drug and coloured drugs (flowers).

Drugs stored in the usual containers-sacks, bales, wooden cases, cardboard boxes and paper bags—reabsorbs 10–12% or even more of moisture, plastic sacks will effectively seal the contents, above all it is also important to protect the drugs against insects attack.

Production of Drugs

Since time immemorial, man has gathered plant and animal resources for medical, cosmetics and culture use, from wild resources as mushrooms (morels, matsutake, truffles) and medicinal plants like ginseng, black cohosh and goldseal, etc. Even today, the trend is continue and hundreds of millions of people, mostly in developing countries, are engaged in gathering the plants and plant products from wild source for their earning by selling into market, with the result, some wild species are over exploited, hence number of agencies including WHO, are recommending that wild species be brought under cultivation system.

Medicinal plants production through cultivation can reduce pressure on harvested wild population and it may also lead to environmental degradation and loss of genetic diversity as well as loss of incentives to conserve wild population. As per survey report estimate that 21% of the world flora is threatened that is about 1500 medicinal species and about 72,000 plant are used medicinally.

Following are the high threatened species which can be propagated for marketing at high price to make the cultivation profitable.

Species are: *Garcinia afzelii*, *Panax quinquefolius*, *Saussurea costus*, *Prunus africana*, and *Warburgia sautaris*.

Medicinal and Aromatic Plants under Cultivation

In survey carried out for the Rainforest Alliance, from the companies involved in trade and production of herbal remedies and botanical products, **volume wise** on an average 60 to 85% material was cultivated, whereas **species wise** data is different, e.g. in Germany out of the 1543 species traded, only 50 to 100 species (3–6%) are exclusively sourced from cultivation. In India more than 400 plants species used for the production of medicines by the Indian herbal industry, 45 to 50 species are currently under cultivation in the different part of the country (Uniyal, et al. 2000). In China about 5000 medicinal plants have been identified and about 1000 are more commonly used, but only 100–250 species are cultivated (He and Ning 1997). In Hungary, only 49 species are cultivated for commercial production (Bernath 1999), in Europe as a whole only 130 to 140 medicinal and aromatic plants are cultivated.

Advantages of Cultivation over the Wild Harvest

Reliable Identification

Material collected from wild source often adulterated with unwanted plant material, sometimes with harmful plant species but chances of adulteration are meager with the cultivated plant raw materials.

Regular Supply

Wild harvested material dependent on many uncontrolled factors leading to irregular supply of plant materials, whereas cultivation can guarantees a steady source of raw materials.

Guaranteed price over times and Quantity

Wholesaler and pharmaceutical industry people can agree with the quantity and price over time with the cultivators.

Economic Development of Medicinal Plant Species as Crop

The selection and development of genotype with commercially desirable traits from wild could be possible for the economic development of plant species as crop.

Assured Quality Product

Controlled post harvest handling is possible, hence, quality control can be assured and standards can be maintained as per the requirement of consumers.

Biodynamic Certification

Cultivators give guarantee for the organic or biodynamic certificate of the products which is not possible with wild collection.

Challenges

Technical Problems with Species

Cultivation is not always possible with all the species because of certain biological features or other ecological requirements, e.g. slow growth rate, some special soil requirements, interaction with the pollinators and other surrounding species, low germination rate and susceptibility to pests.

Competition with wild Raw Material

Long-lived species is the main concern of the growers for short lifespan plant species.

There is a challenge from the commercial wild gatherers who has procured the material from wild resources.

Social and Biological Factors

The social and biological factors also play role in the economic viability of medicinal plants cultivation. As the domestication of previously wild collected species require the investment of capital for years of investigation while few species (cost-effective) are possible to cultivate.

CULTIVATION OF MEDICINAL PLANTS

Number of drugs are obtained almost exclusively from cultivated plants, e.g. cardamom, ginger, cinnamon (Ceylon), linseed, fennel, cinchona, opium and spearmint oil, producing aromatic plants, etc. while some drugs are obtained both from wild as well-cultivated plants, e.g. ginseng, aconite, goldseal, black cohosh, *Panax quinquefolius*, *Saussurea costus*, *Prunus africana*, and *Warburgia salutaris*.

Propagation of Medicinal Plants

Plants propagation, is the multiplication of plants, through **sexual** (seed propagation) and **asexual** (vegetative) propagation methods.

Sexual (Seed) Propagation Method

To ensure the quality of seed for uniform germination, the seeds should be collected, when perfectly ripened, as the germination of seed is possible, only when the embryo is fully matured. Seeds with immature embryo, remains dormant, until the embryo develops completely within the seed, hence take some more time under normal conditions for proper germination. Seeds behave differently, therefore, before selection, healthy perfect seeds are utmost important. Long storage of all seeds usually affect germination rate.

The environment and storage conditions effect the germination ability of the seeds. As seeds start the process of losing their viability from the point of their harvesting. Hence proper conditioning and storage conditions are required, to maintain their viability for long period.

Seeds kept frozen with low moisture can last for years and even decades with excellent germination rate.

Seeds Treatment

Seeds are treated chemically with fungicides or biocontrol agents to eradicate seeds born diseases, to break the dormancy and to harden the seed to withstand drought. Seeds treatment is also required for fertiliser inoculation before sowing in field.

Some seeds have hard seed coat, e.g. seeds of wild indigo (*Tephrosia purpurea*), castor seed having waxy impermeable hard seed coat, needs **Scarification of seeds** to fasten the germination.

Seeds are mixed with sand and hand pounded, this will smoothen the seed coat and facilitate rapid germination. Another way of improving the germination of the seeds with hard coat is by soaking them in hot water. Steeping the seeds of wild indigo in boiling water for 2 to 3 minutes will facilitate early germination, this is known as **soaking seeds in hot water**.

Sowing time of seeds: Time of sowing the seed also affect the germination rate hence it should also be checked from the monograph, as time of seed sowing may affect the active constituents.

Seeds sowing method: Seeds planting depth should be 1–2 times their diameter. Small seeds are scattered or planted thickly in rows, larger seeds to be planted to 2–3 inches depth. Medium size seeds are shown on the surface covered with thin layer of shredded peat moss (*Sphagnum moss*).

Vegetative Propagation (Asexual Cultivation) Methods

Natural Vegetative Propagation

A method of plants reproduction in which vegetative part, like the stem (sub-aerial and underground stem), root and leaves develop into new plant under favourable conditions is known as vegetative propagation.

Underground stems or fragments of new plant for underground stem develop roots and buds, which gradually grow up into vegetative propagation, e.g. underground stem: **bulbs** (squill, onion): **corm** (colchicum, saffron), **tuber** (jalap, potato and aconite) and **rhizome** (ginger).

Sub-aerial stem: The nodes of sub-aerial stems develop new stem at the upper surface and adventitious roots on the lower surface which can grow as a new plant, e.g. runner or offset (colocasia, chamomile and mint), sucker or stolon (liquorice, valerian and garden chrysanthemum).

Artificial Vegetative Propagation

The plants which do not naturally develop vegetative organs, it can often be produced by artificial means like by **cutting, layering, grafting** and **budding,** and by **cell culture**.

Cutting: It is the method of plant propagation, based on the capability of the severed part,

to develop roots when put into moist place, the healthy branch bearing the bud is planted in the moist soil, cutting will develop roots and grow into new independent plant (Fig. 4.1).

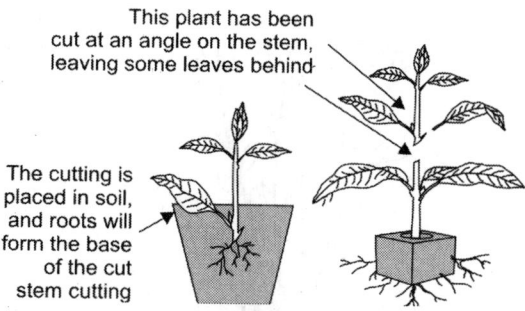

This plant has been cut at an angle on the stem, leaving some leaves behind

The cutting is placed in soil, and roots will form the base of the cut stem cutting

Fig. 4.1: Stem cutting

This method is also possible with root part, in the root cutting method, root is severed, preferably at the plant end and the cut tip of the root be exposed to air, while inserting into the plant medium. The exposed tip will start growing into new plant, e.g. jasmine, curry patta (Fig. 4.2).

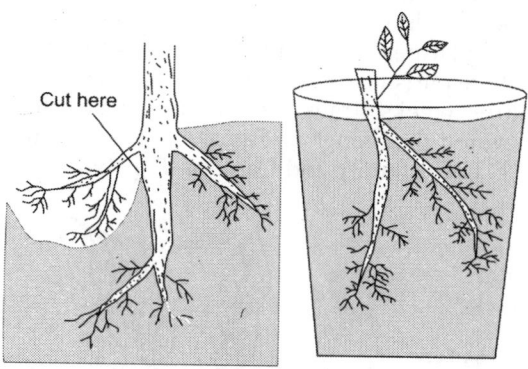

Cut here

Fig. 4.2: Root cutting

Success of the method can also be extended to hard-wood plant by the use of rooting hormones and by the employment of **mist propagation**.

Layering: In this method a branch or shoot of the plant is induced to develop roots, before it is severed/cut from the plant source. It is done by bending the shoot towards the ground and covered with moist soil and tip of the shoot kept out of the soil with artificial support in upright position. After some days roots will develop, the branch is then severed and planted in field, a new plant will grow (Fig. 4.3).

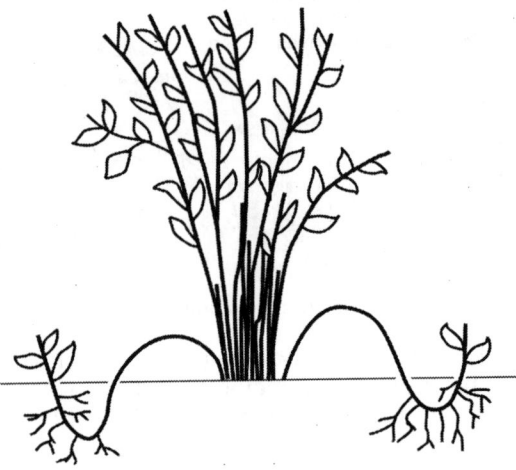

Fig. 4.3: layering

Gootee: It differ from layering in which the branch is not bent to the soil but the injured and the slit portion of the branch is enclosed in moist peat, surrounded by moss and the whole part enclosed in polythene, after two to three weeks times the roots will develop, severed the branch and grow as a new plant, e.g. citrus family and Cascara (Fig. 4.4).

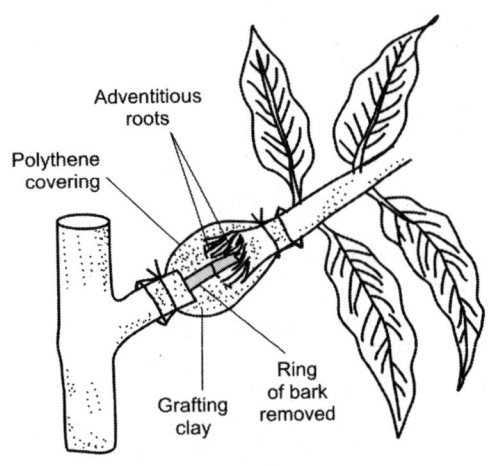

Adventitious roots

Polythene covering

Grafting clay

Ring of bark removed

Fig. 4.4: Gootee

Grafting: This is common method to develop new varieties. In this method of propagation, the two cut surface, usually of different but closely related plants are united in such a way that they grow together. The rooted plant is known as **stock,** the cut-off branch is the **scion** or **Graft,** e.g. *Cinchona ledgeriana* scion are grafted with *Cinchona succirubra* root stock to get a variety of cinchona bark rich in quinidine alkaloids (Fig. 4.5).

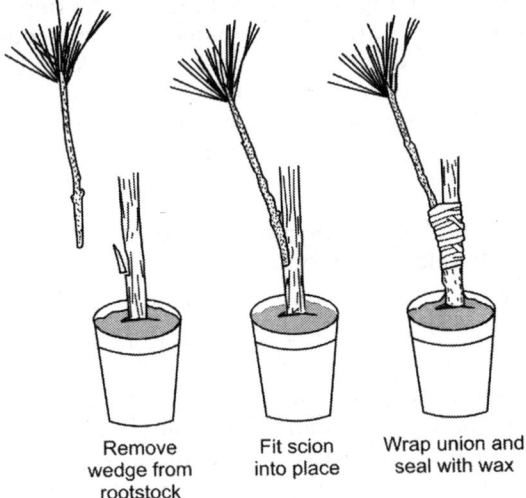

Remove wedge from rootstock

Fit scion into place

Wrap union and seal with wax

Fig. 4.5: Grafting

Budding: In this method a piece of bark of scion bearing a bud is inserted into T-shaped cavity made into the bark of stock plant and united together tightly to grow into a new branch, this method is common for the improvement in the citrus species (Fig. 4.6).

Plant Tissue and cell culture (micropropagation)

Micropropagation is a technique for vegetative propagation, involving the production of callus culture from explants, taken from meristematic zones of the healthy plant. New plants are then developed from callus by manipulation of growth hormones (auxin and cytokinin).

The basis for plant tissue and cell culture is that each plant cell, irrespective of the organ

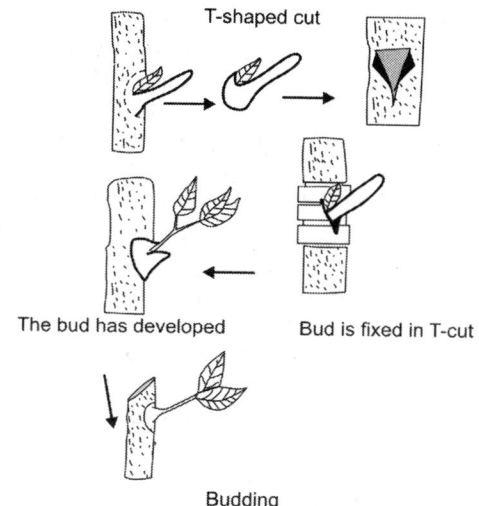

T-shaped cut

The bud has developed

Bud is fixed in T-cut

Budding

Fig. 4.6: Budding

from which it derives, contain all genetic information relating to the whole plant (Totipotency).

It was only few decade back, when this method of plant propagation was developed. By suitable manipulation of the hormone contents of the medium, the development of shoot, roots and complete plants from callus culture is possible for the propagation of new plants (micro propagation).

Method: Micropropagation consists of the following steps:

First step: Selection and preparation of healthy mother plant having meristematic tissue, followed by sterilisation and cutting of explants for the initiation of cell culture.

Second step: In occultation of explants on the sterile, nutrient shoot media under aseptic environment.

Third step: Maintenance of culture for the production of shoot and their multiplication by constant division of the shoots.

Fourth step: Rooting, the shoots are transferred onto a root promoting nutrient media.

Fifth step: Hardening the newly developed plants (offspring) under controlled environment and transfer them to field (*see* detail in tissue culture).

Factors Affecting the Cultivation of Medicinal Plants

1. *Environmental factors*: Temperature, rainfall, altitude and light.
2. Soils.
3. Growth regulators.

Environmental factors: Temperature, rainfall, duration of daylight, and altitude are the environmental factors playing very important role in the growth and development of the plants. Generally, the too drastic change in the environmental conditions, plants are not able to withstand but there are exceptions, e.g. opium which can withstand the drastic change in the conditions without effecting the concentration of alkaloids.

Temperature: The metabolism and development of the plant is affected by the variation of temperature, in general, the highest temperature is experienced near the equator and major effect is noticed in the month of summer, on the plants having volatile oils; as the formation of volatile oil enhanced at higher temperature but at the same time there is loss in oil contents at very high temperature. Fixed oils producing plants are also affected by the variation in temperature as fixed oils produced at lower temperature contains fixed oils with higher contents of fatty acids, with higher number of double bonds than the oils formed at higher temperature. Other example is of the plants producing the alkaloids (solanaceae), hence temperature variation should be minimum possible as per the monograph of the plant under cultivation.

Rainfall: Continuous rain can lead to the loss of water soluble components of plants from leaves and roots by leaching from the plants producing alkaloids, glycosides and volatile oils.

However the rainfall is main source of groundwater. The mineral from the soil get dissolved in water and then absorbed by the plants.

For the production of secondary metabolites optimum level of humidity (water) is the prerequisite, low water fall induce abiotic stress leading to negligible production of secondary metabolites exception is the production of anthraquinone glycoside production of *cassia angustifolia* (Tinne velly senna). In which case the short-term drought increase the production of glycosides contents.

Rainfall variation have devasting effects particularly widely grown (cultivated) medicinal plants, where they are predominantly rain-fed. Hence while collection care should be taken as well while selecting the species of plant to be propagated. *Artificial application of water* to overcome the deficiency of rainfall will influence the entire growth process from seedling, root growth, nutrient utilisation, plant growth, yield and overall quality of the production.

Altitude: Plants having unusual sensitivity to altitude can grow well but with much lower yield of phytoconstituents, e.g. *Cinchona succirubra* grow well at higher altitude (1000 to 3000 m), but also grow well at lower altitude, without the production of alkaloids. **Pyrethrum** gives best yields of flower heads and pyrethrins at high altitude on or near the equator while **sugar cane** is the plant of lowland. Therefore, while selecting the plants for cultivation, monograph instructions to be followed well otherwise the yield will be of low quality. However, the vegetative propagation is more lush under irrigated conditions at lower altitude.

Daylight and radiation: The amount and intensity of light vary from plant to plant; in the wild state, generally the plants will be found in the area, where the shade requirement is more. Research finding have found that the alkaloids or glycosides contents of *Belladonna* spp, *Stramonium* and *Cinchona ledgeriana* have more contents of alkaloids in plants grow in sunshine than the plants grown in shade.

The intensity and length of light also affects the chemistry of the yield, e.g. **Peppermint** leaves collected from the crop of long-day exposure contain menthone, menthol and traces of menthofuran, whereas the plants grown under the short day conditions contain menthofuran as a major components of the volatile oil. Other example is of the long length exposure of light is of the dimerisation of the indole alkaloids: catharanthine and vindoline leading to vinblastine.

Type of radiation, is also important for the metabolism, e.g. flavonoids and anthocyanins are known to be influenced by UV-radiation.

Soils: Soil is highly complex systems, with many components playing diverse functions due to the activity of soil organism. It is a mixture of weathered or eroded rocks, nutrients, living organism, organic matter (humus), water and air. A soil in optimum conditions, contain approximately 45% solid material, 5% organic matter and 50% pore space (air 25% and water 25%). Water holding capacity of the soil, depends on the particle size of the soil components. Variation in particle size, ranging from **clay** (2–20 µm) have high water holding capacity, more than 40% but less air circulation; **sandy soil** (20 µm– 2 mm), water retaining power is very poor but higher air circulation capacity, **gray soil** (2– 20 mm) particle size, the mucilage producing plants contain less mucilage when grown on soil with high moisture contents, e.g. *Althaea officinalis*.

pH: The pH of soil also influence plant growth, on the bases of pH, soil is of three types: **neutral, acidic** and **alkaline**. Soil rich in humus and low in lime is acidic, high in lime make it alkaline pH, neutral pH is most suitable for the growth in plants which is rich in humus and consist of coarse fine particles.

Particular plant species have their own soil pH tolerance, there is no marked influence of pH within tolerance range (e.g. *Datura stramonium* pH range is 6.0–8.2; *Majorana hortensis* 5.6–6.4) for alkaloids and essential oils, e.g. *Mentha piperata*. pH 6 and 8.2 with soil rich in organic matter acidic soil having pH less than 5.5 liming is required.

Calcium is essential element for the development of most plants and ample supply of lime is favourable for most plants, but the caliphobous plants such as *Pirtts pinuster* and *Digitalis purpurea* are the exception in this respect.

Nitrogen containing fertilisers, increases the size of alkaloid producing plants (solanaceous drugs) and their production. The influence of nitrogen on the production of glycosides and volatile oils contents is variable, it is assumed that it is because of the general effect of the nitrogen on the plant's metabolism; as the silymarin contents of the fruits of *Silybum marianum* has shown increased with nitrogen fertiliser.

Trace amount of **manganese** and **molybdenum** also has effect on the growth of secondary metabolites, e.g. the development of *Digitalis grandiflora* and *D. purpurea* has been effected in the presence of trace elements with respect to their glycosides yields.

Soil microflora: Animals that are one centimetre or more but smaller than earthworm are typical members of microflora, play a pivotal role in the quality of soil conditions and in stimulating plant growth, microorganism are beneficial in increasing the soil fertility and plant growth as they are involved in several biochemical transformation and mineralisation activities. **Fungi** and **bacteria** are the fundamental for the soil ecosystem functioning.

Weeds, pest and diseases: Weeds are unwanted plant growth, continued threat to cultivated plants. At the first stage of cultivation its growth is faster than the desired plant, if not removed in time it takeover the entire crop, it has to be managed manually.

Insects (aphides, thrips, cutworms and mites) causes harm to the vegetative parts of the plants. The *worms of nematodes*, attack the underground parts, many fungal diseases such as browning of leaves and roots also cause great loss to cultivation. The management to check their growth is physical, chemical and biological; the most important one is the biological control as the chemical leave a toxic residue in the plant production.

Mutation

A constant alteration of genetic material, which can be transferred to new generation of cells or plants are called **mutation**, it causes change in genome, in amount or structure. It can take place spontaneously or can be induced by the treatment with mutagens (high temperature, radiation and chemicals), the mutagens directly effect on DNA or mRNA structure. Mutation is of two types based on the origin; **Genes mutation** and **Chromosomal** mutation.

Gene mutation: Change in the structure of individual gene by two ways, frame-shift mutation and substitution mutation. Frame mutation caused by the addition or deletion of nitrogenous bases in the DNA or mRNA, whereas in substitution mutation base pair replaced by a different one (transition and transversion).

Chromosomal mutation: It is caused by the change in structure of chromosomes (chromosomal aberrations) or by the change in number of chromosomes is known as genomatic mutation (ploidy).

Mutagenic treatment is influenced by the factors like oxygen tension within the tissue, temperature and pH. The chemical mutagens can be applied in the similar way as to colchicines to seeds, whole plant, isolated organ; growing point, etc. However, to obtain single mutation in plant, irradiation of pollen grains is often advantageous. Less work has been done on medicinal plants with comparison to commercial and vitality important cereals. The study on opium poppy (*Papaver somniferum*), in which irradiation done with ^{60}Co has produced a variety, having morphine content of 0.52% as compared with 0.32% in the starting original variety, other examples are, various species of *Datura* raised from irradiated seeds, showing difference in relative production of alkaloids synthesised and production of sweet lupins variety (almost free from bitterness) by the treatment with ethylmethane sulphonate solution to X-ray induced early maturing mutant of *Lupinus digitatus* (Family Fabaceae).

Polyploidy

Polyploidy is an chromosomal mutation, caused by the change in number of chromosomes in group, instead of pairs, they are in three, four or higher numbers; these are polyploidy individuals—**triploid, tetraploid,** octaploid, etc. Polyploids are derived from the multiplication of chromosomes of an single species (**Autoploid**), or as a result of multiplication of the chromosomes following hybridisation between two species (**alloploids**). Polyploidy can occurs naturally in some organism, e.g. *Primula kewensis* formed from the infertile hybrid *P. verticillata* and *P. floribunda* or it can be induced artificially in many plants by suitable treatment with chemicals (colchicines alkaloid), radioactive substances and by exposure with alternate heat and cold shocks. Other examples of natural polyploidy are various varieties of mint, valerian, and calamus. The oil component of *Acorus calamus*, the sweet flag, varies with ploidy, the 2n variety, contain no detectable toxic β-asarone as preferable.

Polyploidy change the properties of the organisms, all or some organs are enlarged. Typical effects of polyploidy, compared with the diploid state are: larger flowers, pollen grains and stomata. The contents of active constituents may also be affected in positive or negative direction and qualitative change may also occur.

The change must be determined by trial and error in each case. It has been demonstrated that plants of family Solanaceae (*Atropa, Datura*) with the chromosome number 4n produce larger amounts of alkaloids than the diploid but the relative proportions of the main alkaloids are not affected. Another example is of *Digitalis lanata*, the contents of lanatosides A and B in relation to other lanatosides is higher in the 4n forms. In the case of *Cinchona succirubra* the percentage of quinine reported to increase from 0.53% (2n) to 1.12% (4n) whereas in (1n) variety is only 0.27% of quinine is reported.

Newly formed polyploids usually require a number of generations to stabilise themselves and chemical treatment for the induction of artificial polyploidy, sometimes fail to give a uniform plant regarding chromosome numbers.

HYBRIDISATION

Hybridisation is the process of interbreeding between individuals of different species (**interspecific hybridisation**) or genetically divergent individuals from same species (**intraspecific hybridisation**), offspring produced by hybridisation may be fertile, partially fertile, or sterile.

Joseph G. Kolreuter was the first botanist to report on interspecific hybridisation, on the bases of his experiment on tobacco in 1760, he concluded, that the interspecific hybridisation in nature is rare unless there is disturbance in their habitat. Human has used the intraspecific hybridisation between strains of a single species, for the development of high-yielding crops, in 21st century, over 90% of crops of corn grown is of hybrid origin.

The number of hybrid drugs are also well known, e.g. *Cinchona*. The commercial mints are hybrids and must therefore be propagated vegetatively. The cultivated peppermint (*M. piperita*), is probably, a hybrid derived from *M. aquatic* and *M. spicata* and it is the *M. aquatic* responsible for the menthofuran component of the oil, which is characteristic of peppermint.

In the genus *Datura*, the effect of hybridisation on chemical composition has been reported, where hybrid derived from *D. ferox* and *D. stramonium* has shown the results differently, the aerial organ of the *D. stramonium*, normally contain hyoscyamine and hyoscine in the ratio of 2 : 1 at the flowering period: and those of *D. ferox* contain hyoscine with some meteloidine. The F_1 plant of the cross consist of plant larger than anyone of the parents, and containing hyoscine as the principle alkaloid with the small quantity of other components. Another example is of the *Digitalis* hybrid, in which scientist has demonstrated the lanatoside formation, was dominant to purpurea glycoside formation (*D. purpurea* and *D. lanata*: *D. purpurea* and *D. lutea*) hybrid were formed with lanatoside A (principle glycoside), lanatoside B and E. Small amount of glucogitaloxin. No lanatoside C or purpurea glycoside A.

PLANT GROWTH REGULATORS

Plant growth regulators or phytohormones are the organic substances produced naturally, in higher plants, which together exert a complex interaction, to meet the needs of the plant. Five groups of plant hormones are well-established: they are the **auxins, gibberellins, cytokinins, abscisic acid** and its derivatives and **ethylene**. Plant growth regulators include synthetic compounds as well as naturally occurring hormones.

They are biosynthesised at one site and transported another site, where they exert a specific physiological action, in very low concentration, and regulate cell enlargement, cell division, cell differentiation, organogenesis, senescence and dormancy.

Auxins: These are growth promoting substances, generally resembles to indole-3-acetic acid (IAA) (Fig. 4.7a). The compound now considered to be major auxin of plants (natural) and found particularly in actively growing tissues and has the ability to stimulate the elongation of coleoptiles.

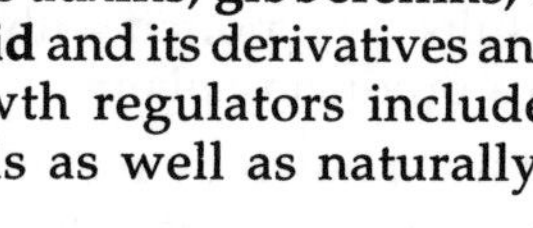

Indole 3-acetic acid

Fig. 4.7a: Indole 3-acetic acid

Synthesis take place at the apex and transported towards the base through polar transportation.

The synthetic auxins include indole 3 butyric acid (IBA), (Fig. 4.7b) naphthalene-1-acetic acid (NAA). And 2,4-dichlorophenoxyacetic acid (2,4-D) (Fig. 4.7c).

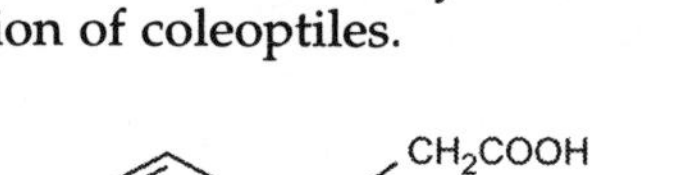

Indole butyric acid

Fig. 4.7b: Indole butyric acid

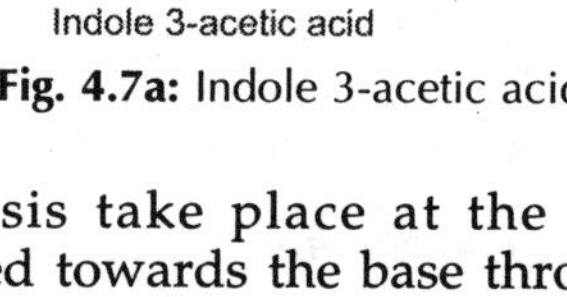

Fig. 4.7c: 2,4-Dichlorophenoxy acetic acid

These substances were first reported by Duch workers, who isolated two growth regulating acids (auxins A and B) obtained from human urine and cereal products respectively.

Functions of Auxins

1. Cell division and elongation in the shoot and differentiation of xylem tissue and phloem tissue in the secondary growth of stem.
2. Apical dominance in many plants, i.e. the apical bud dominates over the growth of lateral bud immediately below the apical bud and does not allow the growth.
3. *Root initiation*: In higher concentration auxin inhibit the elongation of the roots but induces more lateral branches of roots, this property is being used in micro propagation to promote the root formation and also in propagation by cutting method.
4. *Secondary metabolite formation*: It is reported that when seedling and young plants of *Mentha piperita* are treated with derivative of NAA has increased the yield of the oil by 30–50%, in the matured plants and containing more menthol contents. Another example is of increase in alkaloids production in tissue culture study has been reported with tropane alkaloid of Datura species and indole alkaloids of *Rauwolfia serpentina*, ergot and ipomea, etc. by using NAA and 2,4-D auxins.
5. *Prevention of abscission*: Natural auxin prevent the formation of abscission layer, and thus, prevent the fall of premature leaves, flowers and fruits.
6. *Callus formations*: Its cell division property is used for the maintenance of callus culture.
7. *Weedicide*: In higher concentration 2,4-D and 2,4,5 –T are useful as weedicide.
8. *Parthenocarpy*: Auxin can induce the parthenocarpy.

Gibberellins

This group of plant growth regulator was discovered by Japanese workers, in the connection with the rice seedling infected by fungus (foolish seedling), disease by *Gibberella fujikuroi*, plants grow taller, thin and pale in colour with less yield. On investigation, it was found, the compound responsible for the infection was Gibberellins, which later were distinguished as GA_1, GA_2, GA_3, etc. GA_3 commonly referred to as Gibberellic acid produced commercially by fungus cultivation.

Gibberellins are biosynthesised in leaves and accumulated in large quantities in immature seeds and fruits of some plants.

Functions of Gibberellins

1. *Elongation of internodes*: The major effect of the hormone is on the growth of the plant, is the elongation of internodes and because of this property, this hormone is used to overcome the genetic dwarfism, e.g. dwarf peas or dwarf maize, and to increase the size of plants which are producing rosettes of leaves (*Digitalis*, *Hyoscyamus*).
2. *Root growth*: It inhibits the root growth at higher concentration.
3. *Bud dormancy*: Gibberellins are used to break the bud dormancy and to sprouts the tuber for early germination.
4. *Seeds germination*: It overcome the light sensitivity of certain seeds for germination, seeds treatment with gibberellins decrease the germination period in the dark condition otherwise they needs the exposure of light or red light for the germination, e.g. is tobacco seeds, etc.
5. *Enzyme α-amylase synthesis*: Gibberellins are required for the synthesis of α-amylase enzyme in the endosperm of cereal grains, required for the hydrolysis of starch to simple glucose for the growing embryo.
6. *Secondary metabolites production*: Gibberellin has been used *in vitro* for the increase of secondary metabolites, e.g. volatile oils and terpenoids producing plants (*Mentha piperita*, citrus, *Eucalyptus*, *Foeniculum*), spraying with the GA show change in the morphological characters, but the results of general study show negative effect on the percentage of oil contents with exception to some plants, e.g. in the case of *Anethum*, GA treatment has shown the appreciable change in the volatile oil with no significant change in ascaridol contents.

Alkaloid containing plants has also shown negative effects on the yield of alkaloids, similarly, results are reported with glycosides and fixed oils producing plants.

Cytokinins: It is known by name of the cells division hormones. The cell division not only confined to cell division in a tissue they also regulate the pattern and frequency of organ production, as well as position and shape.

Cytokinin is found at the growing root tips, shoot buds and growing fruits and also present in the coconut water (liquid endosperm), chemically they are purines derived from tRNA first naturally occurring cytokinin was identified from the young maize (*Zea mays*) and hence named zeatin (Fig. 4.8) and kinetin was another cytokinin discovered by Miller and Skoog.

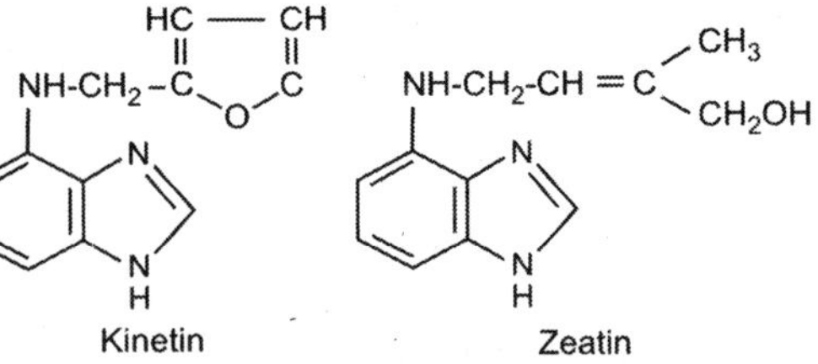

Fig. 4.8: Kinetin and zeatin

Functions of Cytokinins

Cell division: Found in a higher amount in meristematic tissue.

Morphogenesis: Cytokinin promotes cell division by stimulating the process of mitosis and in the presence of auxin, it promotes cell differentiation in callus tissues. In tissue culture, cytokinin in high concentration and auxin in low concentration promote shoot buds in tissue cultures.

Apical dominance: Cytokinin and auxin acts antagonistically in the control of apical dominance. It promotes production of female flowers. It increases the resistance to low and high temperature and diseases. The cytokinins can mediate axillary bud release from apical dominance.

Delay in senescence: It delays the senescence of plant organs by controlling protein synthesis and mobilisation of resources, this phenomenon is called the **Richmond Lang effect**. They help to produce chloroplast in leaves. These are also called **anti-ageing hormones**.

Growth Inhibitors

Natural growth inhibitors are the regulating substances present in plants, which retard the stem elongation, bud opening, seed germination and development of dormancy. They are abscisic acid (ABA) and ethylene.

Some pure flavonoids, coumarins and cinnamic acid are also able to inhibit coleoptiles section elongation, stem and bud opening and seed germination.

Abscisic acid (ABA) is the major inhibitor of growth in plants and is antagonistic to all three growth promoters especially of gibberellic acid (GA). It is mainly produced in mature leaves but is also synthesised in stem, fruits and seeds and transported to other parts through vascular system.

Chemically, it is dextrorotatory cis-sesquiterpene; it has structural similarity with carotenoids and it has been demonstrated that some xanthophylls particularly violaxanthine produce germination inhibition on exposure to light (Fig. 4.9).

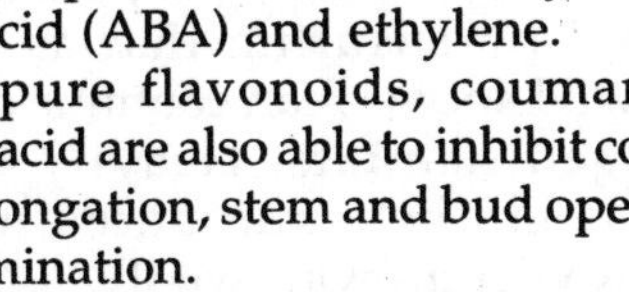

Fig. 4.9: Abscisic acid

Functions of ABA

- Promotes bud dormancy in seeds during winter, and thus, help seeds to withstand, desiccation and unfavorable conditions.
- *Transpiration*: It helps to close down stomata during drought or during the period of water shortage.
- Play major role in the development of seeds, maturation and dormancy.
- Induce synthesis of carotenoid in green oranges making them yellow.

Ethylene

Ethylene is the only gaseous hormone produce, while fruits ripening and during leaves abscission. It is synthesised in plant from S-adinosyl methionine. It is marketed under the name of ethrel, as a source of ethylene response in plants, a high concentration of auxin leads to the formation of ethylene.

Rich source are shoot apex and senescing tissue, stimulated by physiological stresses, including wounding, anaerobic conditions, chilling diseases and drought.

Functions

- Helps in fruit ripening.
- Induction of leaves abscission.
- Inhibition of stem elongation but increase in girth and horizontal plant growth.
- At low concentration, ethylene induce rooting and growth of lateral root hairs.
- It helps in the production of female flower in genetically male plant.
- Helps in breaking the dormancy of storage organs and induce germination in peanut seeds.
- Inhibition of shoot growth.
- Promote senescence of leaves and flowers.
- Altering gravitropism in roots and stems.
  (For further detail see page 109–110).

CONSERVATION OF MEDICINAL PLANTS

Globally intensified alternative healthcare practices has given rise to a great demand for herbal medicines. India is a hub of herbal industry for wild-collected plant species. Almost 90% of the medicinal plant are provided by forests in India's for around 25,000 plant based formulations and 8000 manufacturing units with an annual requirement of 2000 tonnes of raw material. This growth, in demand of traditional, plant-based medicines has resulted in indiscriminate collection and overharvesting of medicinal plants from the wild, resulting in rapid decline in the numbers of wild species and has threatened the status of several high-value medicinal plant species.

Many of these species may face extinction if the plants are not conserved and cultivated for the market needs. Therefore, approaches for cultivation, sustainable harvesting and protection against existing threats should be developed for the conservation of medicinal plants.

There are policy provisions for people's access rights to natural resources, necessary for their survival. This has shown to be positively linking human development with biodiversity conservation.

India is party to The Convention on Biological Diversity (CBD), which was approved in 1992 at the Rio Earth Summit. Along with 190 Parties, Government of India have agreed to commit to protect biodiversity, develop sustainably and engage in the equitable sharing of benefits from the use of genetic resources. The conservation of biodiversity is recognised as the foundation of sustainable development.

India is also party to The World Trade Organisation's (WTO) agreement on Trade-Related Aspects of Intellectual Property Rights (TRIPS), 1994. WTO layout rules to deal with the commercial use of traditional knowledge and genetic material by communities or countries other than the place of origin, especially when these are the subject of patent applications. Promoting fair and equal sharing of the benefits coming out of commercialisation of genetic resources is one of the fundamental objectives of the CBD. One of the probable ways to implement it is by authorising the independent rights of the state over its biological resources that encourages conservation and propagation of medicinal plants. Medicinal plant con-servation, must therefore, operate within several spheres; drawing together disparate groups and mutually acknowledging different stakeholder interests in order to succeed.

Medicinal plant conservation is extremely challenging, due to the fact that the taxa occur in a wide range of geographic regions and habitats. However, it is largely believed that the conservation of medicinal plants and biodiversity can be retained through an integrated approach of *in situ* and *ex situ* conservation strategies.

Definition

Conservation of medicinal plants is the process of management of medicinal plants and their habitats through protection of wild-medicinal-plants, based on sustainable harvesting, in order to obtain the greatest benefit for the present generation and maintaining the potential for future.

Broadly, there are two methods for the conservation of plant genetic resources namely *in situ* and *ex situ*.

In situ Conservation

It is achieved, both by setting aside areas as natural reserves and national park (protected areas) and by ensuring that as many as possible wild species, can continue to survive in managed habitats. Heavily depleted species should be reintroduced into areas where they were growing wildly. As per WHO recommendations, every country should have Botanic gardens in each and every state, if possible in every district headquarter, having scientific research program and documentation of plant grown; the botanic garden should be open to general public for the information, regarding their propagation, and the general properties, economic values and its scope and trade possibilities. To improve the techniques of sustainable harvesting and production, government should disseminate information regarding the harvesting, processing and storage the medicinal plants.

The Ministries of Agriculture and Health should coordinate a programme to establishes nurseries, where the medicinal plants are cultivated to make available the seeds, seedling and/or sampling to individuals and communities for cultivation in home gardens (WHO).

Governments of the countries should have the provisions to provide economic and social incentives for maintaining natural habitats and wild species through the park managers.

Ex situ Conservation

Ex situ conservation involves in the conservation of the medicinal plants out-side the native or natural habitats, where genetic variation are maintained, away from the original wild source. It will fulfil the requirement of present or future economic and social needs.

Drawback: The major drawback of the *ex situ* conservation is of the narrow range genetic variation than that occur wild, hence species reserved *ex situ* can suffer genetic erosion and depend on continued human care. Therefore, the *ex situ* conservation must not be replaced but should complement the *in situ* conservation.

As per WHO guidelines, priority for *ex situ* conservation should be given to species, the habitats of which has been destroyed or cannot be safeguarded. It should also be used to bulk-up population of depleted or locally extinct plants for restocking in nature.

Ex situ conservation can be achieved through the following methods:

1. **In vitro regeneration:** This method involve the maintenance of plant/ex-plant growth, in sterile environment in such a way that their regeneration potential, and genetic stability be maintained. This method is suitable for those species whose seeds cannot be preserved or usually unstable, e.g. shoot tips, root-tips or auxillary buds are cultured on nutrient media containing more concentration of cytokinin than auxin.

   The chances of genetic variation in integrated plants, produced from cell-culture are more.

2. **Cryopreservation:** It is storage of tissue and cell culture at low temperature, in some cases as low as $-196°C$. Basically cryobanks are used for the storage of germplasm for long-term preservation under the nitrogen atmosphere. This method was developed for the production of synthetic seeds, i.e. Somatic embryo, encapsulated in a hydrolysable gel.

3. **Seeds bank:** In seeds bank the seeds are stored at a low temperature ($-20°C$), this will protect the seeds viability for longer period, even for 100 years, but the viability to be checked in between at regular intervals otherwise old should be replaced with new one.

Where the species cannot be stored in seed bank. The trees or shrubs are grown in rows and labelled (Field genebank) but major drawback is of the space.

FURTHER READING

1. Book review: Commercial cultivation of medicinal plants *https://www.downtoearth. org.in›news›book-review-commercial-cultivat.*
2. Chatterjee SK. Cultivation of medicinal and aromatic plants in India—Acta: *https://www. actahort.org›books*
3. Chen SL, et al. Conservation and sustainable use of medicinal plants: problems, progress, and prospects. Chin Med. 2016;11:37. *https://www. ncbi.nlm. nih.gov›pmc›articles›PMC 4967523.*
4. Cultivation of Medicinal Plants in India and Government Support *https://www. agricultureinformation. com›forums›threads›cultivation-o...*
5. Guidelines on the conservation of medicinal plants. The world health organization (WHO) (1993).
6. Gunnar Samuelsson 1992. A Textbook of Pharmacognosy 4th revised edition.
7. History and Chinese herbology-Herbalism WWW.prada-outletco/History-of-Chinese-herbology.htttml
8. IUCN: The World Conservation Union WWf: (1993) World Wide Fund for Nature www. cbd.int.
9. Jarayal GS, Uniyal M. 2003. Aushadiya Padapo Ka VyavasayicKrishikaran (Commercial Cultivation Of Medicinal Plants). Published by Indian Society of Agri-business Professionals, New Delhi.
10. Jean Bruneton. Pharmacognosy, Phytochemistry, Medicinal Plants, Lavoisier publication, England. UK 1995.
11. Kalia AN. Textbook of Industrial Pharmacogonsy. (2005). CBS Publishers and Distributors, New Delhi.
12. Nireesha GR, et al. Lyophilization/freeze drying. An review. International Journal of Novel Trends in Pharmaceutical Sciences, 2013;3(4):87–99.
13. Old Discussion Threads. 2009. Cultivation of Medicinal Plants in India and Government Support. URL: https://www.agricultureinformation. com/forums/forums/archives-old-discussion-threads.109/
14. Prepared by Andhra Pradesh State Forest Department. Manual designed and developed by B S. Somashekhar and Manju Sharma, Foundation for Revitalisation of Local Health Tradition Bangalore (March 2012).
15. Purohit SS, Vyas SP. Medicinal Plant Cultivation. Agrobios India Publication, 2004.
16. Trease and Evans 16th Edition Pharmacognosy.
17. Wallis J, TE &. Churchill A. 1960. Textbook of Pharmacognosy. 4th ed. Little, Brown and Co.
18. WHO guidelines on good herbal processing practices (GHPP).
19. WTO and TRIPS Agreement is available at www.wto.org
20. WWW, biology discussion.com

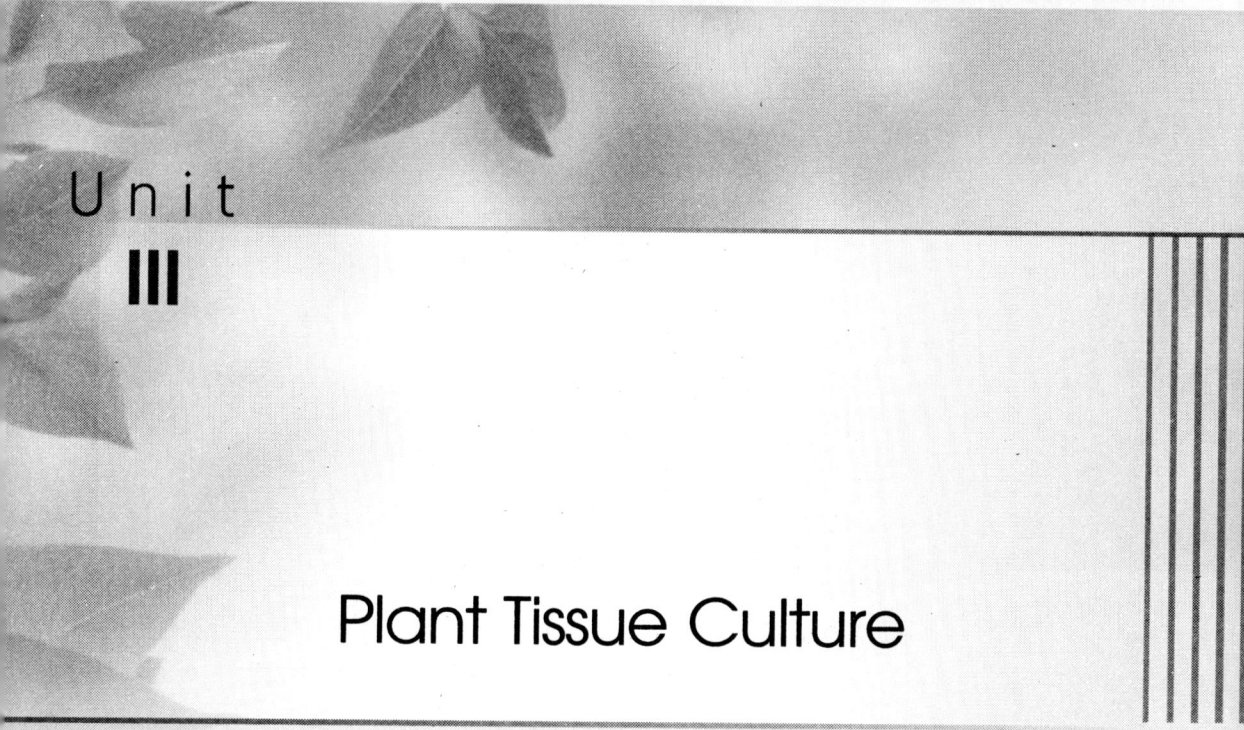

Plant Tissue Culture

5. Plant Tissue Culture and Edible Vaccines

Chapter

5

Plant Tissue Culture and Edible Vaccines

INTRODUCTION

Tissue culture is *in vitro* cultivation of plant cell or tissue under aseptic and controlled environmental conditions, in liquid or on semisolid well-defined nutrient medium for the production of primary and secondary metabolites or to regenerate the plant. This technique provides alternative solution to problems arising due to current rate of extinction and decimation of flora and ecosystem.

The whole process requires a well-equipped culture laboratory and nutrient medium. This process involves various steps, *viz.* preparation of nutrient medium containing inorganic and organic salts, supplemented with vitamins, plant growth hormone(s) and amino acids. Sterilisation of explant (source of plant tissue), glassware and other accessories; inoculation and incubation.

ADVANTAGES OF TISSUE CULTURE TECHNIQUE OVER THE CONVENTIONAL CULTIVATION TECHNIQUES

1. **Availability of raw material:** Some plants are difficult to cultivate and are also not available in abundance. In such a case, the biochemicals/bioproducts from these plants cannot be obtained economically in sufficient quantity. Indiscriminate collection of plants also leads to deforestation, natural imbalance and sometimes may lead to extinction of a particular species. Hence, tissue culture is considered a better source for regular and uniform supply of raw material, manageable under regulated and reproducible conditions in the medicinal plants industry for the production of phytopharmaceuticals.

2. **Fluctuation in supplies and quality:** The production of crude drugs is subject to variation in quality due to changes in climate, crop diseases and seasons. The method of collection, drying and storing also influence the quality of crude drug. All these problems can be overcome by tissue culture techniques.

3. **Patent rights:** Naturally occurring plants or their metabolites cannot be patented as such. Only a novel method of isolation can be patented. For R&D purpose, the industry has to spend a lot of money and time to launch a new natural product but cannot have patent right. Hence, industries prefer tissue culture for production of biochemical compounds. By this method, it is possible to obtain a constant supply and new methods can be developed for isolation and improvement of yield, which can be patented.

4. **Political reasons:** If a natural drug is successfully marketed in a particular country of its origin, the government may prohibit its export to up-value its own exports by supplying its phytochemical product, e.g. *Rauwolfia serpentina* and *Dioscorea* spp. from India. Similarly, the production of opium in the world is governed as such by political consideration. In such case, if work is going on the same

drug, it will be either hindered or stopped. Here also, plant tissue culture is the solution.

5. **Easy purification of the compound:** The natural products from plant tissue culture can be easily purified, because of the absence of significant amounts of pigments and other unwanted impurities. With the advancement of modern technology in plant tissue culture, it is also possible to biosynthesise those chemical compounds which are difficult or impossible to synthesise.

6. **Modifications in chemical structure:** Some specific compounds can be achieved more easily in cultured plant cells rather than by chemical synthesis or by micro-organism.

7. **Disease free and desired propagule:** Plant tissue culture is advantageous over conventional method of propagation in large scale production of disease free and desired propagules in limited space and also the germplasm could be stored and maintained without any damage during transportation for subsequent plantation.

8. **Crop improvement:** Plant tissue culture is advantageous over the conventional cultivation technique in crop improvement by somatic hybridisation or by production of hybrids.

9. **Biosynthetic pathway:** Tissue culture can be used for tracing the biosynthetic pathways of secondary metabolites using labelled precursor in the culture medium.

10. **Immobilisation of cells:** Tissue culture can also be used for plants preservation by immobilisation of cell further facilitating transportation and biotransformation.

HISTORICAL DEVELOPMENT OF PLANT TISSUE CULTURE

Although the feasibility of aseptic culture of **cells, tissues and organs** on defined nutrient medium had been recognised at the beginning of the century. But it is only few decades ago that modern developments in the cultivation of plants cell as a callus or as a suspension liquid culture actually came into existence. It is only in the last **two decades** its implication have been realised and in particular pharmaceutical importance of this modern technique was appreciated. But according to noted biologist the discovery of tissue culture could be considered with the **Henri-Louis Duhamel du Monceau's** (1756) pioneering experiment on wound healing in plants, demonstrated spontaneous callus formation on the decorticated region of the Elm plant. Further contribution to plant tissue culture could be attributed with the **Haberblandt's** hypothesis (1902) that a cell is capable of autonomy and have potential for totipotency (the potential of cell to develop into an organism by regeneration is termed **totipotency** by Morgan) hence the isolated plant cell should be capable of cultivation on artificial medium.

The development of multicellular or multi-organed body of a higher organism from a single cell (zygote) support the totipotent behaviour of a cell. But **Haberblandt and co-worker** have tried to demonstrate the hypothesis but could not succeed. In 1904, another physiologist **Hannig** started research work, by taking embryogenic tissue instead of single cells, for *in vitro* cultivation in an artificial medium consisting of mineral salts and sugar solution. He excised nearly matured embryos of some crucifers (*Raphanus sativus*, *R. landra*, *R. caudatus* and *Cochlearia donica*) and successfully cultivated them up to maturity. Thus, it became an important area of investigation, using an *in vitro* technique.

Simon (1908) obtained more promising results as he achieved success in the regeneration of bulky callus, buds and roots from popular stem segments, and thus, he succeeded in establishing the basis for **callus culture** and to some extent also micro-propagation.

In vitro, technique of culture was carried out further by many biologists. In 1922, **Kotte** (Germany) and **Robbin** (USA) simultaneously conceived a new approach to tissue culture and reported that true *in vitro* culture could be made easier by using meristematic cells (**root tips or buds**). **Kotte** carried out number of experiments, and successfully, cultivated small excised root tips of pea and grew the culture for two weeks by using a variety of nutrients containing salts of Knop's solution, glucose and several nitrogenous compounds (such as asparagine, alanine and yeast extract). **Robbin** working independently maintained maize root tip culture for longer period, by subculturing, but growth gradually diminished and ultimately culture was lost.

White (1934–39) carried out the *in vitro* technique of tissue culture by changing the nature of media. He replaced the yeast extract in a medium containing inorganic salts and sucrose, with three vitamins (pyridoxine, thiamine and nicotinic acid) and was able to maintain the root tip culture, hence **White's** synthetic media later proved to be one of the basic media for cell and tissue culture.

The number of workers continued efforts to develop a complete media, this will be discussed later on under the media composition.

Gautheret (1934) successfully cultured cambium cells of some tree species (*Acer pseudoplatanus, Ulmus campestre, Robinia pseudoacacia* and *Salix caprea*) on the surface of the media (Knop's solution containing glucose and cysteine hydrochloride) solidified with agar and observed that after six month, proliferation of callus was ceased but on addition of auxin enhanced the proliferation of cambial culture and making it possible to prepare subculture.

Van Overbeek *et al* (1941) used coconut milk (embryo sac fluid) for **embryo development** and callus formation in Datura, which proved to be turning point in the development of **embryo culture**, which later on proved to be helpful in the development of several hybrids.

Loo (1945) got success in developing whole plant from **stem tip culture**. He obtained excellent cultures from stem tips of Dodder and Asparagus, subsequently, **Ball** (1946) able to identify the exact part of the shoot meristem, which give rise to whole plant. This method is now being used in plant propagation at industrial scale throughout the world.

Muir (1953) demonstrated that on transferring the callus tissues of these two plants into liquid medium, and on subsequent, **agitating on a shaking machine**, it is possible to breakdown the callus tissue into single cell and small cell aggregates, which on subculturing into fresh liquid medium can multiply while remaining in the medium under constant shaking. **Muir and associates** (1954) reported that the pieces of callus of *Tagetes erecta* and *Nicotiana tabacum* can be cultured in the form of cell suspension.

Van Overbeek *et al* (1941) had suggested earlier that liquid endosperm (coconut milk) is a good medium for embryo culture. Later in 1955 **Skoog** and collaborator finally isolated adenine derivative from the embryo sac known as **kinetin**, which helps in the proliferation of embryo.

Skoog and Miller (1957) proposed the concept of hormonal control of organ formation. They demonstrated that root and bud initiation were conditioned by balance between auxin and kinetin in addition to other ingredients of the define medium. High proportions of auxin promoted rooting, whereas proportionately more kinetin initiated bud or shoot formation.

Bergmann (1960), developed **plating technique** for cloning a large number of isolated single cells. He demonstrated the technique by using **callus culture** of *Nicotiana tabacum* and *Phaseolus vulgaris* and reported population of nearly 90% of free cells. In the same year, i.e. 1960 **Jones et al** used hanging drops of free cells for the **microculture propagation**. This technique proved useful to have continuous observation of cell growth in the culture.

In 1960, **Cocking** introduced **protoplasmic plant tissue culture**. He succeeded in isolating the protoplasts of plant tissue by using cell wall enzymes like cellulase, hemicellulase, pectinase and protease. The enzyme was extracted from fungus *Trichoderma viride*. Earlier **Michel** (1939) had demonstrated the role of sodium nitrate in fusion of protoplasts. In the same year, **Steward and co-worker** had successfully raised a large number of plantlets from carrot root suspension culture. In year 1960, **Moral** initiated **micropropagation** technique and produced virus free orchid, *Cymbidium*.

Steward and co-worker in 1966, raised large number of plantlets from carrot root suspension culture via **somatic embryogenesis**. Actually **Rienert** (1968) introduced somatic embryogenesis in callus, cultured on a semisolid medium. This phenomenon of somatic embryogenesis for the production of plantlets was later reported in many species. All these discoveries contributed to the establishment of totipotency power of the cells under suitable environment, thereby accomplishing the theory introduced by **Haberblandt**.

In 1970, **Power et al** demonstrated the intra- and inter-specific fusion between the protoplasts of different plant roots; subsequently, in 1972 **Carlson et al** succeeded in obtaining the first interspecific **somatic hybrid** by protoplasts fusion of *Nicotiana* species (*N. glauca* and *N. longsdorfi*). In 1981, **Vilnken**, brought new approach of electrical fusion of protoplasts. Later **Gamborg and Neabors** (1987) described a number of variations in protoplasts fusion.

During last two decades, procedures for culture of **somatic cells, pollens and protoplasts** have been refined and many new developments in regenerating plants from such cultured cells have been made. Protoplast fusion has been used to obtain novel somatic hybrid plants among several sexually incompatible species and to produce hybrids, difficult to obtain through conventional methods. Defined tissue culture procedures have made it possible to introduce foreign DNA and cloned genes into cultured cells, protoplasts and plant organs from diverse biological systems and to regenerate transgenic plants (Table 5.1).

BASIC REQUIREMENTS FOR A TISSUE CULTURE LABORATORY

For the successful achievement of any type of tissue culture technique, a tissue culture laboratory should have the following general basic facilities.
- Equipment and apparatus
- Washing and storage facilities
- Media preparation room

- Sterilisation room
- Aseptic chamber/area of transfer of culture
- Culture rooms or incubators fully equipped with temperature, light and humidity control devices
- Observation or recording area well-equipped with computer for data processing.

Equipment and Apparatus

Culture Vessels and Glassware

Many different kinds of vessels may be used for growing cultures. Callus culture can be grown successfully in large test tubes (25 × 150 mm) or wide mouth conical flasks (Erlenmeyer flask). In addition to the culture vessels, glassware such as graduated pipettes, measuring cylinders, beakers, filters, funnel and Petri dishes are also required for making preparations. All the glasswares should be of pyrex or corning.

Equipment

- Scissors, scalpels and forceps for explant preparation from excised plant parts and for their transfer.
- A spirit burner or gas micro-burner for flame sterilisation of instruments.
- An autoclave to sterilise the media.
- Hot air oven for the sterilisation of glassware, etc.
- A pH meter for adjusting the pH of the medium.
- A shaker to maintain cell suspension culture.
- A balance to weigh various nutrients for the preparation of the medium.
- Incubating chamber or laminar airflow with UV light fitting for aseptic transfer of explants to the medium and for subculturing.
- A BOD incubator for maintaining constant temperature to facilitate the culture of callus and its subsequent maintenance.

Washing and Storage Facilities

First and foremost requirement of the tissue culture laboratory is provision for fresh water supply and disposal of the waste water. Space for distillation unit for the supply of distilled and double distilled water and de-ionised

Table 5.1: Brief review of historical developments in plant tissue culture technology

Year	Authors	Results	Species
1892	Klercker	First attempts to isolate protoplasts mechanically	
1902	Haberblandt	First cultivation experiments with isolated plant cells; cell growth, but no cell division obtained	Tradescantia
1904	Hannig	Establishment of embryo culture for the first time	Cochleria Raphanus
1909	Kuster	First observation of fusing cells	
1922	Kotte, Robins	In vitro cultivation of root tips, no permanent cultures obtained	Zea, Pisum
1924	Dieterich	Embryo rescue - "artificial premature birth"	Linum
1925	Laibach		
1934	White	First permanent root cultures beginning in 1934 - terminated in 1968!	Lycopersicum
1934	Gautheret	First permanent callus culture using B-vitamins and auxins	Daucus, Nicotiana
1934	Nobecourt		glauca × N. langsdorffi
1942	Gautheret	Observation of secondary metabolites in plant callus culture	
1946	Ball	Micropropagation: First development of stem tips and subadjacent	Tropaeolum
1952	Morel and Martin	Regions: Plantsfree of viruses	Lupinus, Dahlia
1954	Muir et al	First suspension cultures of single cells or cell aggregates: Nurse culture	Tagetes, Nicotiana, Daucus, Picea, Phaseolus
1955	Mothes and Kala	First reports of secondary metabolite production in liquid media	
1956	Routien and Nickell	US patent No. 2747334 for the production of substances from plant tissue culture	Phaseolus
1958	Wickson and Thimann Reinert Steward et al	Establishment of axillary branching Somatic embryogenesis in tissue cultures	Daucus
1959	Tulecke and Nickell	First report of large-scale (1341) culture of plant cells: Carboy system	Ginkgo, Lolium, Rosa, Ilex
1960	Bergmann	Cell clones obtained from single cultures cells plated in an agar medium	Nicotiana Phaseolus
1960	Jones et al	Hanging drop culture in conditioned medium	Nicotiana
1960	Cocking	Method for obtaining large numbers of protoplasts from plant tissue	Lycopersicon
1965	Morel	Clonal multiplication of horticulture plants (orchids) through tissue culture: Protocorm formation	Cymbidium
1965	Vasil and Hilderbrandt	Regeneration of a plant from one single cell cultivated in a hanging droplet	Nicotiana
1966	Kohlenbach	First cell division and culture of differentiated mesophyll cells	Macleaya

(Contd...)

Table 5.1: Brief review of historical developments in plant tissue culture technology *(Contd...)*

Year	Authors	Results	Species
1967	Kaul and Staba	Reports of the yields of certain products in cell culture equal to those in intact plants	*Ammi*
1967	Bourgin and Nitsch; Guha and Maheshwari	*In vitro* production of haploid plants from immature pollen within cultured anthers	*Nicotiana* *Datura*
1970	Carlson	Isolation of auxotrophic mutants from cultured cells	*Nicotiana*
1971	Nagata and Takebe	Regeneration of plants from cultured protoplasts	*Nicotiana*
1972	Carlson et al	First interspecific somatic hybrid plant from fused protoplasts	*Nicotiana*
1977	Noguchi et al	Cultivation of tobacco cells in 20 000 1 reactors	*Nicotiana*
1978	Melchers et al	First intergenetic somatic hybrid plant from fused protoplasts	
1978	Zenk	Manifold increase in product yields by selection over parent plant documented for a variety of plant metabolites	
1979	Brodlius et al	Alginate beads used to immobilize plant cells for biotransformation and secondary metabolite production	
1981	Shuler	Use of hollow fibre reactor for secondary metabolite production	
1983	Mitsui Petrochemical Ind. Ltd	First industrial production of secondary plant products by suspension cultures	*Lithospermum*

water. Acid and alkali resistant sink or wash basin for apparatus/equipment washing. The working table should also be acid and alkali resistant.

Sufficient space is required for placing hot air oven, washing machine, pipette washers and the plastic bucket or steel tray for soaking or drainage of the detergent bath or extra water.

For the storage of dried glassware separate dust proof cupboards or cabinet should be provided. It is mandatory to maintain cleanliness in the area of washing, drying and storage.

Media Preparation Room

Media preparation room should have sufficient space to accommodate chemicals, lab ware, culture vessels and equipment required for weighing and mixing, hot plate, pH meter, water baths, bunsen burners with gas supply, microwave oven, autoclave or domestic pressure cooker, refrigerator and freezer for storage of prepared media and stock solutions.

Sterilisation Room

For the sterilisation of culture media, a good quality ISI mark autoclave is required and for small amount domestic pressure cooker, can also serve the purpose. For the sterilisation of glassware and metallic equipment hot air oven with adjustable tray is required.

Aseptic Chamber/Area for Transfer of Culture

For the transfer of culture into sterilised media, contaminant free environment is mandatory. The simplest type of transfer area requires an ordinary type of small wooden hood, having a glass or plastic door either sliding or hinged fitted with UV tube. This aseptic hood can be conveniently placed in a quiet corner of the laboratory.

These days, modern laboratory have laminar airflow cabinet having vertical or horizontal airflow, arrange over the working surface to make it free from dust particles/ microcontaminants.

The air coming out of the fine filter (a 0.3 µm HEPA filter) is ultraclean (free from fungal or bacterial contaminant) and having adequate velocity (27±3 m/min) to prevent microcontamination of the working area by worker sitting in front of the cabinet.

Inside the cabinet, there is arrangement for bunsen burner and a UV tube fitted on the ceiling of the cabinet (to make area free from any live contamination).

The advantage of working in the laminar airflow cabinet is that the flow of air does not hamper the use of bunsen burner, and moreover, the cabinet occupies relatively small space within the laboratory (Fig. 5.1).

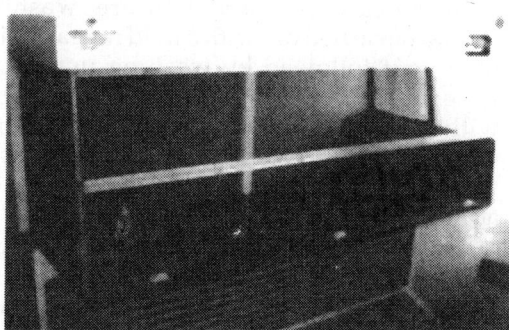

Fig. 5.1: Laminar air flow

Incubation Room or Incubator

Environmental factors have great effect on the growth and differentiation of cultured tissues. Therefore, it is very much essential to incubate all types of cultures in well-controlled environmental conditions, like temperature, humidity, illumination and air circulation. A typical incubation chamber or area should have both light and temperature controlled devices managed for 24 hours period. Air conditioners or room heaters are required to maintain the temperature at 25 ± 2°C. Light is adjusted in the terms of photoperiod duration (specified period for total darkness as well as for higher intensity light). Further, the requirement for humidity range of 20–90% controllable to ±3% and uniform forced air circulation can be achieved.

The incubation chamber or room should have the provision for storing the culture vessels (flask, jars and Petri dishes). Shelves should be designed in such a way, so that the culture vessels can be placed in the shelf or trays in such a way, that there should not be any hindrance in the light, temperature and humidity maintenance. A label having full detail about date of inoculation, name of the explant, medium and any other special information should stuck on each tray and rack to ensure identity and for maintaining the data of experiment.

In the case of suspension culture arrangement for shaker should also be made.

These days BOD incubators (Fig. 5.2) with all the requisite environmental condition maintenance are available in the market, they occupy less space and manageable with small generator or automatic invertor in the case of electricity failure to maintain the necessary light and temperature conditions. Failure of electricity may ruin important experiment and in the case of suspension culture the whole culture may get damaged due to stoppage of the shaker.

BOD incubators required to maintain the culture conditions should have the following characteristics:

- Temperature range 2–40°C
- Temperature control ±0.5°C

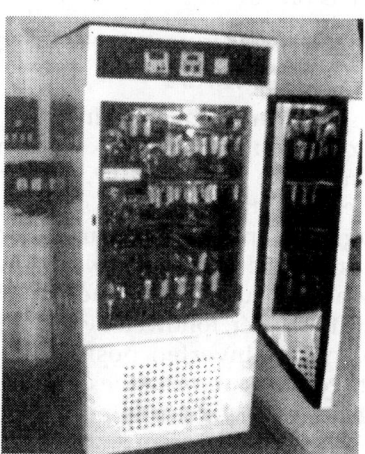

Fig. 5.2: BOD incubator

- Automatic digital temperature recorder
- Twenty-four hours temperature and light programming
- Adjustable fluorescent lighting up to 10,000 lux.
- Relative humidity range 20–98%
- Relative humidity control ±3%
- Uniform forced air circulation
- Shaker
- Capacity up to 0.7 m^3 of 0.5 m^2 shelf space.

Data Collection and Recording of the Observation

The growth and maintenance of the tissue culture in the incubator should be observed and recorded at regular intervals. All the observations should be done in aseptic environment, i.e. in the laminar airflow. Whereas, for microscopic examination separate dust free space should be marked for microscopic work. All the recorded data should be feed in computer.

GENERAL PROCEDURE INVOLVED IN PLANT TISSUE CULTURE

In vitro culturing of plant tissue involves the following steps:
- Sterilisation of glassware tools/vessels.
- Preparation and sterilisation of explant.
- Production of callus from explant.
- Proliferation of cultured callus.
- Subculturing of callus.
- Suspension culture.

Sterilisation of Glassware Tools/Vessels

Cleaning of Glassware

All the glassware to be used in tissue culture laboratory should be of pyrex or corning. To make them free from any dirt, waxy material or bacteria, all the glassware should be kept overnight, dipped in sodium dichromate-sulphuric acid solution. Next morning, glassware should be washed with fresh running tap water, followed by distilled water and placed in inverted position in plastic bucket or trays to remove the extra water. For drying the glassware, it is placed in hot air oven at high temperature about 120°C for ½–1 hour (Fig. 5.3).

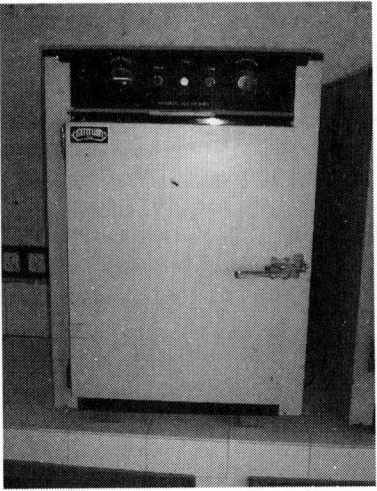

Fig. 5.3: Hot air oven

In the case of plastic labware, washing should be carried out with a mild non-abrasive detergent followed by washing under tap water or the plasticware after general washing with dilute sodium bicarbonate and water followed by drainage of extra water, rinsed with an organic solvent such as alcohol, acetone and chloroform.

Washed and dried glassware or plasticware should be stored in dust proof cupboards.

To prevent reinfection following sterilisation, empty containers are wrapped with aluminium foil. Stainless steel, metals tools (knives, scalpels, forceps, etc.) are also wrapped with the aluminium foil and pads of cotton wool are stuffed into the opening of the pipettes, which are either also wrapped in aluminium or placed in an aluminium or stainless steel box.

The period of sterilisation usually ranges between 1 and 4 hours.

Note: The object with different thermal expansion coefficients may not be mixed together during the treatment period of at least 30 minutes. The accuracy of calibrated instruments is often reduced.

Preparation of Explant

Explant can be defined as a portion of plant body, which has been taken from the plant to establish a culture. Explant can be obtained from plants, which are grown in controlled environmental conditions. Such plants will be usually free from pathogens and are homozygous in nature. **Explant may be taken from any part of the plant like root, stem, leaf, or meristematic tissue like cambium, floral parts like anthers, stamens, etc.**

Age of the explant is also an important factor in callus production. Young tissues are more suitable than mature tissues. A suitable portion from the plant is removed with the help of sharp knife and the dried and mature portions are separated from young tissue. When seeds and grains are used for explant preparation, they are directly sterilised and put in nutrient medium. After germination, the obtained seedlings are to be used for explant preparation.

Surface Sterilisation of Explant

For the surface sterilisation of the explant, **chromic acid, mercuric chloride (0.11%), calcium hypochlorite, sodium hypochlorite (1–2%) and alcohol (70%)** are used. Usually, the tissue is immersed in the solution of sterilising agent for 10 seconds to 15 minutes and then they are washed with distilled water. Repeat the treatment with **sodium hypochlorite for 20 minutes** and the tissue is finally washed with sterile water to remove sodium hypochlorite. Such tissue is used for inoculation.

The explants are sterilised by exposing to aqueous sterilised solution of different concentration as shown in Table 5.2. In the case of leaf or green fresh stem, the explant needs pretreatment with wetting agent (70–90% ethyl alcohol, tween 20), 5–20 drops in 100 ml of purified water or some other mild detergent to be added directly into the sterilisation solution to reduce the water repulsion (due to waxy secretion).

Procedure to be followed for respective explant is as follow:

Seeds

Step 1: Dip the seeds into absolute ethyl alcohol for 10 seconds and rinse with purified water.

Table 5.2: Surface sterilising agent

Name of chemical	Concentration (%)	Exposure (minute)
Bromine water	1–2	2–10
Benzalkonium chloride	0.01–0.1	5–20
Sodium hypochlorite	0.5–51	5–30
Calcium hypochlorite	9–10	5–30
Mercuric chloride	1–2	2–10
Hydrogen peroxide	3–10	5–15
Silver nitrate	1–2	5–20

Step 2: Expose seeds for 20–30 minutes to 10% w/v. aqueous calcium hypochlorite or for 5 minutes in a 1% solution of bromine water.

Step 3: Wash the treated seeds with sterile water (three to five times) followed by germination on damp sterile filter paper.

Fruits

Step 1: Rinse the fruit with absolute alcohol.

Step 2: Submerge into 2% (w/v) solution of sodium hypochlorite for 10 minutes.

Step 3: Washing repeated with sterile water and remove seeds of interior tissue.

Stem

Clean the explant with running tap water followed by rinsing with pure alcohol.

Submerge in 2% (w/v) sodium hypochlorite solution for 15–30 minutes.

Wash three times with sterile water.

Leaves

Clean the leaf explant with purified water to make it free from dirt and rub the surface with absolute ethyl alcohol.

Dip the explant in 0.1% (w/v) mercuric chloride solution, wash with sterile water to make it free from chloride and then dry the surface with sterile tissue paper.

Production of Callus from Explant

The sterilised explant is transferred aseptically onto defined medium contained in flasks. The flasks are transferred to BOD incubator for maintenance of culture. Temperature is adjusted to 25 ± 2°C. Some amount of light is necessary for callus (undifferentiated amorphous cell mass) production. Usually, sufficient amount of callus is produced within 3–8 days of incubation.

Proliferation of Cultured Callus

If callus is well-developed, it should be cut into small pieces and transferred to another fresh medium containing an altered composition of hormones, which supports growth. The medium used for production of more amount of callus is called proliferation medium.

Subculturing of Callus

After sufficient growth of callus, it should be periodically transferred to fresh medium to maintain the viability of cells. This subculturing will be done at an interval of 4 to 6 weeks.

Suspension Culture

Suspension culture contains a uniform suspension of separate cells in liquid medium. For the preparation of suspension culture, callus is transferred to liquid medium, which is agitated continuously to keep the cells separate. Agitation can be achieved by rotary shaker system attached within the incubator at a rate of 50–150 rpm. After the production of sufficient number of cells sub-culturing can be done.

CULTURE MEDIA

Nutritional requirements for optimal growth of a tissue culture may vary with the species. Even tissues from **different parts of a plant may** have different requirements for proper satisfactory growth. As such no single medium can be suggested as being entirely sufficient for the satisfactory growth of all types of plant tissues and organs, hence with **every new system**, it is essential to work out a medium by hit and trial that would fulfil the specific requirements of that particular tissue. List of several culture media developed by scientists to culture diverse tissues and organs are Gautheret (1942), White (1943), Haberblandt et al (1946), Haller (1953), Nitsch and Nitsch (1956), Murashige and Skoog (1962),

Eriksson (1965) and B5 (Gamberg et al, 1968) (Table 5.3).

Media Composition

To maintain the vital functions of a culture, the basic medium consisting of inorganic nutrients (macronutrients and micronutrients) must be supplemented with organic components (amino acids, vitamins), growth regulators (phytohormones) and utilisable carbon (sugar) source and a gelling agent (agar/phytogel), as per the requirement of the object.

Inorganic Nutrients

Mineral elements play very important role in the growth of a plant. For example, magnesium is a part of chlorophyll molecule, calcium is a component of cell wall and nitrogen is an important element of amino acids, vitamins, proteins and nucleic acids. Iron, zinc and molybdenum are parts of certain enzymes.

Essentially, about **15 elements** found important for whole plant growth, have also been proved necessary for the growth of tissue(s) in culture. Elements required in the life of a plant greater than 0.5 mmol l^{-1} are referred as **macronutrients** and those less than 0.5 mmol l^{-1} as **micronutrients**.

Macronutrients: The macronutrients include six major elements: nitrogen (N), phosphorus (P), potassium (K), calcium (Ca), magnesium (Mg), and sulphur (S) present as salts that constitute the various above-mentioned defined media. The concentration of the major elements like calcium, phosphorus, sulphur and magnesium should be in the range of 1–3 mmol l^{-1}, whereas the nitrogen in the media (contributed by both nitrate and ammonia) should be 2–20 mmol l^{-1}.

Micronutrients: The inorganic elements required in small quantities but essential for proper growth of plant cells or tissues are: boron (B), copper (Cu), iron (Fe), manganese (Mn), zinc (Zn) and molybdenum (Mo). Out of these, iron seems more critical as it is used in chelated forms of iron and zinc, in preparing the culture media, as iron tartrate and citrate are difficult to dissolve. The concentration

Table 5.3: Composition of some plant tissue culture media

Constituents	Media (amount in mg l^{-1})						
	White (1963)	Heller's (1953)	MS (1962)	ER	B (1968)	Nitsch (1951)	NT
Micronutrients							
$MnSO_4 \cdot 4H_2O$	5	0.1	22.3	2.23	–	25	22.3
$MnSO_4 \cdot H_2O$	–	–	–	–	10	–	–
$ZnSO_4 \cdot 7H_2O$	3	1	8.6	–	2	10	–
$ZnSO_4 \cdot 4H_2O$	–	–	–	–	–	–	8.6
$CuSO_4 \cdot 5H_2O$	0.01	0.03	0.00025	–	0.025	0.025	0.025
$CoSO_4 \cdot 7H_2O$	–	–	–	–	–	–	0.03
$Fe_2(SO_4)_3$	2.5	–	–	–	–	–	–
$FeSO_4 \cdot 7H_2O$	–	–	27.8	27.8	–	27.8	27.8
KCl	65	750	–	–	–	–	–
KI	0.75	0.01	0.83	–	0.75	–	0.83
H_3BO_3	1.5	1	6.2	0.63	3	10	6.2
$Na_2MoO_4 \cdot 2H_2O$	–	–	0.25	0.025	0.25	0.25	0.25
MoO_3	0.001	–	–	–	–	–	–
$CoCl_2 \cdot 6H_2O$	–	–	0.025	0.0025	0.025	–	–
$AlCl_3$	–	0.03	–	–	–	–	–
$NiCl_2 \cdot 6H_2O$	–	0.03	–	–	–	–	–
$FeCl_3 \cdot 6H_2O$	–	1.00	–	–	–	–	–
EDTA							
$Zn \cdot Na_2EDTA$	–	–	–	15	–	–	–
$Na_2EDTA \cdot 2H_2O$	–	–	37.3	37.3	–	37.3	37.3
Vitamins							
Nicotinic acid	0.05	–	0.5	0.5	1	5	–
Pyridoxine HCl	0.01	–	0.5	0.5	1	0.5	1
Thiamine HCl	0.01	–	0.10	0.5	10	0.5	1
Glycine	3.0	–	2.0	2.0	–	2	–
Folic acid	–	–	–	–	–	0.5	–
Macronutrients							
NH_4NO_3	–	–	1650	1200	–	720	825
HNO_3	80	–	900	1900	2527.5	950	950
$NaNO_3$	–	600	–	–	–	–	–
$Ca(NO_3)4H_2O$	300	–	–	–	–	–	–
$CaCl_2 \cdot 2HO$	–	75	440	440	150	–	220
$CaCl_2$	–	–	–	–	–	166	–
$MgSO_4 \cdot 6H_2O$	750	250	370	370	246.5	185	1233
$(NH_4)_2SO_4$	–	–	–	–	–	–	–
KH_2PO_4	–	–	170	340	–	68.0	68.0
$NaH_2PO_3 \cdot H_2O$	19	125	–	–	150	–	–
Growth regulators							
Inositol	–	–	100	–	100	100	100
2,4-D	–	–	0.1	1.0	–	–	–
IAA	–	–	1.0	30.0	–	–	–
Kinetin	–	–	0.04	10.0	0.02	0.1	–
NAA	–	–	–	1.0	–	–	–
Myo-inositol	–	–	100.0	–	100.0	–	–
pH	–	–	5.7	5.8	5.5	–	–
Sucrose	2%	–	3%	4%	2%	2%	1%

MS—Murashige and Skoog (1962), ER—Eriksson, B—Gamberg et al (1968), NT—Nagata and Takebe (1971).
Note: Growth regulators and complex nutrient mixtures described by various authors are not included.

generally prescribed for all these elements are in traces:

Cu	0.1 mmol l^{-1}
Fe	1 mmol l^{-1}
Mo	5 mmol l^{-1}
Zn	1.5–30 mmol l^{-1}
Mn	20–90 mmol l^{-1}
B	2–5100 mmol l^{-1}

These are added to culture media depending upon the requirement of the objective.

In addition to these elements certain media are also enriched with cobalt (Co), iodine (I) and sodium (Na) but exact cell growth requirement is not well-established.

The composition of some plant tissue culture media reveal that the chief difference in the composition of various commonly used tissue culture media lies in the quantity of various salts and ions. Qualitatively, the inorganic nutrients required for various culture media appear to be fairly constant.

The active factor in the medium is the ions of different types rather than the salt (mineral salts on dissolving in water undergo dissociation and ionisation). A single ion may be contributed by more than one salt. For example, in **Murashige and Skoog's** medium NO_3^- ions are contributed by NH_4NO_3 as well as KNO_3 and K^+ ions are contributed by KNO_3 and KH_2PO_4.

White's medium, one of the earliest plant tissue culture media includes all the necessary nutrients and was widely used for root culture. The experience of various investigators has, however, revealed that quantitatively the inorganic nutrients are inadequate for good callus growth (**Murashige and Skoog's** 1962), hence most plant tissue culture media, that are **now being widely** used (Table 5.3) are richer in mineral salts (ions) **as compared to White's medium. Aluminium and nickel used by Heller's** (1953) could not be proved to be essential, and therefore, were dropped by subsequent workers, but **sodium, chloride and iodide** are indispensable.

In **Heller medium**, special emphasis was given to iron and nitrogen. In the **original White's medium**, iron was used in the form of $Fe_2(SO_4)_3$ but **Street and co-workers** replaced it by $FeCl_3$ for root culture because of the impurities due to Mn and some other metallic ions. However, $FeCl_3$ also did not prove to be an entirely satisfactory source of iron. In this form iron is available to the tissue culture at or around pH 5.2 and within a week of inoculation, the pH of the medium drift from 4.9–5.0 to 5.8–6.0, and the root culture started showing the iron deficiency symptoms. To overcome this difficulty, in most medium, iron is now used as FeEDTA, in this form iron remains available up to a pH of 7.6–8.0. However, unlike root, callus cultures can utilise $FeCl_3$ to pH 6.0 by secreting natural chelates. FeEDTA may be prepared by using $Fe_2(SO_4)_37H_2O$ and $Na_2EDTA \bullet 2H_2O$.

Inorganic nitrogen is supplied in the medium in the forms as nitrates and ammonium compounds, when nitrate is used alone the pH of the medium shifted toward alkalinity, to check this drift small amount of ammonium compound is added along with nitrate.

Following are the deficiency symptoms of the some of the elements shown by callus tissues:

• **Nitrogen:** Spectacular appearance of anthocyanins; vessels are not formed.
• **Nitrogen phosphorus and potassium:** Cell hypertrophy and a reduction of cambium tissue.
• **Sulphur:** Very apparent chlorosis
• **Iron:** Cessation of cell division
• **Boron:** Retardation of cell division and cell elongation.
• **Manganese or molybdenum:** Effect cell elongation.

Organic Nutrients

Nitrogenous substances: Most cultured plant cells are capable of synthesising essential vitamins but not in sufficient amount. To achieve best growth, it is essential to supplement the tissue culture medium with one or more vitamins and amino acid. Among the **essential vitamins, thiamine** (vitamin B$_1$) has been proved to be essential ingredient. Other vitamins, especially pyridoxine (vitamin B$_6$), nicotinic acid (vitamin B$_3$) and calcium pentothenate (vitamin B$_5$) and inositol are also known to improve growth of the tissue culture material. As shown in Table 5.3, there is variation in the quantities of essential vitamins used by various standard media.

Numerous **complex nutritive mixtures** of undefined composition, like **casein hydrolysate, coconut milk, corn-milk, malt extract, tomato juice and yeast extract** have also been used to promote growth of the tissue culture, but these substances specifically fruit extracts may affect the reproducibility of results because of variation in the quality and quantity of growth promoting constituent in these extracts.

Carbon Source: It is essential to supplement the tissue culture media with a utilisable source of carbon to the culture media. **Haberblandt** (1902) attempted to culture green mesophyll cells, probably with the idea that green cells would have simple nutritive requirement, but this did not prove to be true. In fact even fully organised green shoot in cultures also did not show proper growth and proliferation without the addition of suitable carbon source in the medium.

The most commonly used carbon source is **sucrose** at a concentration of 2–5%. **Glucose and fructose** also known to be used for good growth of some tissues. **Ball** (1953, 1955) demonstrated that autoclaved sucrose was better than filtered sterilised sucrose. Autoclaving may do the hydrolysis of the sucrose, thereby, converting it into more efficiently utilisable sugar such as **fructose**. In general, excised **dicotyledonous roots** grow better with sucrose, whereas monocots do best with **dextrose** (glucose). Some other forms of carbon that plant tissues are known to utilise include **maltose, galactose, mannose, lactose and sorbitol**. It has been reported that some tissues can even **metabolise starch** as the sole **carbon source**, e.g. tissue cultures of Cymbidium, Sequoia and maize endosperm.

Growth Regulators (Hormones)

In addition to the nutrients, it is generally necessary to add one or more growth hormones, e.g. **auxin, cytokinins and gibberellins** to support better growth of tissues and organs. However, the requirement of these hormones varies considerably with their endogenous levels.

i. Auxins: In tissue culture auxin induces **cell division** and also **stimulate root formation/differentiation**. Both natural IAA (Indole-3-acetic acid) and synthetic IBA (Indole-3-butyric acid) NAA (Naphthalene acetic acid) NOA (Naphthoxyacetic acid), 2,4-D (2,4-dichlorophenoxy acetic acid) and 2,4,5-T (trichlorophenoxyacetic acid) are used.

Among auxins, IBA and NAA are widely used for rooting. In interaction with cytokinin, the auxins are used for shoot proliferation. 2,4-D and 2,4,5 T are very effective for the induction and growth of callus. IAA inhibits the bud formation and also play role in embryogenesis.

Auxins are generally dissolved in either ethanol or dilute NaOH.

Although, the synthetic forms are relatively stable, IAA is considered to be rapidly inactivated by certain environmental factors, e.g. light.

ii. Cytokinin: Chemically cytokinins are *adenine derivatives* and have been employed in **tissue culture** work to promote the formation of adventitious buds and shoots from undifferentiated cells. In **cell cultures** they have been shown to promote the biosynthesis of berberine (*Thalictrum minus*), condensed tannins (*Onobrychis viccifolia*) and rhodoxanthin (*Ricinus*).

Cytokinin (adenine or kinetin) in the medium leads to the promotion of bud differentiation and development. **Kinetin is 30,000 times more potent than adenine. Kinetin** is originally detected as an artificial rearrangement product of the autoclaving process of herring sperm

DNA (6-furfurylaminopurine), while **kinetin** is only rarely used for callus induction aside from specific experimental purposes.

Other cytokinins which influence the induction of shoot buds include 6-benzylaminopurine (BAP) or 6-benzyladenine (BA), 6-γ-γ-dimethylaminopurine (2-iP), 6-tetrahydropyrane-adenine and zeatin. **Zeatin and 2-iP** are naturally occurring cytokinins while BA and kinetin are synthetically derived. **6 BAP** (6-benzyl-amino-purine) and **zeatin** are very commonly used to induce and maintain growth of callus and cell suspension cultures.

Cytokinins are generally dissolve in dilute HCl or NaOH.

Zeatin isolated from maize embryos at the milky stage. It is 6-substituted adenine derivative, 6-(4-hydroxy-3-methyl-2-butenyl)-amino-purine obtained from maize associated with zeatin riboside (1β-D-ribofuranose) and with phosphate ester of this compound.

iii. *Gibberellins:* There are over 20 known gibberellins, of these, GA$_3$ is usually used to increase the **shoot elongation** in tissue culture. As compared to auxins and cytokinin, **gibberellins are used very rarely**. It is reported to stimulate normal development of plantlets from *in vitro* formed adventive embryos. GA is readily soluble in cold water up to 1000 mg^{-1}.

Solidifying Agents for Solidification of the Media

Due to improved oxygen supply and support to the culture growth, solid media are often preferred to liquid cultures. For this purpose, substance with strong gelling capacity is added into the liquid media. These reversibly bind water, and thus, ensure the humidity of the medium desired for culturing depending on the concentration.

Gelling Agent Used to Solidify Liquid Media

- Agar
- Sodium alginate
- Carrageenan
- Gelatin
- Hydroxyethylcellulose
- Polyacrylamide
- Starch
- Silica gel

The most commonly used substance for this purpose is the phycocolloid agar-agar obtained from red algae (*Gelidium gracilaria*). It is generally used at a concentration of 0.8–1.0%, with higher concentration, medium become hard and does not allow the diffusion of nutrients into the tissues medium. However, agar is not an essential component of the nutrient medium. Single cell and cell aggregates can be grown as suspension cultures in liquid medium containing inorganic, organic nutrients and other growth factors. Such culture should, however, be regularly aerated either by bubbling sterile air or gentle agitation. In nutritional studies, the use of agar should be avoided because of the impurities present in all the commercially available agar-agar especially of Ca, Mg, K, Na and trace elements.

Agar (Agarose) is extraordinary **resistant to enzymatic hydrolysis** at incubation temperature and only a few bacteria exist which are capable of producing degrading enzyme, agarase. This resistance to hydrolysis is the fundamental importance to the use of agar-agar in cell culture medium. It is also neutral to media constituents, and thus, do not react with them.

pH

pH of the medium is generally adjusted between 5.0 and 6.0 before sterilisation. In general pH higher than 6.0 give fairly hard medium and pH below 5.0 does not allow satisfactory gelling of the agar.

Media Preparation

For media preparation, there are two possible methods, i.e.:

i. To weigh the required quantity of nutrient, dissolved them separately and mixed at the time of medium preparation.

ii. To prepare the stock solution separately for macronutrients, micronutrients, iron solution and organic components, store them in the refrigerator till not used, e.g. **Murashinge and Skoog's** media stock solution is prepared as under:

Procedure

All the ingredients may be grouped into following four groups:

Stock Solution Ingredients Amount (mg/L)

Group I

• NH_4NO_3	1650
• KNO_3	1900
• $CaCl_2 \cdot 2H_2O$	440
• $MgSO_4 \cdot 7H_2O$	370
• KH_2PO_4	170

Group II

• KI	0.83
• H_3BO_3	6.2
• $MnSO_4 \cdot 4H_2O$	22.3
• $ZnSO_4 \cdot 7H_2O$	8.6
• $Na_2MoO_4 \cdot 2H_2O$	0.25
• $CuSO_4 \cdot 5H_2O$	0.025
• $CoCl_2 \cdot 6H_2O$	0.025

Group III

• $FeSO_4 \cdot 7H_2O$	27.8
• $Na_2EDTA \cdot 2H_2O$	37.3

Group IV

• Inositol	100
• Nicotinic acid	0.5
• Pyridoxine HCl	0.5
• Thiamine HCl	0.1
• Glycine	2

Concentration of the ingredients: For the preparation of stock solution the **Group I** ingredient are prepared 20 × concentrated solution. **Group II** 200 × concentrated, **Group III** Iron salts (200 × concentrated) and **Group IV** organic ingredient except sucrose (200 × concentrated).

Solution preparation: For the preparation of stock solution, each component (analar grade) should be weighed and dissolved separately in glass distilled or demineralized water and then mix them together.

Stock solution may be prepared at the strength of 1 mmol l^{-1} or 10 mmol l^{-1}. All the stock solutions are stored in refrigerator till used.

For iron solution dissolve $FeSO_4 \cdot 7H_2O$ and $Na_2EDTA \cdot 2H_2O$ separately in about 450 ml distilled water by heating and constant stirring. Mix the two solutions, adjust pH of the medium to 5.5 and final volume adjusted 1 L with distilled water.

Semisolid media preparation: Required quantities of agar and sucrose are weighed and dissolved in water by 3/4th volume of medium, by heating them on water bath.

Adequate quantities of stock solution (for 1L medium 50 ml of stock solution of Group I, 5 ml of stock solution II, III and IV groups) and other special supplements are added and final volume is made-up with double distilled water. After mixing well, pH of the medium is adjusted to 5.8 using 0.1 N NaOH and 0.1 N HCl.

Note: *These days dry powdered media are available in the market. The available powder is to be dissolved in 3/4th volume of distilled water and after adding sugar, agar and other desired supplements, the final volume is made-up with distilled water pH is adjusted and the medium autoclaved.*

Sterilisation of Culture Media

Culture media packed in glass containers or vessels are sealed with cotton plugs and covered with aluminium foils and are autoclaved at pressure of 2–2.2 atm at 121°C for 15–40 minutes (time to be fixed from the time when temperature reaches the required temperature). The exposure time depends on the volume of the liquid to be sterilised as given below.

Minimum Autoclaving Time for Plant Tissue Culture Media

Volume of the media per vessel (ml)	Minimum autoclaving time (min)
25	20
50	25
100	28
250	31
500	35
1000	40
2000	48
4000	63

Minimum autoclaving time include the time required for the liquid volume to reach the sterilising temperature (121°C) and 15 minutes at this temperature. Time may vary due to difference in autoclaves.

Moreover, the actual success of sterilisation can be tested using a **bioindicator**, commonly spores of the bacterium Bacillus stearothermophillus are used as such as a test organism. Together with culture medium and a pH indicator in ampoules sealed by melting, both autoclaved material and non-autoclaved controls are incubated for 24–48 hours at 60°C. If the spores are dead, the colour of the pH indicator in the solution remains unchanged indicating no change in pH (Fig. 5.4).

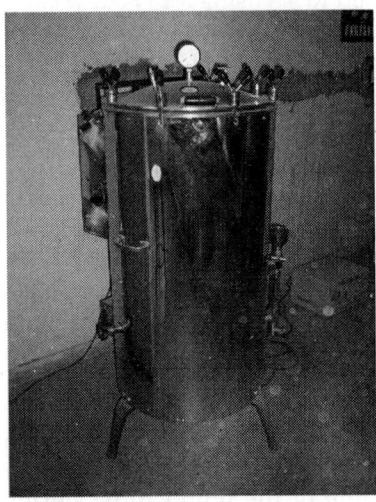

Fig. 5.4: Autoclave

TYPES OF PLANT TISSUE CULTURES; THEIR ESTABLISHMENT AND MAINTENANCE

Plant tissue culture is a general term to culture the isolated plant organs (particularly of isolated roots, but to a lesser extent of stem tips, immature embryo, leaf primordia, flower structures and even the cells and the protoplasts) under aseptic environment.

Types of Cultures

Root tip culture: Tips of the lateral roots are sterilised, **excised** and **transferred** to fresh medium. The roots continue to grow and provide several roots, which after **seven days**, are used to initiate stock or experimental cultures. Thus, the root material derived from a **single radicle** could be multiplied and maintained in continuous culture, such genetically uniform root cultures are referred to as a clone of isolated roots.

Leaves or leaf primordia culture: Leaves (800 µm) may be detached from shoots, **surface sterilised** and placed on a solidified medium where they will remains in a **healthy conditions** for a long periods. Growth rate in culture depends on their stage of maturity at excision. **Young leaves have more growth potential** than the nearly mature ones.

Shoot tip culture: The excised shoot tips (100–1000 µm long) of many plant species can be cultured on relatively simple nutrient media containing growth hormones and will often **form roots and develop into whole plants.**

Complete flower culture: Nitsch in 1951 reported the successful culture of the flowers of several dicotyledonous species, the flowers remain healthy and develop normally to produce mature fruits. Flowers (2 days after pollination) are excised, sterilised by immersion in 5% calcium hypochlorite, washed with sterilised water and transferred to culture tubes containing an agar medium. Often fruits, which develop are smaller than their natural counterpart; but the size can be increased by supplementing the medium with an appropriate combination of growth hormones.

Anther and pollens culture: Young **flower buds** are removed from the plant and surface sterilised. The anthers are then carefully excised and transferred to an appropriate nutrient medium. Immature stage usually grow abnormally and there is **no development of pollen grains from pollen mother cells.** Anther at a very young stage (containing microspore mother cells, or tetrads) and late stage (containing binucleate starch filled pollen) of development are generally ineffective and hence for better response always select mature anther or pollen.

Mature anther or pollen grains (microspora) of several species of gymnosperms can be induced to form callus by spreading them out on the surface of a suitable agar media.

Mature pollen grains of angiosperms do not usually form callus, although, there are one or two exceptions.

Ovule and embryo culture: Embryo is dissected from the ovule and put into culture media.

Very small globular embryos require a delicate balance of the hormones. Hence mature embryos are excised from ripened seeds and cultured mainly to avoid inhibition in the seed for germination. This type of culture is relatively easy as the embryos require a simple nutrient medium containing mineral salts, sugar and agar for growth and development.

The seeds are treated with 70% alcohol for about **two minutes**, washed with sterile distilled water, treated with surface sterilising agent for specific period (Table 5.2), once again rinsed with sterilised distilled water and kept for germination by placing them on double layers of pre-sterilised filter paper, placed in Petri dish moistened with sterilised distilled water or placed on moistened cotton swab in Petri dish. The seeds are germinated in dark at 25–28°C and small part of the seedling is utilised for the initiation of callus.

Apart from above-mentioned cultures, there are two more methods for culturing of plant tissues/cells:

• Protoplast culture

• Hairy roots culture.

Protoplast Culture

Protoplasts are the naked cells of varied origin without cell walls, which are cultivated in liquid as well as on solid media. Protoplasts can be isolated by mechanical or enzymatic method from almost all parts of the plant: roots, tubers, root nodules, leaves, fruits, endosperms, crown gall tissues, pollen mother cells and the cells of the callus tissue but the most appropriate is the leaves of the plant.

Fully expanded young leaves from the healthy plant are collected, washed with running tap water and sterilised by dipping in 70% ethanol for about a minute and then treating with 2% solution of sodium hypochlorite for 20–30 minutes and then washed with sterile distilled water to make it free from the trace of sodium hypochlorite.

The lower surface of the sterilised leaf is peeled off and stripped leaves are cut into pieces (midrib).

The peeled leaf segments are treated with enzymes (**macerozyme** and then treated with cellulase) to isolate the protoplasts.

The protoplasts so obtained are cleaned by centrifugation and decantation method. Finally, the protoplast solution of known density (1×10^5 protoplast/ml) is poured on sterile and cooled down molten nutrient medium in Petri dishes. Mix the two gently but quickly by rotating each Petri dish. Allow the medium to set and seal Petri dishes with paraffin film. Incubate the Petri dishes in inverted position in BOD incubator. The protoplasts, which are capable of dividing undergo cell divisions and form callus within 2–3 weeks. The callus is then subcultured on fresh medium. **Embryogenesis** begins from callus when it is transferred to a medium containing proper proportion of auxin and cytokinin, the embryos develop into plantlets which may be transferred to pots (Fig. 5.5).

Hairy Roots Culture

The name "hairy root" was mentioned in the literature by **Steward** et al (1900). A large number of small fine hairy roots covered with root hairs originate directly from the explant in response to *Agrobacterium rhizogenes* infection are termed "hairy roots". These are fast growing, highly branched adventitious roots at the site of infection and can grow even on a hormone-free culture medium.

Many plant cell culture systems, which did not produce adequate amount of desired compounds is being reinvestigated using hairy root culture methods. A diversified range of plant species has been transformed using various bacterial strains. One of the most important characteristics of the transformed roots is their capability to synthesise

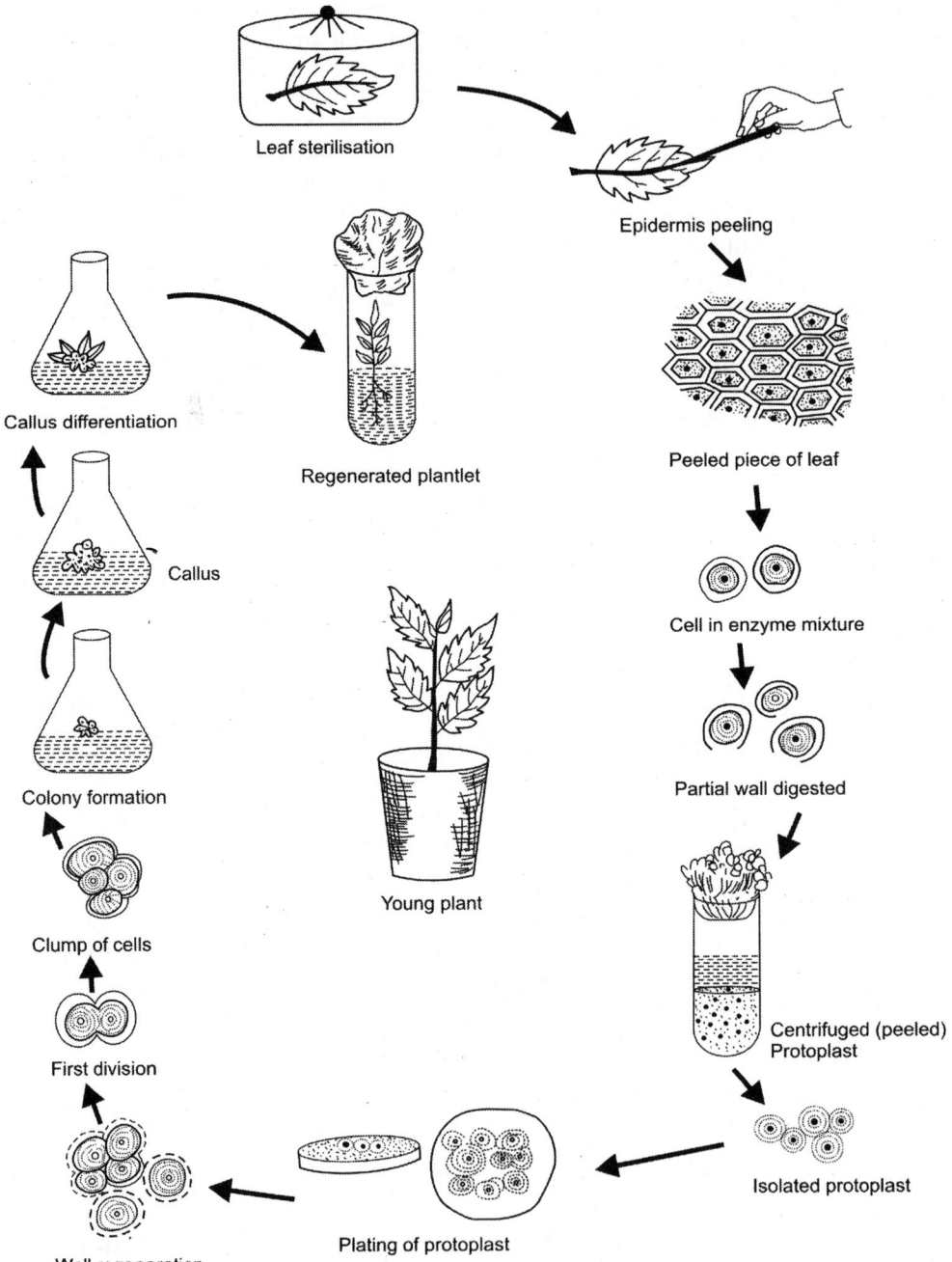

Fig. 5.5: Schematic diagram showing the isolation, culture and regeneration of young plant from leaf protoplast

secondary metabolites specific to that plant species from which they have been developed. Growth kinetics and secondary metabolite production by hairy roots is highly stable and are of equal level and even they are higher to those of field grown plants (Fig. 5.6).

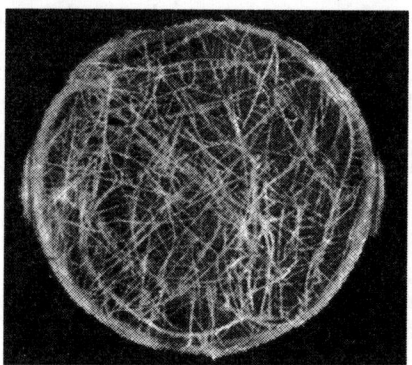

Fig. 5.6: Hairy roots

ESTABLISHMENT AND MAINTENANCE OF VARIOUS CULTURES

For the growth establishment and maintenance of various types of plant tissue cultures, there are three main **culture systems**, selected on the basis of the objective.

   i. Growth of **callus** masses on solidified media (**callus culture** also known as **static culture**).

  ii. Growth in liquid media (**suspension culture**) consists of mixture of single cells or cell aggregates.

 iii. **Protoplast culture.**

The protoplast culture can be grown as:

• Callus culture (static tissue culture)
• Suspension culture.

Callus Culture

Callus is an amorphous aggregate of loosely arranged parenchyma cells, which proliferate from mother cells. Cultivation of callus usually on a solidified nutrient medium under aseptic conditions is known as **callus culture**, unlike tumor tissue, the cell division take place periclinically (Fig. 5.7a and b).

Initiation of Callus Culture

a. Selection and preparation of explant (also see at p.105)

Selection: For the preparation of callus culture, organ or culture is selected such as segments of root or stem, leaf primordia, flower structure or fruit, etc.

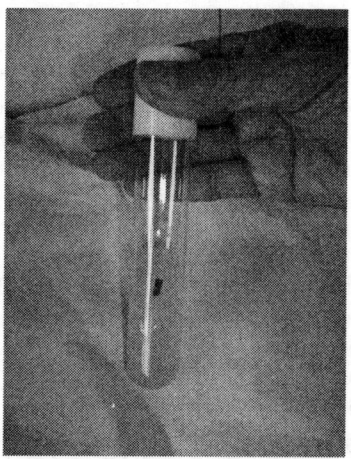

Fig. 5.7a: Initiation of callus culture

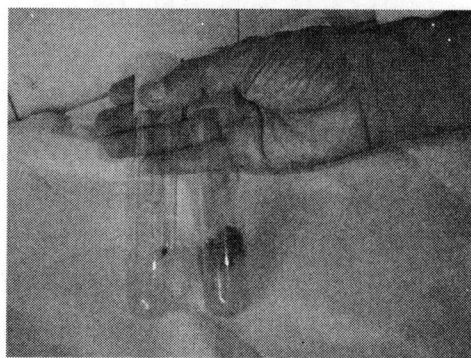

Fig. 5.7b: Development of callus culture

Preparation

   i. Excised parts of the plant organ are first washed with tap water, then sterilised with 0.1% of mercuric chloride ($HgCl_2$) or 2% w/v, sodium hypochlorite (NaOCl) solution for 15 minutes.

     In the case of plant organ containing waxy layer, the material is either pretreated with wetting agents [ethanol 70–90%; tween 20 (polyoxyethylene-sorbitan-monolaurate); 1–20 drops into 100 ml distilled water]; or other detergents are added to the sterilisation solution to reduce the water repulsion.

  ii. Washed the sterilised explants with sterile glass distilled water and cut aseptically into small segments (2–5 mm).

b. Selection of culture medium

The organ is to be cultured in well-defined nutrient medium containing inorganic, organic nutrients and vitamins. The culture of the medium depends on the species of the plant and the objective of the experiment. The MS medium is quite suitable for **dicot tissues** because of relatively high concentration of nitrate, potassium and ammonium ions in comparison to other media (Table 5.3).

Growth hormones (auxin, cytokinin) are adjusted in the medium according to the objective of the culture. For example, **auxins, IBA and NAA** are widely used in medium for rooting and in combination with cytokinin for shoot proliferation. 2,4-D and 2,4,5-T are effective for good growth of the callus culture. This is also quite favourable for monocot tissues or explant.

The selected semisolid nutrient is prepared. The pH of the medium is adjusted (5.0–6.0) and poured into culture vessels (15 ml for 25 × 150 mm culture tubes or 50 for 150 ml flasks) plugged and sterilised by autoclaving.

c. Transfer of explant

Surface sterilised organs (explant) from stem, root or tuber or leaf, etc. is transferred aseptically into the vessel containing semisolid culture medium.

d. Incubation of culture

The inoculated vessels are transferred into BOD incubator with autocontrolled device. Incubate at 25–28°C using light and dark cycles of each 12 hours duration. Nutrient medium is supplemented with auxin to induce cell division. After 3–4 week callus should be about 5 times, the size of the explant. Many tissue explants possess some degree of polarity with the result that the callus is formed most early at one surface. In stem segment, callus is formed particularly from that surface, which *in vivo* is directed towards the root.

The unique feature of callus is its ability to develop normal root and shoot, ultimately forming a plant. Commercially important secondary metabolites can also be obtained from static culture by manipulating the composition of media and growth regulators (physiological and biochemical conditions) but on the whole it is a good source for the establishment of suspension culture.

Callus is formed through three stages of development. They are:

a. Induction
b. Cell division
c. Cell differentiation.

Induction: During this stage metabolic activities of the cell will increase; with the result, the cell accumulates organic contents and finally divide into a number of cells. The length of this phase depends upon the functional potential of the explant and the environmental conditions of the cell division stage.

Cell division: This is the phase of active cell division as the explant cells revert to meristematic state.

Cell differentiation: This is the phase of cellular differentiation, i.e. morphological and physiological differentiation occur leading to the formation of secondary metabolites.

Maintenance

After sufficient time of callus growth on the same medium following changes will occur, i.e.:

• Depletion of nutrients in the medium
• Gradual loss of water
• Accumulation of metabolic toxins.

Hence for the maintenance of growth in callus culture it becomes necessary to **subculture the callus** into a fresh medium. Healthy callus tissue of sufficient size (5–10 mm in diameter and weight 20–100 mg) is transferred under aseptic conditions to fresh medium. Subculturing should be repeated after every 4–5 weeks (Fig. 5.7b).

Many callus cultures, however, remain healthy and continue to grow at slow rate for much longer period without subculturing, if the incubation is to be carried out at low temperature 5–10°C below the normal temperature (16–18°C). Normally, total depletion takes about 28 days.

Callus tissue may appear of the following different colours:

- **White:** If grown in dark due to the absence of chlorophyll.
- **Green:** If grown in light.
- **Yellow:** Due to development of carotenoid pigments in greater amounts.
- **Purple:** Due to the accumulation of antho-cyanins in vacuole.
- **Brown:** Due to excretion of phenolic substance and formation of quinones.

Callus culture may vary widely in texture appearance and rate of growth. Some callus growth are heavily lignified and hard in texture while others are fragile.

The cells in callus tissue vary in shape from spherical to elongated.

Suspension Culture

Suspension culture contains a uniform suspension of separate cells in liquid medium. For the preparation of suspension culture, callus fragments is transferred to liquid medium (without agar), which is agitated continuously to keep the cells separate. Agitation can be achieved by rotary shaker system attached within the BOD incubator at a rate of 50–150 rpm. After sufficient number of cells are produced, subculturing can be done in fresh liquid medium.

Single cells can also be obtained from fresh plant organ (leaf).

Initiation of Suspension Culture

Isolation of single cell

a. **From callus culture:** Healthy callus tissue is selected and placed in a Petri dish on a sterile filter paper and cut into small pieces with the help of sterile scalpel.

Selected small piece of callus fragment about 300–500 mg and transferred into flask containing about 60 ml of liquid nutrient media (i.e. defined nutrient medium without gelling agent), the flasks is agitated at 50–150 rpm to make the separation of the cells in the medium. Decant the medium and resuspend residue by gently rotating the flask, and finally, transfer 1/4th of the entire residue to fresh medium, followed by sieving the medium to obtain the degree of uniformity of cells.

b. **From plant organ:** From the plant organ (leaf tissue) single cell can be isolated by any of the following methods:
   - Mechanical method
   - Enzymatic method

Mechanical Method: The surface sterilised fresh leaves are grinded in (1:4) grinding medium (20 μmol sucrose; 10 μmol $MgCl_2$, 20 μmol tris-HCl buffer, pH 7.8) in glass pestle mortar. The homogenate is passed through muslins (two layers) cloth. Then washed with sterile distilled water, centrifuge with culture medium, sieved and placed on culture dish for inoculation.

Enzymatic Method: Leaves are taken from 60 to 80 days old plant and sterilised by immersing them in 70% ethanol solution followed by hypochlorite solution treatment. Then washed with sterile double distilled water, placed on sterile tile and peeled off the lower surface with sterile forceps.

Cut the peeled surface area of the leaves into small pieces (4 cm^2). Transfer them (2 g leaves) into an Erlenmeyer flask (100 ml) containing about 20 ml of filtered sterilised enzyme solution (macerozyme 0.5% solution, 0.8% mannitol and 1% potassium dextran sulphate).

Incubate the flask at 25°C for 2 hours, during incubation, change the enzyme solution with the fresh one at every 30 minutes.

Wash the cell twice with culture medium and place them in culture dish.

Growth Pattern of Suspension Culture

Cell suspension culture is generally initiated by transferring an established (undifferentiated) callus tissue to a liquid nutrient medium, in flask culture vessel, which is agitated continuously during culture period. Agitation serves both, to aerate the cultures and to disperse the cell in medium. The composition of the medium for the establishment of suspension culture could be the same as for the callus culture except for the addition of agar. **After transferring the cells** into a suitable liquid medium they divide after **lag phase** and **linearly increase** their population. The soft callus, generally, forms a suspension culture without much difficulty. The release of cells and tissue fragments from less friable callus masses and the maintenance of good degree of cell separation may often be promoted by the presence of liquid medium of a high auxin concentration, an appropriate balance between yeast extract and auxin or between auxin and kinetin. After sometime depending upon the nutrient level and the rate of cell division, it comes to **stationary phase** (Fig. 5.8).

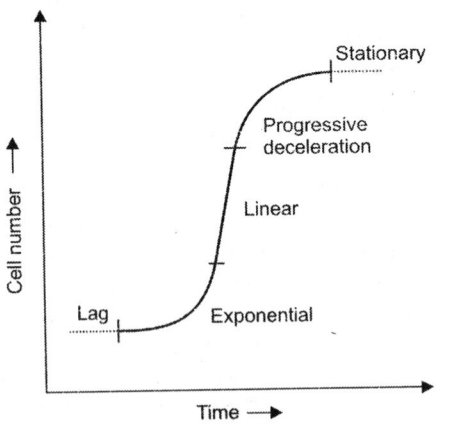

Fig. 5.8: Curve showing the growth pattern in the suspension culture

Stationary phase: The suspension culture are usually incubated at 25°C in darkness or low intensity fluorescent light at this stage, cell cultures are sub-cultured by dilution of stock culture 5–10 times (v/v) depending upon the growth of cells. The growth of suspension, culture is higher than callus culture, and therefore, it requires rapid sub-culture (7–21 days) as compared to callus culture (4–8 weeks).

The incubation period from culture initiation to the stationary phase is determined primarily by:

  a. Initial cell density

  b. Duration of lag phase

  c. Growth rate of cell type.

The cell density used to subculture is critical and depend largely on the type of suspension culture to be maintained. The low initial cell density will prolong the lag phase and exponential phase of growth. At an initial cell density of 9–15×103 ml, the cell will generally undergo eight fold increase in cell number before entering the stationary phase. Normal incubation time of stock culture is 21–28 days, while for sub-culture it is 14–21 days.

There are several **parameters** for measuring growth of cultured cells such as measurement of fresh and dry weight, cell mass, cell number, mitotic index or indirectly by the conductivity of the medium (King et al, 1973).

  i. **Fresh weight:** The value of callus cultures, frequently determined as total weight of callus medium layer and Petri dish. However, in this method, there are variations due to evaporation via the medium's surface. Hence, more exact values are obtained by determining the weight after complete separation from the culture medium. This is possible when the material is cultured on separate layers of cellulose or nylon.

  ii. **Dry weight:** It requires repeated drying, usually at 60°C to the point of constant weight, up to fresh weight of 500 mg, a linear relationship between fresh and dry weight is assumed. This method excludes error due to varying endogenous water contents.

  iii. **Cell mass:** It may be determined by densification by centrifugation (Ca 2000 g, 5 min.) of a particular percentage of the volume (4–7 ml) in graduated conical centrifuge tubes. In order to avoid error, due to water absorption by the cells, the so-called packed cell volume (PCV) must be recorded immediately following the separation process.

  iv. **Cell number:** To determine the number of cell per unit volume, existing cell clumps or aggregates must be separated into isolated cell (callus culture and in most suspension cultures). This is commonly done using chrome-trioxide alone or in combination with hypochlorous acid. Possible alternative are EDTA and pectinase.

Procedure: Cell aggregates are treated with 5–15% chromic acid or pectinase. To 1 volume of cell suspension culture may be added 2 volumes of 8% chromic acid, trioxide solution and mixture is heated at 70°C for 2–15 minutes. The mixture is cooled and then agitated vigorously for 10 minutes on a shaking machine.

The suspension is now centrifuged, the chromic acid is poured off and the pellet resuspended in 8% saline solution. After 10–15 minutes free cells are counted on a haemocytometer. Heating is avoided if an enzyme is used to disrupt the aggregates.

v. **Conductivity:** A continuous record measurement of conductivity of medium represents a speedy convenient, and manageable on line monitoring for the determination of the growth phase of a suspension culture without affecting the sterility. It is directly related with ion concentration in the culture.

As long as the pH of the medium remains above 3 (C^{H+}<10–3 ml/L) the concentration of hydrogen ions does not affect conductivity.

Maintenance of Suspension Culture

Maintenance of suspension culture can be done by following three ways (Fig. 5.9):

i. **Batch suspension culture:** In this technique, the cells are allowed to multiply in liquid medium, which is continuously agitated to break-up cell aggregates. The system is "**closed**" with respect to additions or removal of culture, except for circulation of air. In this technique to commence the growth again on the stationary phase, more amount of nutrient medium is added to the original culture or the cells are to be transferred into fresh medium. Each fresh medium containing culture (suspension) constitutes a batch. Such cultures are grown again and again for the purpose of experiment to achieve certain

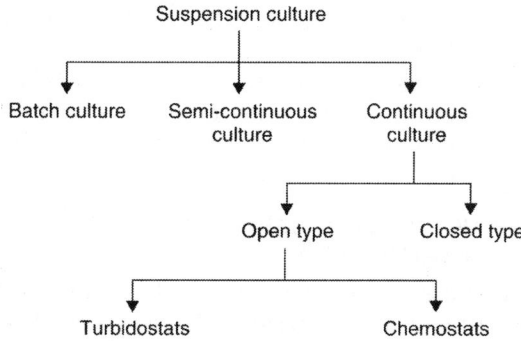

Fig. 5.9: Schematic diagram showing the maintenance of suspension culture

specific objectives. In batch culture, there is no steady state of growth, hence it is not ideal for commercial production of secondary metabolites.

ii. **Semi-continuous suspension culture:** In this very type, the system is **open**. It is designed for periodic removal of culture and addition of fresh medium. Hence, the **growth** is continuously maintained.

iii. **Continuous suspension culture:** Here, the volume of culture remains constant and fresh medium and culture are continuously added and withdrawn respectively. The important feature of the continuous culture is the proliferation of cell occurs under constant conditions. In this very suspension culture technique, a steady state is achieved by adding medium in which single nutrient has been adjusted so as to be growth limiting.

Continuous culture is **closed** and **open** type.

In the **closed** type, addition of fresh medium is balanced by the outflow of spent medium. The cell passing through the outgoing medium are separated mechanically and reintroduced into the culture for the continuous growth of the cell biomass.

Open continuous system involves regulated new medium and balancing harvest of equal volume of culture. The open system is further of two types depending upon regulation technique: **chemostat and turbidostat**.

In chemostat, the desired rate of growth is maintained by adjusting the level of concentration of nutrient by constant inflow of fresh medium.

In turbidostat, on the contrary, the input of medium is intermittent, and it is mainly required to maintain the cell density in the culture.

APPLICATIONS OF TISSUE CULTURE IN PHARMACOGNOSY

Plant tissue culture technology has been used in almost all the field of biosciences. The desirable products produced by plant tissue cultures are as diversified as is industry itself. Its applications include:

- Production of Phytopharmaceuticals
- Biochemical Conversions
- Clonal Propagation (Micropropagation)
- Production of Immobilized Plant Cells.

Production of Phytopharmaceuticals

The use of plant tissue culture for the production of phytopharmaceuticals was started in 1959 when Wenstein et al studied Agave, for the production of steroids using tissue culture method. Dioscorea was reported to contain industrially useful steroids by 1966, but it was 1969 when Kaul reported the production of 1.2% dry weight diosgenin by tissue culture of *D. sylvatica.*

During the last two decades advancement in tissue culture technology such as **development of hairy root cultures, immobilised plant cell systems, and technique to enhance the excretion of desired product into medium** has resulted in promising findings for a variety of medicinally important substance from several medicinal plants. Even the callus and suspension cultures are also capable of synthesising secondary metabolites and yields are comparable to the intact plant (Tables 5.4 and 5.5). There are report about few cell line producing secondary metabolites far in excess of that found in intact plants. For example:

Berberis for jatrorrhizine, **lithospermum** for shikonin; **coleus** for rosamarinic acid production and coptis for berberine.

During the last few years, plant tissue culture of several medicinal plants has been initiated and in many cases interesting compound with high yields of secondary metabolites are produced. For example, ten times more production of anthraquinone derivative from *Cassia tora* (6%) as compared to the crude drug. A twenty times more production of anthraquinone content in suspension culture of *Morinda citrifolia* and similar results were obtained from the suspension culture of *Galium* species. The suspension culture of *Dioscorea deltoidea* could produce up to 1.5% dry weight content of diosgenin. The cell culture of *Dioscorea deltoidea* yielded 26 mg/g dry weight of diosgenin, whereas the plant produce only 20 mg/g of diosgenin. The *Catharanthus roseus* cell culture yielded four times more ajmalicene and serpentine than the whole plant. The production of ginsenoside (21% of dry weight) from the cell culture of *Panax ginseng* has also been reported. The selected cell lines of *Euphorbia millic* produce seven times as much anthocyanin as the original calluses.

Nowadays, pharma industry is using plant tissue culture as source of variety of pharmaceuticals, which includes **alkaloids, terpenoids, glycosides and steroids** (Tables 5.6 and 5.7).

Industrial Production of Secondary Metabolite

It has been possible to establish large-scale production of biomass containing useful secondary metabolites by defining nutritional requirements and ensuring proper environmental conditions for their growth.

Secondary metabolism products compete with primary metabolism for precursors and potential bottlenecks for the former may involve those enzymes linking the primary and secondary pathways, as tryptophan dicarboxylase converting tryptophan to tryptamine in the formation of Indole alkaloids and cyclase enzymes involved in the synthesis of cyclohexanoid monoterpenes from geranyl pyrophosphate.

With cell cultures, as distinct from whole plants, particular genes may be repressed and need to be activated by suitable elicitors (Table 5.5).

Table 5.4: Phytopharmaceuticals of pharmaceutical significance

Compound	Plant species	Culture type
Ajmalicine	Catharanthus roseus	S
Anisodamine (6-hydroxy-hyoscyamine)	Anisodus tanguticus (bioconversion)	S
Anthocyanins	Euphorbia milli	S
Anthraquinones	Cassia angustifolia	C
	Cassia obtusifolia	C
	Cassia tora	C
	Galium mollugo	S
	Morinda citrifolia	S
	Rubia species	S
Atropine	Atropa belladonna	Hairy root
Berberine	Coptis japonica	C & S
Betacyanins	Chenopodium rubrum	S
Caffeine	Coffea arabica	C
Carboline alkaloids	Phaseolus vulgaris	S
	Peganum harmala	S
Cardenolides	Digitalis purpurea	S & C
	Digitalis lanata	S (biotransformation)
Cinnamoyl putrescines	Nicotiana tabacum	S (reduction of phosphate)
Codeine	Papaver somniferum	S
Digoxin (Biotransformation)	Digitalis lanata	S
Diosgenin	Dioscorea composita	C
	Dioscorea deltoidea	S
	Solanum xanthocarpum	S
	Trigonella foenum-graecum	S
L. dopa	Mucuna ruriens	S
Ginsenosides	Panax ginseng	S
Glycyrrhizin	Glycyrrhiza glabra	S
Harringtonine and homoharringtonine	Cephalotaxus	S
Hyoscyamine	Hyoscyamus niger	S root culture
	Duboisia leichhardtii	
Indole alkaloids	Ipomoea violacea	C & S
	Rivea corymbosa	
Isoprenoids (vol. oil)	Pelargonium fragrans	C & shoot proliferation
Morphine	Papaver sominiferum	S
Naphthoquinone	Lithospernum erythrorhizon	C & S
Nicotine	Nicotiana tobacum	S
Papain	Carcia papaya	C
Phenolics	Pinus resinosa	C
Protoberberines	Thalictrum, Coptis japonica & Berberis	S
Psoralen	Ruta Graveolens	S
Quinoline alkaloids	Cinchona ledgeriana	C & S
Quinine & quinidine	Cinchona ledgeriana	Root culture

(Contd...)

Table 5.4: Phytopharmaceuticals of pharmaceutical significance *(Contd...)*

Compound	Plant species	Culture type
Reserpine	*Rauwolfia serpentina*	S
	Alstonia constricta	C
Rosamarinic acid	*Coleus blumei*	C & S
Scopolamine	*Duboisia leichhardtii*	Root culture
Serpentine & other monomeric alkaloids	*Catharanthus roseus*	C & S
Shikonin	*Lythospermum erythrorhizon*	C & S
Steroidal glycoalkaloids	*Solanum acculeatissimum*	C
	Salanum khasianum (Organogenesis)	C
	Solanium xanthocarpum	C
Trigonelline	*Trigonella foenum-graecum*	S
Tropane alkaloids	*Datura innoxia*	S
	Datura innoxia (regeneration)	S
	Datura stramonium	C & S
	Hyoscyamus niger	S
	Scopolia parviflora	C
Ubiquinone 10	*Nicotiana tabacum*	S
Undecanone & other volatile components	*Ruta gravealens*	C
Verbascoside	*Syringa vulgaris*	S
Vinblastine	*Catharanthus roseus*	C (differentiation)
Vindoline	*Vatharanthus roseus*	S
Visnagin	*Ammi visnaga*	S
Xanthotoxin	*Ruta graveolens*	S

C: Callus; S: Suspension.

Elicitors are the compounds (phytoalexins) produced in normal plants in response to stress; induce the accumulation of secondary products. When cell cultures are subjected to such elicitors, some genes are derepressed (activation), resulting among other things in the formation of secondary metabolites, which are found in the entire plants.

For the production of secondary metabolites in large amounts, the plant cells should be grown in bioreactor, in the form of suspension culture (continuous), having proper effective aeration, optimum heat, light and pH adjustment necessary for optimum production and isolation of natural substances. Some times callus cultures are also used for secondary metabolite production.

As mentioned earlier, different classes of secondary metabolites are produced by plant cell cultures. Some suspension cultures were reported to produce product at a level, which is equal or higher than plant itself.

Factors Affecting the Production of Secondary Metabolites

Media composition and environmental factors

Variations in the relative **hormonal contents** of the growth medium affect the metabolism, e.g. **cytokinins** have been found to enhance secondary metabolites accumulation in a number of tissue cultures—Indole alkaloids (*C. roseus*) condensed tannins (*Onobrychis* species), Coumarins (*Nicotiana* species), Rhodozanthin (*Ricinus* species), Berberine (*Thalictrum minus*).

Mixture of naphthalene, acetic acid and **kinetin** has affected the concentration of ginkgolides in the cell culture of *Ginkgo biloba* in medium, as the production medium not only support the level of growth required to

Table 5.5: Induced production of metabolites in cell cultures by various elicitors

Elicitor	Plant-cell suspension culture	Effect
High light intensity	Coffea arabica	Stimulation of caffeine production
Colchicine	Valeriana wallichi	Sixtyfold increase in valepotriates with six new compounds (not due to higher ploidy level)
Copper sulphate	Lithospermum erythrorhizon	Greatly increased shikonin production
	Various Solanaceae	Induced formation of sesquiterpene phytoalexins of lubimin type
Thiosemicarbazide	Panax ginseng	Promotes biosynthesis of saponins and inhibits phytosterol production
L-Tryptophan (a biosynthetic precursor of quinoline alkaloids)	Cinchona pubescens, C. ledgeriana	Enhanced alkaloid production
Phytophthora megasperma preparation	Tobacco plant	Accumulation of capsidiol
Non-viable conidia of the wilt-producing fungus Vertiicillium dahliae	Gossypium arboreum	One hundredfold increase in gossypol after 120 h incubation
Yeast carbohydrate preparation	Thalictrum rugosum	Up to fourfold enhancement of berberine
Yeasts (free and immobilized)	Ruta graveolens	Increased production of acridone epoxides but not rutacridone
Phytophthora cinnamomi and Aspergillus niger (sterilized mycelia)	Cinchona ledgeriana	Increase in anthraquinone production
Sterilized fungal mycelia (Pythium, Phytophthora, Verticillium), etc.	Pimpinella anisum Petroselinium crispus Ammi majus	Stimulation of coumarin synthesis
	Catharanthus roseus	Production of catharanthine and other major indole alkaloids stimulated
	Cephalotaxus harringtonia	Dramatic increase in alkaloid content
	Cinchona ledgeriana	Increase in anthraquinone production
	Gossypium arboretum	One hundredfold increase in gossypol after 120 h incubation
Yeast, yeast extracts and alkaloid carbohydrate preparations	Escholtzia california	Large and rapid increase or benzophenanthridine
	Thalictrum rugosum	Up to fourfold enhancement of berberine
	Ruta graveolens	Increased production of acridone epoxides but not rutacridone
	Orthosiphon aristatus	Stimulation of rosmarinic acid production

obtain an appropriate biomass but also the secondary metabolite.

Addition of **IAA and zeatin riboside** has effected the concentration of alkaloid biosynthesis (fivefold increase in alkaloid contents of *Cinchona ledgeriana* have been reported, on transferring the cell from 2,4-D, benzyl adenine medium, to a medium containing IAA and Zeatin riboside).

The presence or absence of **phosphate** in a medium, greatly affect the production and accumulation of some secondary products.

Table 5.6: Important plant alkaloids and their pharmacological activities

Alkaloids	Plant source	Culture type	Pharmacological use
Ajmalicine	Catharanthus roseus	Cell suspension	Hypotensive
Atropine	Atropa belladonna	–	Anticholinergic
Berberine	Berberis spp., Coptis japonica	Cell suspension	Antispasmodic, antiprotozoal
Codeine	Papaver somniferum	–	Sedative, analgesic
Colchicine	Colchicum autumnale	Callus culture	Antimitotic
Caffeine	Coffea arabica, Camellia sinensis	–	Stimulant
Camptotecine	Camptotheca acuminata	Cell suspension	Antitumour
Emetine	Cephaelis ipecacuanha	Root culture	Emetic
Ellipticine	Ochrosia elliptica	Cell suspension	Antitumour
Ephedrine	Ephedra gerardiana	–	Spasmolytic
Morphine	Papaver somniferum	Cell suspension	Analgesic, sedative
Papaverine	Papaver somniferum	–	Spasmolytic
Quinine	Cinchona lederiana	Cell suspension	Antimalaria
Reserpine	Rauwolfia serpentina	Cell suspension	Hypotensive
Vinblastine, vincristine	Catharanthus roseus	Shoot culture	Anticancer

Table 5.7: Steroids and saponins produced through tissue cultures

Plant species	Product formation
Sponins	
• Aesculus hippocastamum	Aescin
• Agave sisalana	Hecogenin
• Dioscorea deltoidea	Diosgenin
• Glycyrrhiza glabra	Glycyrrhizin
• Panax ginseng	Ginseng saponins
Cardiac glycosides	
• Digitalis lanata, D. purpurea	Digoxin, digitoxin
• Strophanthus	Quabain
• Ureginea maritima	Proscilariddin
Other steroids	
• Holarrhena antidysenterica	Sitosterol, stigmasterol, cholesterol
• Solanum xanthocarpum	Solasodine
• Withania somnifera	Withanolides

About 50% increase in anthraquinone accumulation was reported in cell culture of *Morinda citrifolia* on increasing the phosphate concentration to 5g/L; paradoxically, the overall accumulation of tryptamine and Indole alkaloids could occur only by shifting *Catharanthus roseus* cells to a medium devoid of phosphate concentration. Similar type of sensitivity has been reported in the cell culture of *Nicotiana tabacum*.

Source of carbon, nitrogen, vitamins and ions have all played significant role in altering the expression of secondary pathways. The addition of sucrose, NO^{3-}, Cu^{2+} or SO_4^{2-} in the culture media above the optimum level have a profound effect on shikonin biosynthesis. Ion concentration and sugar has been reported to have increased the production of Ubiquinone-10 in tabacco cell culture and anthraquinone in *Morinda* suspension cultures.

Precursors

Addition of precursors to the culture medium affect the growth and concentration of secondary metabolites—addition of conferrin (a phenylpropane) to cell suspension culture of Podophyllum hexandrum improved podophyllotoxin production by 128 fold. An increase in quinoline alkaloids has been reported, with the addition of L-tryptophan in the cultures of Cinchona ledgeriana. Cinnamic acid or α-phenylalanine precursors, affect the increase of flavonoids and tropic acid biosynthesis of tropane alkaloids.

Light Intensity

The intensity of light and certain wavelengths of light have been reported to have a stimulating effect on the production of some secondary metabolites in various tissue cultures. It has been reported that **blue light** enhances whereas **red light** decreases diosgenin production in Dioscorea deltoidea callus cultures.

Selection of Cell-lines

To increase the yield of secondary metabolite a tissue culture should be started from an explant of **high-yielding variety of plant** and capable of yielding high secondary metabolites and capable of accumulating higher levels of the desired metabolites. The yield can then be further improved **by selection of cell lines originating from individual protoplast,** taking advantage of the **somaclonal variation.** In the case of Catharanthus roseus cultures; the dimeric alkaloids vinblastine and vincristine (important anticancer drugs), are produced at the end of a complex biogenetic pathway in which monomers are first produced. The latter, as corynanthe, strychnos and aspidosperma type alkaloids can all be produced (0.1–1.5%) in culture using Zeink's alkaloid production medium. Different cell cultures derived from anyone species of plant may vary enormously in their synthetic capacities, so that in above cases, distinct ajmalicine producing and high serpentine producing stains are possible. Example of other plants for which somaclonal variation has been exploited are Nicotiana tabacum and N. rustica (Nicotine), Coptis japonica (berberine) Lavandula vera (biotin) and Thalictrum minus (berberine), a strain giving a 350 fold increase in alkaloid production has been reported.

Genotype of Mother Plant

A range of variability in the amount and type of secondary metabolite has been observed in cell cultures raised from different mother plants and sometimes even from the same mother plant. This is because of the difference between the genotype of mother plant and relative productivity of cell cultures.

Cell cultures are known to show gradual loss of productivity and very little is known about the factors that inhibits the secondary metabolite synthesis in tissue cultures or cause of its re-emergence upon re-differentiation.

High-yielding lines are rather easily distinguished from low-yielding lines where cell synthesises **visible metabolites,** e.g. anthocyanins, quinones, betacyanins and carotenoids. For other compounds, quantitative analysis of cellular accumulation patterns of specific metabolites (rosemarinic acid and cinnamyl putrescines) may be determined by **micro-spectrophotometry**.

Age of Cell Culture

The accumulation of metabolites at any particular instant in the cell culture is the result of a **dynamic balance between rate of its biosynthesis and biodegradation,** in which a variety of metabolisms are involved. Hence, there is no strict particular time in the cell cycle for harvesting the cells in order to obtain the maximum yield of the secondary compounds. Most of the secondary metabolites accumulate during the late stages of growth in tobacco batch cultures although under same conditions certain metabolites in Catharanthus cell cultures accumulate even during the **lag phase.**

Instability of cell line: It is well known that changes in the genetic characteristic of cell occur within a culture so that callus selected for specific biochemical properties may need reselection after a period of time.

Isolation of secondary production: Secondary metabolites synthesis occurs intercellularly. For cultivation and production of active metabolite it is preferable, that the metabolite be excreted into the medium rather than retained within the cells. **For the better excretion, media should be of lower pH.** The biomass then can be separated from the nutrient liquid from which the active constituents are extracted. **Two phase culture system** have been described, i.e. a **Silicone product** is added to the fermentation tank to extract the metabolites and in this way the development of culture is not disturbed.

Second method is the use of **media at low pH,** and application of **DMSO sonication** with continuous ultrasound and electrical treatment inducing permeabilisation of cell in culture.

To date over 30 classes of compounds have been produced in appreciable quantities by plant cell cultures, these include *Digitalis glycosides,* **diosgenin-derived steroid hormone precursors, shikonin, rosemarinic acid, opium alkaloids** (codeine and morphine), **ginsenosides, ajmalicine and other indole alkaloids, including vinblastine and vincristine,** and possibly complex mixtures such as rose and jasmine oil. Mitsui Petrochemical Industries of Japan have been producing shikonin, a red coloured phenolic naphthoquinone compound from cell cultures of *Lithospermum erythrorhizon,* which is used as a dye and as an astringent. A West-German Pharmaceutical company is in process of producing Digitalis glycosides by biotransformation in cell cultures. The worldwide research in commercial production of anti-cancer alkaloids of *Catharanthus* shall be soon a practical reality. The factors that limit the success of plant culture include slow growth of plant cells and low accumulation of metabolites. The desired secondary product is often retained within the cells.

List of phytopharmaceuticals of medicinal and industrial importance produced by plant tissue cultures is given in Tables 5.4, 5.8–5.10 and Fig. 5.10.

Table 5.8: Antitumour agents produced in culture

Plant species	Compound
Baccharis megapotamica	Baccharin
Brucea antidysenterica	Bruceantine
Camptotheca acuminata	Camptotaecine
Catharanthus roseus	Vincristine, vinblastine
Cephalotaxus harringtonia	Harringtonine, homo-harringtonine
Fagara zanthoxyloides	Fagaronine
Heliotropium indicum	Indicine=N-oxide
Maytenus bucchananii, Putterlickia verrucosa	Maytansine
Ochrosia elliptica	Ellipticine, 9-methoxy-E
Podophyllum peltatum, P. hexandrum	Podophyllotoxin
Taxus brevifolia, T. baccata	Taxol
Thalictrum dasycarpum	Thalicarpine
Tripterygium wilfordii	Tripdiolide, tryptolide
Withania somnifera	Withanolide-A, withaferine

Table 5.9: Production of food additives by plant tissue culture

Food activities	Plant species
Colours	
• Anthocyanin	Dacus carota
• Anthocyanin	Euphorbia milli
• Anthocyanin	Vitis vinifera
• Betalaines	Beta vulgaris
• Crocin, crocetin	Crocus sativus
Flavours	
• Onion flavour	Allium cepa
• Capsicum, capsaicin	Capsicum annuum
Frutescens	
• Safranal	Crocus sativus
• Vanilla, vanillin	Vanilla planifolia
Sweetner	
• Stevioside	Stevia rebaudiana
• Thaumatin	Thaumatococcus danielli

Biochemical Conversion (Biotransformation)

The conversion of small part of a chemical molecule by means of biological systems is

Table 5.10: Insecticides of plant origin

Plant species	Insecticides
Azadirachta indica	Azadirachtin
Derris elliptica, Tephrosis vogelii, Lonchocarpus utilis	Rotenoids
Chrysanthemum cinerariaefolium, Tagetes erecta	Pyrethrins
Nicotiana rustica, N. tabacum	Nicotine
Quassia amara	Quassin

termed biotransformation. It is a process in which the substrate can be modified. For example, *Digitalis lanata* cell cultures have a ability to effect hydroxylation, acetylation, glycosylation, etc. It is reported that *D. lanata* strain 291 can convert β-methyl digitoxin into β-methyl digoxin. Cell suspension culture of *Strophanthus gratus* affects various biochemical conversions of digitoxigenin.

Monoterpene bioconversions are reported with mentha cell culture. It can convert (–) menthone to (+) neomenthol and pulegone to isomenthone.

Podophyllum peltatum in semi-continuous culture can produce anticancer drugs by biotransformation of synthetic dibenzyl butanolides to lignans suitable for conversion to etoposide.

In some tissue culture stereospecific biotransformation is also reported, which is important for the isolation of optically active compound from racemic mixture.

Example of cell culture of Nicotiana tabacum selectively hydrolyse R-configurational form of monoterpenes like bornyl acetate and isobornyl acetate.

Apart from the above-mentioned bio-chemical conversions many other, like saponifications, esterification, epoxidation, oxidation, methylation and isomerisation are also reported.

Clonal Propagation (Micropropagation)

Clonal propagation (micropropagation) is the technique to produce entire plant from single individual by asexual reproduction, constitute a clone. This fact can be commercially utilised to produce high yielding crops of the desirable characters in a short period of time, which otherwise show variation when grown using seeds. For example, *Foeniculum vulgare* (fennel) shows wide variations in the yield and composition of the volatile oil and by this technique it has been reported to have uniform clones of fennel with narrow variation in the volatile oil composition, in comparison to the normal cultivation.

Somaclonal Variation

In clonal propagation, clones are produced from tissue culture with uniform characters but few clones may show variations among the population of clones, which were not present in the parent cells. This formation of variant clones from cultured tissue is called

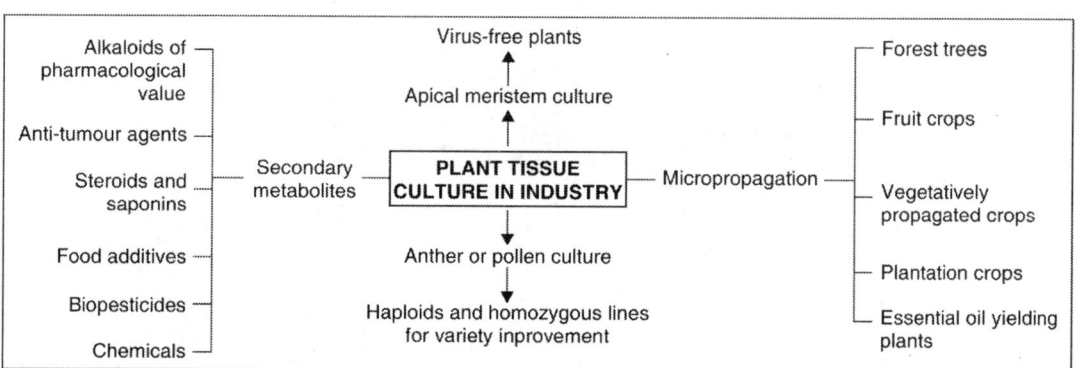

Fig. 5.10: A schematic presentation of role of plant tissue culture in industry

Somaclonal variations: Variants are of two types:

1. Desirable Variants and 2. Undesirable Variants

Desirable variants can be used for the improvement of crops. The clone showing high productivity can be used for commercial purposes.

Immobilisation of Plant Cells

The immobilisation of plant cell or enzymes has increased the utility of plant cell biotechnology for production of **pharmaceuticals**. The plant cells can be immobilised by using **matrices** such as alginates, polyacrylamides, agarose and poly-urethane fibres. The immobilised plant cells can be utilised in the same way as immobilised enzymes to effect different reactions.

Immobilised cell systems may be used for bioconversions such as **(–)codeinone to (–)codeinine and digitoxin** to **digoxin** or for synthesis from added precursors, e.g. production of ajmalicine from tryptamine and secologanin. The suspension cultures of *Anisodus tanguticus* have been reported to convert hyoscyamine to anisodamine in good quantity. Subsequently, the cultures convert anisodamine into scopolamine. The biotransformation reactions such as glycosylations, hydroxylation, acetylation, demethylation, etc. have been successfully attempted in immobilised cell systems. The hydroxylation or glycosylation of cardiac glycosides in cultures of *Digitalis lanata* and *Daucus carota* have also been reported.

Immobilised plant cells can be used for tracing the biosynthetic pathways of secondary metabolites and also can be used for carrying out biotransformation or biochemical reactions.

EDIBLE VACCINES

Edible vaccines are the vaccines which can be administered orally. It consists of plant's antigenic proteins in the form of components of fruits, roots and seed products. It is also available as concentrated vaccine in the form of food, pills or pudding, etc. It is obtained from transgenic plants. The desired gene is being transferred into the cells of plant, bacteria and yeast by transformation methods (Bombarding process or *Agrobacterium tumefaciens* infection). The recombinant plant cell or viruses with desired genes are then incorporated into plants where they subsequently multiply. The plants products in the form of fruits, roots, seeds or leaves are used for immunisation (Fig. 5.11).

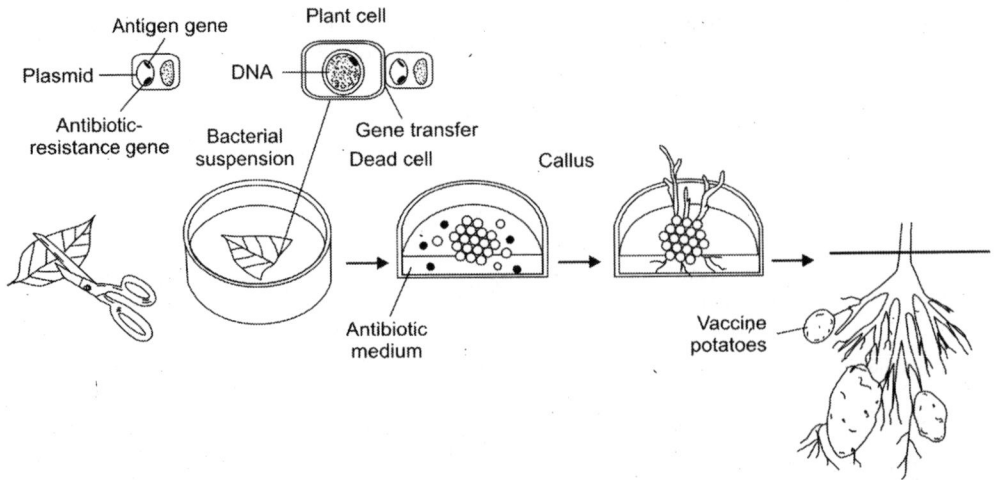

Fig. 5.11: Development of edible vaccine

Plant viruses can also be used to manufacture the edible vaccine in which the virus are genetically engineered to produce the desired proteins which are subsequently incorporated into plants. The **chimeric virions** (virus like particles) are then isolated from the matured plants/plant products, purified and used for immunisations. Examples of plants products used are potatoes, tomatoes, soya beans, lettuce, rice, wheat and other crops. Edible vaccine is presently in use for number of human and animal diseases like cholera, measles, foot and mouth disease of animals. It has been reported that diabetes mellitus can also be controlled by feeding transgenic plants engineered to produce diabetes related proteins.

The edible vaccines are safe to use as they do not contain killed or attenuated disease causing organisms unlike classical vaccines. They are **resistant to gastric juice** and secretions as the vaccine is encapsulated in cells having rigid cell wall which provide protection from gastrointestinal tract (GIT) to intestine, where it gets released. In intestine, the antigens comes in contact with lymphoid tissue of mucosa's cell of intestine to further deliver to immune system thus, the edible vaccine stimulate both surface and humoral immunity against the pathogens.

Brief history: The concept of edible vaccine was developed by **Amtzen in 1990s** (Head of plant biology at Arizona State University). Idea clicked to him after attending a conference at New York organised by WHO. The earliest demonstration of edible vaccine was the expression of a surface antigen from the bacterium *Staphylococcus mutant* in tobacco (dental carries) which prevents dental carries by stimulating mucosal immunity. The first human trial for edible vaccine took place in 1997 for anti-diarrhoea potatoes vaccine, produced by Boyce Thompson institute at cornell university, Ithaca, NY, USA.

Current status: At least 20 to 30 preparations are being expressed in plants, e.g. hepatitis B vaccine, vibrio cholera (potato) vaccine.

Advantages: Oral route of administration, no need of medical personnel, economical, less manufacturing cost, no refrigeration required, no storage problem as it can be stored at the site of patient.

Drawbacks: Consistency to dosage form varies from fruit to fruit, plant to plant and generation to generation.

Selection of the best plant is difficult

Stability in plant product not known.

Foods like potatoes not eaten raw hence cooking might weaken the efficacy of vaccine.

Dosage evaluation is difficult.

Recent development: Edible plants could be used to deliver antigens for active immunisation or to deliver monoclonal secretory antibodies to provide passive immune therapy.

FURTHER READING

1. An Introduction to Plant Tissue Culture: Advances and Perspectives *experiments. springernature. com/ý*
2. Bhatia S. 2015. Plant Tissue Culture, Modern Applications of Plant Biotechnology in Pharmaceutical Sciences, ScienceDirect.
3. Edible vaccine-an overview/science direct topics. www.sciencedirect.com:topic
4. Edible vaccines-sri Ramachandra university. www.sriramachandra.edu.in
5. History-edible vaccinations, nifty 50/NSF-National science. www.nsf.gov>edible vaccine.
6. Kalia AN. Textbook of Industrial Pharmacognosy. (2005). CBS Publishers and Distributors, New Delhi.
7. Loyola-Vargas VM, Ochoa-Alejo N. 2018. An Introduction to Plant Tissue Culture: Advances and Perspectives Methods In Molecular Biology, Book: Plant Cell Culture Protocols. Springer Protocols.
8. P Lal, et al. Edible Vaccines: Current Status and Future. Indian Journal of Medical Microbiology. 2007;25 (2):93–102.
9. Plant Tissue Culture: an overview Science Direct Topics. *https://www.sciencedirect.com>biochemistry-genetics-and-molecular-biology*
10. Pocket K No. 14 Tissue Culture Technology. 2004. http://www.isaaa org/kc
11. Tissue Culture Technology/ISAAA.org *https://www.isaaa.org>resources>publications>pocket*

Pharmacognosy in Various Systems of Medicines

6. Role of Pharmacognosy in Allopathy and Traditional Systems of Medicines

7. Introduction to Secondary Metabolites

6 Role of Pharmacognosy in Allopathy and Traditional Systems of Medicines

The word pharmacognosy is derived from two Greek words *'pharmakon'* a drug and *'gignosko'* to acquire knowledge. It includes cultivation, harvesting, collection, storage, preservation, isolation, standardisation, biological evaluation safety and purity of drugs obtained from natural origin. In 18th century the term pharmacognosy and pharmacodynamics were probably first coined by Johann Adam Schmidt (1759–1809) in his handwritten manuscript published in Vienna in 1811 (posthumously) entitled **Lehrbuch der Materia Medica**. Then it was appeared again in 1815 in a small work by C.A. Seydler entitled **Analecta Pharmacognostica**.

Pharmacognosy is closely related to Botany and Chemistry. Its fundamental importance is for the pharmacopoeial identification and quality control of the medicinal plants based on the active therapeutic phytoconstituents (chemistry of plants). The modern isolation technique and pharmacological screening of the drugs has made the subject of pharmacognosy more important in the novel drug discovery for the inclusion of new plant drug into medicines as purified substances rather than in the form of galanical preparation (**Allopathy**), e.g. the isolation and identification of alkaloids; vinblastine and vincristine from *Catharanthus roseus* as an anti-cancer compound reserpine from *Rauwolfia surpentina* as anti-hypertensive compound, digoxin from *Digitalis purpurea* cardiotonic, ephedrine from *Ephedra sinica*, anti-asthamatic, etc. For these pure compounds isolated from plants and are being used in allopathy medicines needs standard parameters including physical, chemical and chromatographical techniques/ methods, applicable for the identification of purity, quality and safety of drugs (pharmacopoeial standards) and are being established by the pharmacists (pharmacognosists). Modern pharmacognosy involves the broad study of natural products from various sources including plants animals, minerals, bacteria, fungi and marine organisms.

Research into ethnobotany, ethnomedicine and ethnopharmacology has also become an important elements in pharmacognosy.

On the discovery of new drugs from natural sources/plants, generate the interest of global companies to develop its new/novel formulations, against various pharmacological targets including cancer, HIV/AIDs, Alzheimer's, malaria and neuralgia, etc. with the result the local wild sources suddenly become exhausted, e.g. *Coleus forskohlii, Podophyllum* spp., *Ginkgo biloba, Artemesia, Kuth, Arnica montaria,* and *Taxus brevifolia,* etc. Thus, it becomes necessary to search for novel cultivation techniques including cell-cultures technology for the continuous supply of these exhausted drugs to the world market which is the job of pharmacognosists.

The use of single pure compound, including synthetic drugs has its own limitation and are not free from the side effects, hence in recent years the world has shown an immense interest in the traditional systems of medicines, As per WHO, traditional alternative systems of therapeutics includes the diverse health practices, approaches, knowledge and belief incorporating plants, animals and/or mineral based medicines, spiritual therapies, manual techniques and exercises which can be used to maintain well-being, as well as to treat, diagnose or prevent illness.

According to Global Survey reported by WHO the following system of medicines has been included in traditional systems of medicines—Ayurveda, Chinese, Arabic, Unani, and indigenous medicines. As per WHO survey report, Chinese traditional medicines are practised by about 40% of the total health delivery care system, In Chile accounts for around 70% of the total health care account, Columbia account for around 65% of the total healthcare delivered.

Use of Ayurvedic medicines and medicinal plants for healthcare in developed countries are as follow: 48% in Australia, 31% in Belgium, 70% in Canada, 49% in France and 42% in United States of America.

The traditional, complimentary and alternative systems of medicines are popular as these medicines are commonly used to treat or prevent diseases and chronic illness to improve the quality of life. The efficacy of acupuncture in relieving pain and nausea has been acknowledged world-wide.

A National Expert Panel of the United States National Institute of Health concluded in 1997 about the effectiveness of the needle puncture in relieving the acute pain without any side effects. Germany and United Kingdom of Great Britain, and Northern Ireland 70% and 90% respectively use acupuncture as pain relief in clinics.

The traditional medicines has also been in practice in the treatment of life-threatening diseases like malaria and AIDS in Ghana Mali, Nigeria, and Zambia. Herbal medicines are the first line of action in the treatment of more than 60% of children suffering from high fever. Africa and North America's survey report show that up to 75% of people suffering from AIDS /HIV use traditional medicines alone or in combination with other medicines to treat the various symptoms, the reason behind the self-medication with herbal medicine is of the misconception that natural means are safe, they may be unaware about the potential side effects and how and when herbal medicines are safe. Because of lack of quality control and improper use of herbal drugs by the consumers, the cases of toxicity of herbal drugs are reported. For instance in 1996, more than 50 people of Belgium suffered kidney failure after taking herbal preparation containing *Aristolochia fangchi* (toxic plant) in place of *Stephania tetrandra* or *Magnolia officinalis*.

Chemical marker for authentication of herbal formulation (Role of Pharmacognosy in traditional medicines).

The therapeutic efficacy/potency of traditional medicines depends upon the chemical constituents of the plants parts used in the formulations which is directly depends on the quality of raw material, processing technique and storage of the final products. Above all of these factors, the adulteration and substitution of the raw materials also play the major challenges in the manufacture of traditional formulations. To evaluate the medicines for quality, purity, and safety the **pharmacognostical parameters/procedures** play major role. These parameter are physical (physicochemical values, extractive value, ash value, microscopical characters of the whole plant, part or powdered form), organoleptic parameters (colour, odour, taste, size and fracture, etc.), chemical analysis (qualitative and quantitative chemical test, chromatography for chemical profile using chemical marker(s), DNA fingerprinting), Biological evaluation by using *in vivo/in vitro* analysis, toxicological studies for safety, thus play major role in the standardisation of traditional medicines.

Raw material from India and Sri Lanka can gets contaminated with toxigenic fungus, pesticides residue and heavy metals contamination, hence all the traditional medicines are to be validated for standard values for these contaminants.

AYURVEDA

It is one of the oldest written medical system of traditional system of medicines in Indian systems of medicines. Ayurveda literally means science of life; the word Ayurveda is derived from two words 'Ayur' meaning life and 'Veda' meaning science. Hence literally means science of life.

The Ayurveda's based on the philosophy of tridoshas (vatta, pitta, kapha) sapta dhoshas (rasa, rakta, mansa, medo, ashti majja, sukra), trimalas (purusha, mootra, sweda) imbalance of these result disturbance in internal body physiology and emotional factors leading to disease. Therefore ayurvedic treatment is aimed the patient as an organic whole and treatment consist of drugs, food supplements and exercises.

The Ayurvedic formulation consists of complex mixtures including plants and animals derived products, minerals and metals made in the form of panchavidha kashaya kalpana to suite the palatability of the patient and the release of drug in required potency/dose at the target organ.

Presently, there has been new trend in the preparation of formulations from plants under the label of herbal drugs or phytomedicines as single plant extracts or active fraction of the extract. These plants derived products are properly standardised with respect to component profile with the help of TLC/HPTLC, HPLC and GLC, etc. The preparations are also evaluated for their safety, efficacy and pesticide residue hence pharmacognosy play major role in Ayurvedic system of medicine in the quality, safety and efficacy.

Principle of Ayurveda and Siddha

Human body is made up of five basic elements:

1. Prudhvi (earth)
2. Apa (water)
3. Teja (fire)
4. Vayu (air)
5. Akasha (Sky)

Tridosha theory (vitta, pitta and kapha).

According to Tridosha; balance result good health and imbalance leads to illness.

Septadhatu (seven forms): (a) Rasa (lymph), (b) Rakta (blood), (c) Meda (adipose tissue), (d) Mamsa (flesh), (e) Majja (nervine tissue), (f) Shukra (reproduction tissue), (g) Asthi (bones).

Source of raw material: Ayurvedic medicines are based on plants, animal extracts and minerals both as single ingredient drug and compound formulations. The compound formulations are mainly divided into two groups.

1. Kasthausadhi (predominantly of plant origin) such as asavarishtra, asavas, avleha, gutica, churna, and taila.
2. Rasausadhi (predominantly metals and minerals) such as bhasma, pisti, lauha, kapibadkva, Rasayana, etc.

About 25 varieties of compound formulation in which some of the single drugs of animal origin (52) mineral origin (53) and plant origin (351). Detail is available from Ayurvedic Formulary of India published by Govt of India Ministry of Health and Family Welfare.

Dosage form

Swarasa (expressed juice)
Churna (powder)
Kwath churna (coarse powder for decoction)
Asava and Arishta (fermented liquids)
Arka (distilled medicated water)
Avaleha (jam like formulation)
Ghrita (butter based formulation)
Taila (mediated/oil based formulation)
Lepa (for external application)
Malhara (ointment)
Vati/Gutica (tablet/pill)
Panaka (syrup)
Aaschayotana (eyedrops)
Karn bindu (eardrops)
Nasaya (nasal drops)
Bhasma (calcinated ash)
Ras Yoga; herbo mineral formulation.

Ayurvedic pharmacopoeia of India: It is a legalised document of the government of India describing the quality, purity and strength of selected drugs that are manufactured, distributed and sold by the licenced manufacturers, included therein and standards prescribed (under the drug and cosmetic Act, 1940). At present **Seven volumes** has been printed. The first volume contains 80 monographs dealing with pharmacognostical, chemical and Ayurvedic standards of plant drugs used in Ayurveda:

Volume II contains 78 monograph

Volume III contains 100 monograph

Volume IV contains 68 monograph

Volume V contains 92 monograph

Volume VI and VII are in pipelines containing about 160 monograph of drugs.

Ayurvedic medicines are obtained from plants and their parts (stem, leaves, flowers, fruits, seeds and underground parts roots, rhizomes and tubers, etc.). Plants and their parts are used either alone in the form of powder or extracts (aqueous or alcoholic), or in combination (compound formulation), from animals and mineral sources.

The therapeutic efficacy depends upon the chemical constituents, responsible for their pharmacological effects; on the basis of the effects; the drugs (Dravyas) are classified as medicines (Oushdha) or as food supplements (Ahara Dravya).

The chemical constituents varies with the species, origin, environments, altitude, temperature, as well as geographical location and their vernacular nomenclature, e.g. drug Bala (*Sida cordifolia*) is known by numbers of names, atibala (*Abutilon indicum*), nagabala (*Sida spinosa*), mahabala (*Sida rhombifolia*); all these plants are sold in the market under the name of bala. The sida species are also adulterated with *Parvonia odorata* and *Urena lobata*. All the *Sida* species are almost have similar morphological characters but different microscopical characters, starch grains, calcium oxalate crystal and lysogenous cavities, the leaves also have different stomatal index, vein islet numbers and other characters like arrangement of vascular bundles, etc. Above all, the time of collection, drying, processing, transportation their storage, and extraction followed by subsequent manufacturing procedure, also effects the constituents hence the standardisation of the ayurvedic formulation is important factor which include:

authentication foreign mater, organoleptic characters, macro- and micro-scopic characters, extractive value chromatographic profile, assay of marker compounds and pesticide residue, etc. where the pharmacognosy has integrated role in ayurveda system of medicines.

MODERN SYSTEM OR ALLOPATHY

The term 'allopathy' was also invented by German physician Samuel Hehnemann who conjoined 'allos' means apposite and 'pathos' means 'suffering'. It is method of treating disease with remedies that produce effects different from those caused by the disease itself, e.g. using laxative to relieve constipation. It was practiced in America for the period of American revolutionary war till about 1876. It was considered to be harsh medical practice of the which include bleeding, purging, vomiting and administration of highly toxic drugs. Specific type of therapy for specific disease was not too common in 18th century, as the same heroic remedies were used for almost all diseases, i.e. cleaning the digestive tract using purgative, e.g. rhubarb, etc. and enemas of varying formulation.

Prior to 1876 scientific medical emphasis was focused on hygiene and sanitation. After 1876 it was the era of preventive medicine or the use of bacteriological weapons to prevent diseases. From 19th century onwards this modern system of medicine (allopathy) come into practice.

In this system, treatment is based on the symptoms rather than the causes of the diseases. The drugs used has some times very serious side effects in comparison to traditional system of medicines. The treatment in allopathy system of medicines is quite costly in comparison to traditional systems.

It is the system of medication adopted by western countries.

In modern allopathy system of medicine stress is being given on the use of single organic compound, identified and designed to alter the specific protein/enzyme of liver, for the production or elimination, to effect the particular pathway reaction (specific target delivery). The single molecule ingredient for the purpose can be obtained from natural sources as a lead compound or molecule followed by pharmaceutical processing to get the desired dosage form, e.g. quinine (antimalarial drug) from cinchona bark, vinblastine, Vincristin (anticancer drug) from *vinca rosea* roots, ajmalicine (antihypertensive) from *Rauwolfia serpentina*; digitoxin (cardiotonic) from *Digitalis purpurea* leaf, etc. This process of screening, isolation fractionation, identification and purification is the entire role of pharmacognosist.

It is the system of medication adopted by western countries, in this system drugs dosage forms (tablet, capsules, injections, syrup, ointments, jellies, paste and lotion, etc.) are manufactured from synthetic/semisynthetics and from the chemicals derived from natural origin (plants, animals, marines and minerals). The system also uses the modern equipment for diagnosis, treatment, analysis and surgery, etc.

UNANI SYSTEM OF MEDICINES

Unani system was originated in Uunan-ancient Greece. The Greece has adopted the intial concept of medicine (Tibb) from Egypt and Mesopotamia; then adopted by Roman. In middle age the system travelled to Arab world. It was introduced in India around 8th century. Currently, Unani system of medicine along with the homeopathy and other traditional system of medicine including ayurveda, yoga, naturopathy, siddha and Sowa Rigpa comes under the jurisdiction of Department of Ayush under the Ministry of Health and Family Welfare, Government of India, These systems are well recognised and practised in India in public, private and voluntary organisations.

Till march 2013 six volumes of Unani medicines containing 1228 standardised unani formulation has been published in Unani Pharmcopoeia of India. Quality standards of 298 single drugs and 100 compound drugs have also been included.

Unani system of medicines follow all the systems of medicines, i.e. physiology, preventive medicine, pathology, diagnostic, pharmacology and therapeutics.

The principle related to human biology are: Elements (Arkan), humour (Akhlat), temperament (Mizaj) Organ (Ada) pneuma (Arwah) faculties (Quwa) and functions (Afal). Imbalance in temperament and humour, disorganisation and discontinuity of the structure leads to the development of diseases.

Drugs: The drugs used are procured from natural resources (plants, animals and minerals). Medicines are manufactured using modern equipment and by means of good manufacturing technique/processes.

Therapeutics of Unani system of medicines: The treatment in Unani system of medicines depends mainly on Mizaj (temperament) of individual. The whole personality of patient (basic structure, physique, like, dislike, reactions to different factors, etc.) is kept in mind during the treatment. It has **four main types of treatment**:

a. **Regimental therapy** (Ilaj bil Tadbir): In this therapy treatment is done by removing the toxic material from body and by improving the defence system of individual.

b. **Diet therapy** (Ilaj bil Cohiza): This, therapy is done by regulating the quality and quantity of food/diet of the patients.

c. **Pharmacotherapy** (Ilaj bil Daua): In this drugs from natural sources (plants, minerals, animals) are used to cure the disease. The physician/Hakim prescribes the drug on the basis of potency, age, temperament/Mizaj of patient, nature and severity of disease. Drugs are used in different forms like powder, decoction, infusion, jawarish, Jalinoos, khamira, syrup, tablet, etc.

d. **Surgery** (Ilaj bil Yad): The surgery by specialised person is done by using special instruments and techniques. Only minor surgeries are performed these days to cure the diseases.

Standardisation and quality control: Government of India has fully control on the standardisation and quality control of the formulations. It is from the step of procurement to final product as well as the storage, etc.

followed by good manufacturing procedure and stability at self-life of the formulation. As drugs from natural source are used in the therapy of this system and role of pharmacognosy is well-justified.

HOMEOPATHY SYSTEM OF MEDICINES

The word homeopathy derived from the Greek words *"homois"* (similar) and *"pathos"* (suffering). This means the homeopathic medicines produce the symptoms similar to disease. The key principle of the treatment is *simila similibus curentur*, this refer to as like be treated with likes or like cure like, e.g. peel of *Allium cepa* causes eye itching with tears in the eye subsequently followed by sneezing but it is used for the treatment of hay fever and cold.

Urtica urens: It is allergic to human skin and produces burning sensation with redness and at the same times it is used for the treatment of skin diseases.

Brief history: This system of alternative medicines was originated by a German physician **Dr. Christian Friedrich Samuel Hahnemann** (10th April 1755–2nd july 1843) who coined the word homeopathy (*"homois"* in Greek means similar; *"pathos"* means suffering), law of similar. This system was made popular in United States and Europe in 1800 and was made popular among the people by American entrepreneurs, religious leader and literary personalities. However it gains more popularity after the emigration of Dr. Hans Gram a Dutch homeopath in 1825 to United States. He spread it so rapidly that by 1844 institute of homeopathy was organised in America which subsequently came out as a **American first National Medical Society**.

As per Dutch Govt. report on alternative system in 1981 in Netherland, homeopathy was one of the most popular therapeutic system of medicines. Homeopathy is widely spread in Europe as well as in Asian continents, especially in India, Pakistan and Sri Lanka. It was made popular in India because of the support from national leader Mahatma Gandhi ji, as well as, of its effectiveness in treatments of acute infectious

diseases in the subcontinent. Even there was recommendation by the WHO in Journal of World Health Forum for the treatment, in rural areas, lacking infrastructure, equipment and moreover being cheaper and affordable by the poor people of the society with less side effects in comparison to allopathy. WHO cited homeopathy as one of the system of traditional medicines that should be integrated world-wide with the conventional medicines to provide adequate global healthcare (WHO Traditional Medicine Strategy 2002–2005).

This system is being followed by 300 million patients and about 400,000 healthcare providers world-wide (OMHI 2003).

The FDA regulates the manufacturing process and distribution of homeopathic medicines. FDA has also approved the Homeopathic Pharmacopoeia of United States (HPUS).

In India it is recognised system of alternative medicine by Homeopathy Central Council Act 1973.

Medicnes: Source of medicines are plants, mineral, insects and marine (Fishes) pharmacognosy play role in the quality of herbal material used in extraction and scientific validation of the extracts/tincture used in dilution.

Formulation: Alcoholic tinctures prepared by maceration followed by dilution, in which one part is diluted to 100 parts, i.e. add 99 part of solution to one part of tincture that result into 1C potency (1 M is equal to 1000 C).

The standard potencies are 6 C, 30 C, 200 C, 1 M, 10 M, 50 M.

6 C for local symptoms

30 C for acute illness as influenza, diarrhoea and vomiting and for childhood.

1 M or 10 M for strong emotional symptoms, e.g. depression and anxiety, etc.

SIDDHA SYSTEM OF MEDICINES

It is the oldest system of the alternative system of medicines practiced in **South India** especially in **Tamil Nadu**. This system of medicines has close link with the Dravidian culture hence it is also known as **Dravidian system of medicines**. Siddha system of medicines has a close link with Ayurveda (plant extracts), Unani, Acupressure (sensitive points), and Reki (energy field). This system utilise the plant extracts and metal oxides for the preparation of medicines in an environment of spiritual chanting with the belief of inclusion of divine energy in the medicines. The medicines are formulated on the basis of panchabuthas (metal of gold, lead, iron, zinc and copper), the gold and lead are used for the maintenance of the human body, iron being the electricity conductor is the power attractive of the magnetic, zinc for the generation of electricity for the extension of life and copper is being used for the preservation of heat in the body, hence siddha medicines for the rejuvenation and longevity. The aim of siddha system of medicines is to make the human body perfect, imperishable and promote longevity. It is the system which emphasise on the perfect state of health (physical, mental, social, moral and spiritual component of human being). The system is based on *Andapinda Thathuvam*, i.e. the relationship between universe and human body which is inter-linked through Panchabuthas:

1. The structural aspects of human body is said to *Udal Thathus*, i.e. the physical component of the body.
2. Functional unit means *Uyir Thathus* the physiological unit, i.e. **vatham, pitham** and **kapham.**

The functional cooperation of these thathus is essential for the good health.

The system consider the predominance of vatham, pitham and kapham in childhood, adult and old age respectively, whereas ayurveda have reverse version that is kapham is dominated in childhood, vatham in old age and pitham in adult. The use of metals and minerals are more predominant in siddha system comparison to other traditional system of medicines.

The drug used in siddha are classified into **Mooligai/thavaram** (herbal product), **thatu** (inorganic substances) and **jeevam** or **sangamam** (animal products).

Herbal drugs are collected from Himalayas region as well as from tropical region. Korakkar was the first scientist (Siddhar), who used the cannabis (bhang) as a painkiller and skull (animal as well as human) to prepare the bashma for the treatment of mental disease. The siddhar also belief in yogic ashana/disciplines (pranayams) for the general maintenance of health and longevity of life.

Siddhar Nagarjuna introduced the use of heavy metals (salts) particularly, the mercury as preserver of body from degeneration, as the herbal drugs were not available throughout the year. More than 80% of the siddha medicines are prepared from herbal products and others are herbo-metal or herbo-minerals formulations. Raw material is properly purified and standardised by following the pharmacopoeial guidelines.

The finished products are of nano-microne size for rapid absorption and free from toxicity, the dosages size are from 20 to 200 mg.

Dosage forms are classified on the basis of taste (suvai), characters (guna), potency (veerya), class (pirivu), and action (mahimai) and on the basis of their mode of applications into two classes; internal and external applications.

Siddha science is very popular science that always insist for healthy lifestyle and minimum possible medication.

Materia Medica in Siddha

In siddha medicines, mineral and metal based preparations are more in practice in comparison to drug of vegetable origin. The drugs of mineral and metal-based are in the following form/category:

1. **Uppu (Lavanan):** These are water soluble drugs and gets degenerated to vapours, on exposure to fire.
2. **Pashanam:** Water insoluble drugs but gets vaporise on putting on fire.
3. **Uparasam:** Ratnas and uparatnas—drugs based on precious and semi precious stones.
4. **Loham:** Drugs are from metal and metal alloys that do not dissolve in water but melt on heating and solidify on cooling.
5. **Rasm:** Drugs are soft and sublime which gets crystallise or amorphous form on heating.

6. **Gandhakam:** Sulphur like insoluble in water but burn on exposure to fire.
7. Only 35 products have been included and are the formulation similar to ayurvedic formulations.

The Siddha system of medicines is the oldest documented alternate system of medicines in the world. It includes medicines from natural sources (plants, metals, minerals, etc.) but this system is not gaining much popularity except in the South India. The reason behind could be inherent toxicity of raw material used as the medicine in this system. Therefore, there is immediate need to standardise these formulations regarding the quality, toxicity and purification. The study and **implementation of pharmacognosy** in this system can overcome these hurdles and could make this system very popular in rest of the world.

TRADITIONAL CHINESE MEDICINES

Traditional chinese system of medicines (TCM) is a comprehensive medical healthcare system consisting of acupuncture, acupressure, message, yoga exercises, ashan, moxibustion, nutrition, herbal medicines and exercise. This system also believe in the five elements theory of life (water, earth, fire, wood and metal) responsible for the human health and it is a miniature version of surrounding universe, dependent upon two interconnected forces called Yin and Yang; harmony of these two forces support good health whereas imbalances between them resulted disease. The balance is effected by the external factors like emotions and lifestyle.

Traditional Chinese System of Medicine is in practice in Asian region for more than 2000 years, in United States since 1820 but the American population became aware about the TCM system in 1970s through acupuncture only, it also exist in other southern and east Asian countries like Japan and Korea. In Japan it is known by the name Kampa. **Chinese Materia Medica** is important monograph of Chinese traditional medicines and its civilisation. The first book of Chinese Materia Medica was known as **Canon of Materia medica** written in second century BC. This materia medica has monograph for thousands of medicinal substances from plants, animal and mineral sources. Medicines obtained from plant sources have used all parts of plants like leaves, stem, flowers, fruits, seeds, etc. Chinese formulations are mostly combined form of teas, capsules, liquids extract, granules and powders.

Commonly used Chinese herbs are astragalus, ginger, ginseng, cinnamon bark, coptis and ephedra, etc. The Chinese herb Ephedra (mahuang) has been banned by FDA in 2014 for the safe use in dietary supplement.

More than 5000 species of plant are identified in the pharmacopoeia of People's Republic of China (PRC), and the 80% of Chinese traditional drugs are herbal and are of plant origin. Like other tradional system of medicines, the Chinese medicine also has the chances of contamination with toxins, pesticide residue, heavy metals toxicity and substitution with inferior quality of adulterated drugs **hence the classic pharmacognostic parameters play** important role in the evaluation of the formulation for its quality, purity, safety and efficacy of TCM.

FURTHER READING

1. Introduction, The Indian System of Medicine. URL: http://ayush.gov.in/sites/default/files/Introduction_2.pdf
2. Ravishankar B, Shukla VJ. Indian Systems of Medicine: A Brief Profile Afr J Tradit Complement Altern Med. 2007;4(3):319–37.
3. Sen S, Chakraborty R, De B. 2016, Indian Traditional Medicinal Systems, Herbal Medicine, and Diabetes, Diabetes Mellitus in 21st Century. Springer, Singapore.
4. Stepan J. Traditional and Alternative Systems of Medicine: A Comparative Review of Legislation, International Digest of Health Legislation. 1985;36 (2).
5. The Ayurvedic pharmacopoeia of India. 2001–2012. Central Council for Research in Ayurveda and Siddha (CCRAS). Dept. of AYUSH, Ministry of Health & Family Welfare, New Delhi, India.

Chapter

7

Introduction to Secondary Metabolites

Secondary metabolites are the chemical compounds, biosynthesised by plants from primary metabolites (carbohydrates, amino acids and fatty acids), through different biosynthetic pathways. They do not play role in the primary functions of plants like growth, reproduction and photosynthesis. They play defensive role in plant by preventing the attack of herbivores, pathogens and chemical inhibition of competing plant species (allelopathy). Therefore, they are an integral part of the interactions of species in plants and the adaptation of plants to their environment.

Each plant family, genus and species produces characteristic chemical compounds used as taxonomic characters for plant classification. Most of them are used in medicines for human, e.g. (antibacterial, anti-oxidant, anti-inflammatory, analgesic, anti-cancer, cardiotonics, antimalarial, and vitamins, etc.)

BIOSYNTHETIC PATHWAYS

i. Secondary metabolites biosynthesised through **shikimic acid pathway**; are alkaloids, phenols, hydroxycinnamic acid, phenylpropane, coumarins, chromones, xanthones, stilbenes, flavonoids, lignans, neo-lignans, lignins and others. Shikimic acid also synthesise tannins via gallic acid.

ii. **Acetate pathway:** Acetate formed from carbohydrate via pyruvic acid, is the starting material for the biosynthesis of many secondary metabolites through two routes, i.e. **acylpolymalonate pathway**

leading to fatty acids and polyketides and **isopentenyl diphosphate** pathway which biosynthesises terpenes and steroids.

Amino acids formed through trans-ammination used for building peptides and proteins, some amino acids are precursors of other secondary metabolites like alkaloids, isothiocyanate glycosides and cyanogenic glycosides.

ALKALOIDS

They are the largest class of plant secondary metabolites. Alkaloids are cyclic organic compounds, consisting of one or more nitrogen atom in the heterocyclic ring, formed biosynthetically from amino acids **(true alkaloids)**, most of them occur in plants but some are found in animals. Most of them are basic in nature and have marked physiological action on man or animals even in small doses.

Pseudoalkaloids also known as heterocyclic nitrogen containing substances not derived from amino acid precursor but they are derived from the metabolism of acetate, e.g. coniine; terpenoid alkaloids such as aconitine or steroid alkaloids, e.g. paravallarine.

They do not show many of typical characters of alkaloids but give standard quality tests, e.g. conessine, caffeine.

Proto alkaloids are simple physiologically active amines in which nitrogen is not a part of heterocyclic ring, but they are:

Basic in nature, e.g. serotonin, mescaline.

141

Solubility: Alkaloids (bases) are insoluble in water but are soluble in non-polar solvents. But alkaloidal salts are soluble in water (polar solvents) but exceptions are there. Caffeine (base) being readily soluble in hot water and colchicine soluble either in acid, neutral or alkaline water. Similarly with alkaloidal salt, e.g. quinine sulphate is sparingly soluble in water (1 in 1000 parts of water), while one part quinine hydrochloride is soluble in less than 1 part of water. They are bitter in taste hence avoid tasting till not sure.

Classification of Alkaloids

Alkaloids can be classified on the basis of:

i. Basic chemical structure from which they are derived.
ii. On the basis of biosynthesis precursor, from which alkaloids are derived.

Precursor based

i. Ornithine derived alkaloids
ii. Lysine derived alkaloids
iii. Phenylalanine, tyrosine and dihydro-xyphenylalanine-derived alkaloid
iv. Tryptophan derived alkaloids
v. Miscellaneous alkaloids:
  a. Imidazole alkaloids
  b. Purine alkaloids
  c. Reduced pyridine alkaloids
  d. Terpenoid alkaloids
  e. Steroidal alkaloids

I. Ornithine alkaloids

Tropane alkaloids, e.g. hyoscyamine, atropine, hyoscine

II. Lysine-derived alkaloids

Lysine

For example, Lobelia

III. Phenylalamine, tyrosine and dihydro-xyphenylalanine-derived alkaloids.

i. Phenylalanine derivative, e.g. ephedrine
ii. Tyrosine–Benzylisoquinoline derivative, e.g. opium alkaloids
iii. Dihydroxyphenylalanine derivative, e.g. dopamine:
  a. Benzylisoquinoline group, e.g. tubo-curarine; phenylisoquinoline alkaloids, e.g. colchicine
  b. Tetrahydroisoquinoline mono-terpenoid alkaloids and glycosides, e.g. ipecosides, emetine.

IV. Tryptophan-derived Alkaloids, e.g. Ergot and Ergot alkaloids
  – Nux vomica alkaloids
  – Rauwolfia alkaloids, vinca, cinchona

V. Miscellaneous alkaloids
  i. Imidazole alkaloids, e.g. Joborandi leaf, (pilocarpine).
  ii. Purine alkaloids, e.g. caffeine, theo-phylline and theobromine
  iii. Reduced pyridine alkaloids, e.g. Areca nut
  iv. Terpenoids alkaloids, e.g. Aconite root and Taxus spp. (aconitine)
  v. Steroidal alkaloids, e.g. Veratrum, (Jerveratrum alkaloid and Ceveratrum alkaloids)
  Kurchi bark (Kurchicine and Conessine).

On the basis of Chemical Structure

1. Pyridine–Piperidine alkaloids

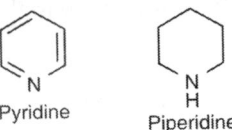

Example: Areca nut (arecoline) Lobelia (lobeline)

2. Tropane alkaloids

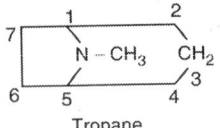

Example: Belladonna leaf, (Atropine) (Hyoscyamine) Hyoscyamus, solanaceous alkaloids

3. Quinoline alkaloids

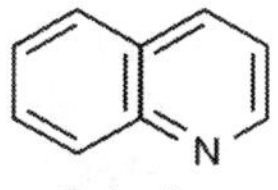

Quinoline

Example: Cinchona bark (Quinine, Quinidine)

4. Isoquinoline alkaloids

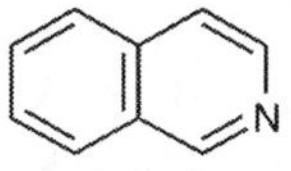

Isoquinoline

Example: Opium (Papaverine) alkaloids, ipecac (emetine); Hydrastis or goldenseal (–)hydrastine); Tubocurarine.

5. Indole alkaloids

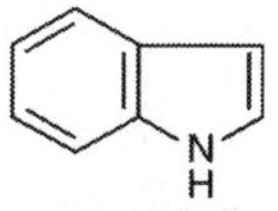

Indole

Example: Rauwolfia spp. (ajmaline, reserpine), Catharanthus or vinca (vincristine, vinblastine) nux vomica seeds (strychnine, brucine); Physostigma (eserine or physostigmine), ergot (ergonovine, ergometrine)

6. Imidazole alkaloids

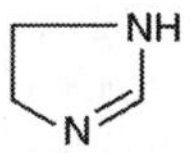

Imidazole

Example: Pilocarpus or Jaborandi (pilocarpine)

7. Steroidal alkaloids

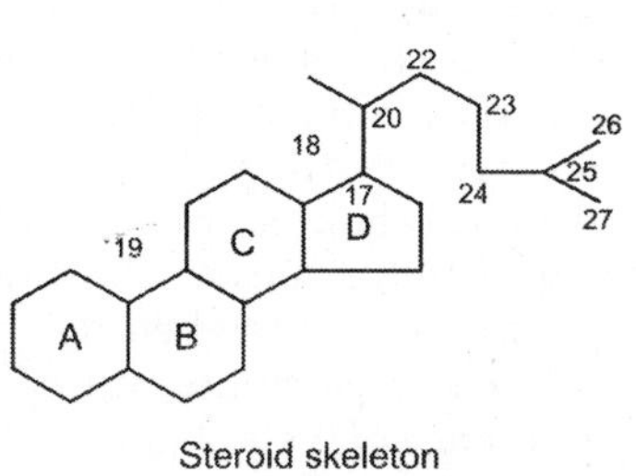

Steroid skeleton

Examples: Veratrum virdi Example (veratramine), potatoes (solanine and chaconine); tomato (tomatine); Solanum spp (solanine).

8. Alkaloidal amines

Examples: Ephedra or ma huang (ephedrine), colchicum seeds (colchicine)

9. Purine basis

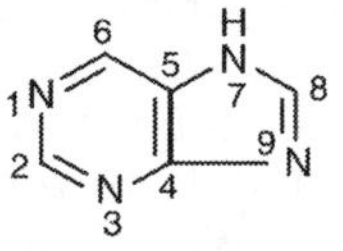

Purine

Example: Coffee seed (Caffeine) cocoa (Theobromine and caffeine)

Physical characters: Alkaloids containing C, H, N only are usually liquid at room temperature (coniine and nicotine) while those containing C, H, N, O are crystalline in nature, e.g quinine.

Colour: Generally alkaloids are colourless but few are coloured, e.g. berberine, serpentine are yellow coloured, the sangunarine salt is brownish red colour.

Distribution: Alkaloids, found in almost all parts of the plant but generally, they are stored in seeds, roots, barks and leaves of Apocyanaceae, Solanaceae, Papaveraceae, Rutaceae and Liliaceae families in the form of their acetate, citrate, oxalate, tartarate and oxalate salt form.

Chemical properties: Aqueous or acid solution of alkaloids gets precipitated with picric acid or tannic acid. Generally, they are **l-rotatory** in nature. Their acidic solution precipitated with Mayer's reagent, Dragendorff reagents, Hager's reagent and Wagner's reagent.

Chemical Tests for Alkaloids

Spot test: About 2–4 g of **fresh plant part** (aerial) grounded in a pestle mortar with small sand and sufficient chloroform to make slurry. Add ammonical chloroform to dilute the slurry, after stirring for 1–2 minutes with glass rod filter the mixture and perform the following test.

Add 0.5 ml of 2 N H_2SO_4 after shaking, separate the aqueous layer by means of dropper. A few drops of the acid extract are then tested with alkaloidal testing reagents: Dragendorff's reagent, Mayer's reagent and Wagner's reagent.

Dried material: Coarsely powdered plant material extracted with 80% methanol/ethanol, by heating in conical flask on water bath for 10–15 minutes. Filter the extract, concentrate by evaporating on water bath. Residue leftover treated with 2% hydrochloric acid (aqueous) by stirring with glass rod. Separate the aqueous layer and washed twice with organic solvents to remove colouring matter, bitter principles, tannins, etc. followed by basification with ammonia solution and extraction with chloroform thrice, and remove the chloroform by distillation, residue dissolved in 2% (v/v) aqueous hydrochloric acid (HCl) and perform test for alkaloids with the alkaloidal reagent—Mayer's reagent, Dragendorff reagent, Wagner's reagent, picric acid and tannic acid.

Mayer's reagent: It is potassium mercuric iodide solution; mix 2 ml of filtrate with 2 ml of reagent; cream coloured ppt.

Dragerdorff's reagent: It is potassium bismuth iodide solution prepared by dissolving bismuth subnitrite in conc. nitric acid (HNO_3) and potassium iodide in water, mix both the solution and supernatant used as reagent. Mix 2 ml of reagent with 2 ml of filtrate. It will give orange red precipitate.

Wagner reagent: It is iodine potassium iodide solution in water. It is prepared by dissolving iodine and potassium iodide in water. This reagent will give reddish brown flocculant precipitate.

Quantitative Analysis

Gravimetric method: This method is based on the fundamental theory that alkaloidal bases are soluble in non-polar solvents (dichloromethane, diethyl ether and chloroform) while alkaloid salts are soluble in polar solvent (water or alcohols). On this basis, the total alkaloids are isolated from the crude drug.

Isolation of total alkaloids

i. **Basification:** The coarse powdered drug is either basified with ammonia solution or diethylamine and the bark drug containing more tannins (cinchona bark) are basified with calcium hydroxide and 5% (w/v) sodium hydroxide solution.

In the case of seeds drugs containing fatty material, e.g. nux vomica or ergot, are to be treated with petroleum ether (40–60°C) to make it free from fatty material.

After basification drug is dried at room temperature and extract with non-polar solvents using chloroform, dichloromethane or diethyl ether. To make it free from non-alkaloidal basic material, residue leftover after the removal of organic solvent dissolve in 2% (v/v) aqueous hydrochloric acid, the undissolved residue/material to be discarded. The acidic aqueous solution, again basified and the free pure alkaloids are extracted with non-polar solvents. After the removal of the organic solvent (at low temp.) the pure alkaloids are dried in vacuum desiccator and weighed. Calculate the percentage value with respect to the weight of the dried drug.

ii. **Acidification method:** Coarsely powdered plant material acidified by treating the material with aqueous 1 M hydrochloric acid; tartaric acid; acetic acid (10%) and 2 N sulphuric acid (H_2SO_4). Keep the drug in contact with aqueous acid from one to four hours, then drain out the aqueous layer and dried at room temperature, followed by drying at 40°C in hot air oven.

The dried acidified coarse powdered material extracted with 80% methanol or ethanol by soxhlet extraction method till the complete exhaustion of the alkaloids. Filter and concentrate the filtrate to syrupy mass, basified with 10% (w/v) sodium hydroxide (NaOH) or sodium carbonate (Na_2CO_3) solution and extracted the aqueous layer with chloroform or dichloromethane, washed chloroform layer thrice with water, dried over anhydrous sodium sulphate, transferred to tared vessel, removed the chloroform by distillation and weighed residue (total alkaloids) and calculate the percentage with reference of weight of the dried drug sample or by dissolving in standard acid and titrating the excess with standard alkali.

Spectrophotometric Method for Estimation of Total Alkaloids

Spectrophotometric Method of Analysis for Total Alkaloids

Bismuth pentahydrate 1 mg dissolved in 5 ml conc. nitric acid; volume made up to 100 ml with distilled water; used as stock solution.

Colorimetric method: Colorimetric method of analysis is performed when the quantity of alkaloidal contents is low or small or when specific colour reaction is available and presence of other components do not interfere.

The BP uses ultraviolet absorption characteristic as standard for a number of alkaloids, e.g. emetine, morphine, reserpine, cocaine, colchicine and tubocurarine chloride.

Narasimhan Sreevidya and Shanta Malhotra (2003) developed spectrophotometric method for the quantitative analysis of total alkaloids precipitated with Dragendorff's reagent, e.g. *Berberis aristata, Solanum nigrum* and *Piper longum* can be estimated by this method. This method is based on the chemical reactions to develop persistant yellow colour, and obey Lambert-Beer's law in the concentration range of 0.06 to 50 µm/ml with λ 435 nm.

In this method the Dragendorff's reagent develop precipitate with alkaloids as (Bil3) (Alk-H1) complex, depending upon contents of alkaloids, amount of bismuth complex is formed. The bismuth alkaloid precipitate in the presence of sulfide in nitric acid media develop yellow colour complex with dilute solution of thiourea $[Bi\{CS(NH_2)_3\}(NO_3)_3]$ which can be measured. The amount of alkaloid present is calculated by multiplying with absorbance factor.

Calibration curve obtained from yellow colour developed by using different dilution of bismuth nitrate pentahydrate stock solution and standard dilute solution of thiourea. Absorbance values of yellow colour are measured at λ_{max} 465 nm against colourless reagent blank.

Bandelin (1950) used aqueous solution of ammonium reineckate to precipitate alkaloids from plant extracts. Alkaloid reineckate precipitates, dissolved in acetone and measured the absorbance at λ_{max} 525 nm.

This method is applicable to sample from 2 to 10 mg of alkaloids or alkaloidal salts. This method provides a useful and rapid method of determining small quantities of various alkaloids in pure form.

Quaternary ammonium salts of certain heterocyclic amine can also interfere. Therefore, precautions to be taken to remove these impurities while extracting the alkaloids from plant by using acid, base technique of extraction.

Francis Duric, et al. (1950) developed acid dye method for the quantitative estimation of alkaloids and others base compounds by colorimetric method.

This method based on the observation that acidic dye combine with many alkaloids, e.g. tropane alkaloids (*Belladonna* and *Hyoscyamus*) to form salts like compounds which are characterised by their solubility in organic solvent. After separation, the dye components are estimated colorimetrically, e.g. bromocresol purple dye used for the estimation of atropine and hyoscyamine. This method is sensitive for the amount ranging from 0.1 to 2 mg per sample.

Titration Involving Precipitate Formation

Alkaloids in general precipitated from acid solution upon addition of Wagner's reagent (potassium iodate) these precipitates are quantitative and have form bases for volumetric titration.

Alkaloids in general produce precipitates when their solutions in various degrees of dilution, (depending upon the particular) are treated with any of the following reagents:

• Phosphomolybdic acid
• Phosphotungstic acid
• Cadmium potassium iodide
• Potassium iodide
• Mercuric potassium iodide.

Method

1. The precipitate dissolved in standard acid and back titrated with standard alkali.

2. Direct titration of the alcoholic solution of the alkaloidal residue with standard acid.

3. Non-aqueous titration to determine the weak base, e.g. caffeine.

Chromatographic Method of Evaluation

Procedure: Extract the alkaloids from dried material by extracting with 10% (v/v) acetic acid in ethanol, by keeping the drug in contact with solvent for 4 hours. Filter, and concentrate the filtrate to one fourth volume. Precipitate the alkaloids by basifying the concentrated extract with concentrated ammonia solution add dropwise to complete the precipitation, centrifuge the residue, wash with 1% ammonium hydroxide (NH_4OH), dissolve the residue in small quantity of chloroform or ethanol.

Chromatography: An aliquot on sodium citrate buffer paper in n-butanol-aqueous citric acid; on silica gel G plate in concentrated methanol: conc. NH_4OH (200 : 3).

Confirm the presence of alkaloids on plate or paper under fluorescence in UV light followed by spraying the testing reagents: Dragendorff's, iodoplatinate or Wagner's, conform the presence of particular alkaloid by compairing the Rf with monograph of alkaloid TLC.

Assay: Dissolve the crude alkaloids in 96% ethanol - 20% H_2SO_4 (1 : 1) so that the conc. of H_2SO_4 remains between 0.2 and 3.0 mm/L.

The alkaloidal solution 1 ml, mixed with 5 ml 60% H_2SO_4 (keep the tube cooled), after 5 minutes add solution of formaldehyde in 60% H_2SO_4, leave to stand for 180 minutes and measure the absorbance at 565–570 nm. Actual amount of alkaloids in crude extract can be determined with reference to absorbance measurement on pure alkaloid solution treated in the same way with formaldehyde in sulphuric acid (H_2SO_4).

GLYCOSIDES

Glycosides are organic compounds obtained from plants, which on hydrolysis yield one or more sugars (**glycone**), along with an alcoholic, phenolic or hydroxyl group of second non-sugars molecule known as **aglycone**. The therapeutic activity is based on aglycone moiety.

When sugar is glucose the substance may be called **glucoside**.

Chemically, the glycosides or heterosides are **hemiacetals** in which hydroxyl of sugar is condensed with the hydroxyl group of non-sugar to form oxide ring (sugar ether).

$$R - \boxed{OH + H} \quad O - X \rightleftharpoons R - OX + H_2O$$
$$\text{Sugar} \quad \text{Non-sugar} \quad \text{Glycoside}$$

Generally, **anomeric carbon** of sugar is attached with OH of non-sugar part. Both alpha and beta glycosides are possible depending on stereo configuration of glycoside linkage. However, β-form occur in plants. In general, plant glycosides are easily hydrolysed with dilute acids or appropriate enzymes exception to **C-glycosides** which are **resistant to usual acid hydrolysis** and require ferric chloride along with acid.

I. Classification

Based on the **linkage of anomeric carbon** of sugar to non-sugar moiety, the glycosides are named:

O-Glycoside, i.e. nucleophilic atom of the non-sugar is oxygen, e.g. salicin.

S-Glycoside, i.e. nucleophilic atom is sulphur such as thiol, e.g. sinigrin.

N-Glycoside, nucleophilic atom is nitrogen, e.g. adinosin.

C-Glycoside, nucleophilic atom is carbon in the form of carbonium, e.g. aloin.

Hydrolysis: Generally, natural glycosides are easily hydrolysed by boiling with mineral acid, exception to C-C glycoside. In most cases glycoside gets hydrolysed with enzymes present in plant itself. These enzymes are exposed on injury to the tissue or on germination process and perhaps other physiological activities of cells bring enzymes in contact. Mostly enzymes are specific for hydrolysis of glycoside, except two enzymes namely **emulsion of almond** kernels and **myrosin** of black mustard seeds which can hydrolyse more than one glycoside. Otherwise **specific enzyme** is required, e.g. rhamnase enzyme is required for the hydrolysis rhamnose.

II. Classification of Glycosides

Based on **chemical nature of aglycone** group, the glycosides are classified as follow:

i. **Steroid group:** Squill, digitalis
ii. **Anthraquinone group:** Aloe, senna, cascara bark, frangula bark, rhubarb
iii. **Saponin group:** Ginseng, dioscorea
iv. **Cyanophore group:** Bitter almond, wild cherry
v. **Isothiocyanate group:** Mustard oil plant
vi. **Aldehyde group:** Vanilla bean
vii. **Lactone group:** Santonin
viii. **Phenolic group:**
- **Flavonol group:** Hesperidin, rutin.
- **Tannins:** Galls, catechu, hamamelis
ix. **Alcohol:** Salicin
x. **Coumarin:** Celery fruit, Tonka bean, umbelliferae Apiaceae.

III. Classification Based on Therapeutic Activity

Cardiac glycoside: Cardiac muscle stimulator, e.g. digitalis glycoside, digoxin, digitoxin, ouabain, scilla, strophanthus.

Laxative group: Anthraquinone, sennoside, cascaroside, aloin, barbaloin, linarin.

Local irritant: Black mustard.

Analgesic and antipyretic: Willow and salix bark (salicin).

Anti-inflammatory: Glycyrrhizin, caffeic acid.

IV. Classification Based on Sugar Moiety

Sugar moiety	Glycoside
Glucose	Glucoside
Rhamnose	Rhamnoside
Digitoxose	Digitoxoside
Glucose + Rhamnose	Glucorhamnoside
Rhamnose + Glucose	Rhamnoglucoside

Qualitative and Quantitative Evaluation of Drug Containing Glycosides

Qualitative Examination

Physical properties:
- Most of the glycosides are soluble in water, alcohol and acetone (polar solvent).
- They are less soluble in organic solvent (generally insoluble).
- Solubility is dependent upon the sugar molecule present in glycosides.
- Steroid molecule of cardiac glycoside can alter the solubility, hence soluble in chloroform.

- Glycoside reduce the Fehling solution (A and B) but on hydrolysis with hydrochloric acid, except C-glycosides which hydrolyse by boiling with mineral acid along with ferric chloride.

Glycosides do not form precipitates with aqueous lead acetate solution.

Chemical test

General

Molisch test: Extract the drug with 70% alcohol, filter, add Molisch reagent: The violet colour indicates the presence of carbohydrates as well as glycosides.

Fehling solution test: Extract the drug with 70% alcohol, filter, to the filtrate, add sulphuric acid, and boil it at 70–100° for half an hour followed by neutralisation with ammonia solution. Filter the extract (test on pH paper). Mix the Fehling solution A and B in a test tube (1 ml each) then add one milliliter of neutralised test solution and boil it again on the water bath: Reducing sugar gives deep blue colour turning to red.

Chemical test specific for cardiac glycoside: All the cardiac glycosides are classified as steroids (sterols) having cyclopentanoperhydrophenanthrene nucleus, an α,β-unsaturated lactone ring (5 or 6 membered) at C17, cis fusion of the C and D ring at C13-C14, α,β-oriented hydroxyl at C14 and at C3, an attachment of one or more sugar usually deoxyhexose. On the basis of lactone ring the cardiac glycosides are of the two types:

Cardenolide: One double bond 5 membered lactone ring.

Furan

Bufadienolide: Two double bond six membered lactone ring.

α-pyrone

Chemical Identification

For detection of steroid nucleus: To the glycosides test solution in acetic anhydride, add few drops of sulphuric acid, positive test gives reddish violet-green colouration.

Test for 2,6-deoxy Sugar

Keller-Killiani test: Glycosides (digitalis and strophanthus) dissolved in acetic acid containing traces of ferric chloride and add concentrated sulphuric acid along the sides of test tube. At the junction of the liquids, reddish-brown colour gradually reduced to blue colour is indicative of positive test.

Legal test: To 1 ml test solution, add 2 ml of pyridine, 2–3 drops of sodium nitroprusside followed by one to two drops of 20% sodium hydroxide. Appearance of pink or red colouration is the positive test for five membered lactone ring (**cardenolide**).

Baljet test: To 2–3 ml of the test solution add 2 ml solution of picrate solution—yellow, orange to deep red colour. This test is for **cardenolide** and negative for **bufadienolide**.

Xanthydrol test: This colour reaction specific for 2,6-dideoxy hexoses. To the test solution add 1% solution of xanthydrol in glacial acetic acid containing 1% hydrochloric acid. Occurrence of red colour because of 2,6-deoxy sugar.

Antimony trichloride test: For presence of α-β-unsaturated lactone ring at C-17.

To the test solution add few drops of antimony trichloride and trichloroacetic acid followed by heating the solution, occurrence of blue or violet colour indicates the presence of α-β-unsaturated lactone ring.

Raymond test: For the presence of **active methylene group**. To the alcoholic extract of glycoside test solution add 0.1 ml of Raymond's reagent (1% solution of m-dinitrobenzene in alcohol) followed by few drops of sodium hydroxide solution (20% (w/v)). Appearance of violet colour indicates positive test for methylene group.

Structure

- Steroidal nucleus must be present
- 3β-OH group involved in glycoside linkage
- 14β-OH group at C-14
- A/B ring junction is cis
- B/C ring junction is trans
- C/D ring junction is cis
- Additional OH groups at C-5, C-11 and C-16 may be present and the presence of lactone ring at C-17

Cardenolide
Fluorescence reaction of cardiac glycoside

The cardiac glycosides in acidic condition, derivatise into dehydro derivative and becomes fluorescent in nature, higher the number of conjugation, increase in fluorescence intensity, e.g. aglycone substitution at C-14, 16 give didehydro derivative with the result trienone has 3 double bonds conjugated with carbonyl group become more intense fluorescent and useful to visualise.

TLC chromatogram: The reaction is temperature dependent and influenced by the respective acid. Reactivity increases from

$$H_2PO_4 \rightarrow CH_3SO_3H \rightarrow H_2SO_4$$

Subsequent use of oxidant increases the fluorescence with different colours. For spot observation phosphoric acid can be used alone or along with ferric chloride or with sulphuric acid.

Quantitative Analysis for Cardiac Glycosides

The reaction between digitoxin and 3,5-dinitrobenzoic acid (**Kedde's** Reagent).

i. Kedde investigated the use of 3,5-dinitro-benzoic acid for the estimation of digitoxin and other cardiotonic glycosides.

0.4% ethanolic solution (52–58%) of reagent mixed with glycosides in dilute ethanol, and 0.1 N sodium hydroxide solution in fixed amount is then added and intensity of colour is measured at a wavelength between 5350 and 5500 Å.

Procedure: The glycosides after extraction with dilute alcohol purified with lead acetate solution are hydrolysed in the presence of hydrochloric acid, the aglycone extracted with chloroform, repeatedly two times for the complete extraction, washing with water, drying over anhydrous sodium sulphate, evaporation under vacuum. The residue dissolved in dilute ethanol, added 3,5-dinitrobenzoic acid and colour develops with sodium hydroxide is measure at wavelength of 540 nm.

ii. The **French Pharmacopoeia** used **Baljet reaction** (picric acid) to estimate the aglycone of foxglove. As per the pharmacopoeia requirement the quantitation of aglycones fraction, i.e. lactone ring of the cardenolide glycosides.

iii. **HPLC:** In these days total quantity of glycosides concentration is being estimated by means of HPLC.

SAPONIN GLYCOSIDES

Saponin glycosides are widely distributed in higher plants. They form colloidal solution in water, and form honeycomb foam on shaking that remain persistent for 20 to 30 minutes.

They have bitter acrid taste. Because of this property drug-containing saponins are sternutatory and irritant to mucous membranes.

They have ability to lower the surface tension of aqueous solution, hence used as emulsifiers in fire extinguishers.

They hemolyse red blood corpuscles (RBC) especially of cold blooded animals. Hence, many saponins are used as fish poisons.

On hydrolysis they yield an aglycone known as a "**sapogenin**" which form readily crystallisable compound upon acetylisation.

In human and other warm blooded animals saponins are not very toxic on oral administration as they are absorbed in the intestines, only to a small extent.

Pharmacologically saponins have antitumour, chemopreventive, antihepatotoxic, antifungal, antiphlogistic, immunomodulating and molluscidal activities.

They also have shown activity on the cardiovascular system, the central nervous system (CNS) and on the endocrinal system.

Classification

Saponin glycoside are divided into two types, based on their chemical structure of the aglycone (sapogenins).

Steroidal saponins: They are derivative of steroids with spiroketal side chains (neutral saponins).

Triterpenoid saponins: They are acidic saponins.

Distribution

Steroidal saponins: They are distributed in monocotyledons angiosperm, i.e.

    Liliaceae family (smilex, asparagus)
    Agavaceae family (agave, yucca)
    Dioscoraceae (diosogenin)
    Fabaceae (fenugreek)
    Solanaceae (tobacco)
    Scrophulariaceae (foxglove)

Steroidal aglycone possess a skeleton with **27 carbons** which comprise six rings; E (**furan**) ring F (**pyran**).

E = Furan ring
F = Pyran ring

Spiroketal steroid (Diosgenin)

Steroidal saponins cause rapid hemolysis whereas triterpenoid have slower effect.

Triterpenoid saponins are predominantly present in dicotyledons, e.g. Leguminosae, Araliaceae, Caryophyllaceae (glycyrrhiza root, quillaja bark, polygala senega roots, panax, and ginseng, etc.).

Pentacyclic triterpenoids
(β-Amyrin)

Classification on the basis of number of sugar chain in their structure. They are **monodesmosidic** having single sugar chain normally attached at C-3.

Bidesmosidic saponins having two sugar chains, often attached with C-3 (ether linkage) and second attached as ester linkage at C-28 (triterpene saponin) or at C-26 an ether linkage (**furostanol saponin**).

Tridesmosidic saponins having three sugar chains.

Physicochemical properties: Due to the presence of lipid soluble aglycone and water soluble sugar chains in their structure they are of amphiphilic nature.

Saponins are surface active compounds with emulsifying, foaming and detergent property.

In aqueous solution they form micelle above a critical concentration called **critical micelle concentration** (CMC), which depend upon temperature, pH and salt concentration. Addition of cholesterol increases their CMC, size and viscosity.

Qualitative Test

Test Solution

All saponins are soluble to some extent in 80% alcohol, they are usually extracted with this solvent to perform chemical tests.

I. Hemolysis test: Test solution is mixed with standardised red blood corpuscle (RBC) suspension, the RBC will hemolyse. This indicates positive test, although steroid saponins will hemolyse rapidly while the **terpenoid saponins** slow in reaction hence not easy to differentiate.

II. Liebermann-Burchard test: To 1 ml test solution in a test tube, add chloroform (10 ml), 2 ml acetic anhydride, after shaking the test tubes add 0.2 ml concentrated sulphuric acid, followed by heating on water bath maintained at 40°C, appearance of blue or blue green colour or red, pink and purple colour for steroidal and triterpenoid saponins, respectively can be used to differentiate the steroidal and triterpenoid on the basis of colour (Table 7.1).

Test for steroid: 2 ml of dry extract dissolve in acetic anhydride heated to boiling, cooled then add 1 ml of concentrated sulphuric acid along the side of the test tubes.

Formation of green colour—steroids

Formation of pink colour indicate triterpenoid.

Salkowski reaction: 2 mg dried extract shaken with chloroform, to the chloroform layer add conc. sulphuric acid alongside of test tube slowly.

Formation of red colouration, indicates the presence of steroids.

Principle: Sterols react as typical alcohol with strong sulphuric acid (H_2SO_4).

Acetic anhydride used as solvent and dehydrating agent.

H_2SO_4 used as dehydrating and oxidising agent.

Quantitative Analysis of Saponins

Extraction of saponins from the crude drug by the following method and dissolved the pure saponins in 80% alcohol.

Quantitative estimation can be done by means of colorimetry, measuring the colour intensity produced by **Liebermann Burchard** test reagent at 430 mm wavelength.

Scheme: Defat the drug material with light petroleum ether, defatted material, extracted with 70% alcohol (ethanol/methanol) by soxhlet extraction process. Filter and concentrate the extract under vacuum, residue suspended in water, extract the aqueous layer with chloroform (twice), remove the chloroform layer, the aqueous layer further extracted with n-butanol (three times), washed the n-butanol extract with water, dried over anhydrous sodium sulphate and evaporate under vacuum. Concentrated extract suspended in diethyl

Table 7.1: Liebermann Burchard test

Hemolysis test	Froth test	Liebermann Burchard test	Group
+ ve	+ ve	Blue or green	Saponin probably steroid
+ ve	+ ve	Red, pink, purple or violet	Probably triterpinoid
+ ve	+ ve	Pale yellow	Saturated steroidal or saturated triterpenoid
+ ve	– ve	Red, pink, purple or violet	Saponin absent diterpene, triterpene, sterols or related polycyclic substance
– ve	– ve	Pale yellow	Saponin, unsaturated terpenes, sterol absent but may contain saturated sterol and saturated terpenes
– ve	+ ve	Pale yellow, red pink, purple or violet	Saponin absent probably free diterpene acids

ether, precipitation will take place, separate the precipitate, it will be **pure saponin**.

Chromatographic Analysis and Spectral Analysis

Sapogenins: Hydrolyse the dried plant tissue with molar hydrochloric acid for 2–6 hours (reflux). Hydrolysed solid matter, extracted with petroleum ether, residue dissolved in chloroform, concentrate and subjected to thin layer chromatography (TLC) on silica gel plate.

Solvent System

Acetone : Hexane

4 : 1

Chloroform : CCl_4 : Acetone

2 : 2 : 1

Spray reagent antimony trichloride in concentrated hydrochloric acid.

Colour reaction—pink to red colour.

Saponins: Being polar, they can be separated on paper chromatograph or on TLC using cellulose plate.

Solvent systems such as:

i. Butanol (saturated with water)

ii. Chloroform : methanol : water

13 : 7 : 2

CYANOGENIC GLYCOSIDES

Cyanogenic glycosides consist of an a-hydroxy nitrile stabilised by a glycoside linkage, to sugar moiety.

$$R_1 \diagdown \quad \diagup CN$$
$$C$$
$$R_2 \diagup \quad \diagdown O - OSE$$

Cyanogenic glycosides

Organic compounds in plants which on hydrolysis liberate hydrocyanide (HCN). It is generally recognised that a small amount of HCN occur free in plants, but the large amount is combined in glycosidic linkage. High concentration of cyanogenetic glycosides have been reported to be present only in seeds of few species of plants of Rosaceae family.

Screening Tests

I. Sodium picrate paper test: Place 2 g of moist shredded plant material or crushed seeds in a small test tube, followed by the addition of four drops of chloroform (to enhance the enzyme activity). A strip of filter paper saturated with sodium picrate solution (5 g Na_2CO_3, 0.5 g picric acid and water to 100 ml). Dry the strip and insert between split cork stopper and then introduce into the neck of the test tube containing reaction mixture while inserting the paper strip not to touch the side of the test tube. Heat the test tube at 42°C for 1–2 hours, change in the colour of strip from yellow to reddish brown indicates the positive test for cyanogenic glycosides.

II. Feigl-Anger paper test: This paper strip is useful for quick semi-quantitative analysis of cyanogenic level of sample. This screening method is particularly useful when large number of field samples are to be checked. Positive test based on colour conversion of the copper reagent to blue-purple in the presence of cyanide.

Method: Whatman No. 541 paper is prepared by dipping into the mixture solution of 0.5% copper ethyl acetate solution in chloroform and 0.5 g tetrabase in 50 ml chloroform (4,4′-methylene-bis-N-N-dimethyl-aniline) sigma.

Using gloves and tweezers dip the paper in solution and dry by hanging on the retort stand. Once dried, store in air-tight ambered glass container.

Procedure is same as for sodium picrate paper.

Quantitative Assay Method

Total Cyanide Determination

Substance: Flax seed, apricot, apple seed and bamboo shoot.

Method: Picrate kit method.

Picrate method: Plant material to be analysed quantitatively weighed out (immediately after grinding in glass pestle mortar) into a small flat-bottom plastic vial or glass vial, add phosphate buffer (0.5 ml of 0.1 M at pH 4–10) followed by exogenous enzyme in the case of cyanoglucoside solution. A picrate paper attached to plastic backing strip (Bradbury et al, 1999) is added, close the vial immediately with screw stopper. After about 16 hours at 30°C, remove picrate paper and immerse in 5 ml water for 30 minutes. Measure the absorbance at 510 nm and total cyanide (ppm) determined by the equation

Total cyanide content (ppm) = 396 × absorbance × 100/Z

where Z = weight (mg) of ground powder or leafy material.

FLAVONOID GLYCOSIDES

Flavonoids are plant pigments based on $C_6C_3C_6$ carbon skeleton, e.g. flavones, isoflavones, flavonones, catechin, leucoanthocyanins, anthocyanins and aurones.

Flavonoids are found in plant kingdom in the form of aglycone as well as heterosides. As **aglycone** they are found in **woody tissues** and **heteroside** in flowers, fruits and to some extent in leaves.

Based on degree of oxidation and saturation of the heterocyclic 'C' ring flavonoid may be classified into following groups:

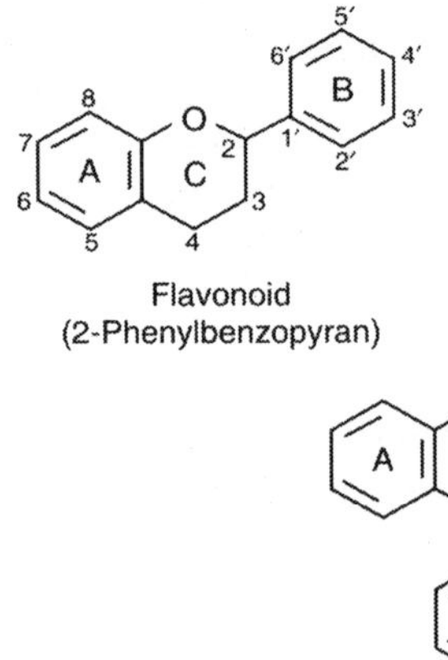

Flavonoid
(2-Phenylbenzopyran)

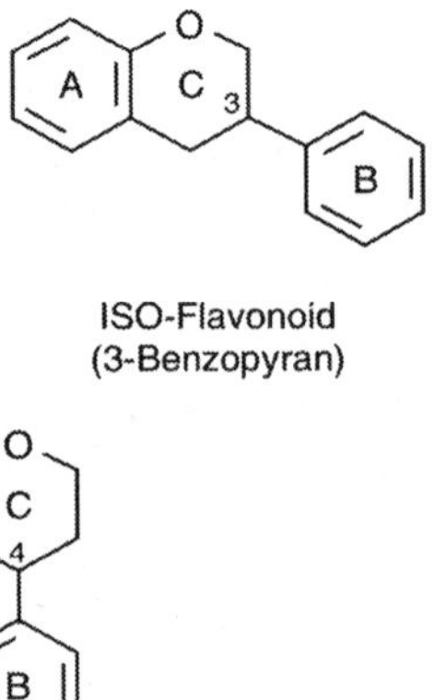

ISO-Flavonoid
(3-Benzopyran)

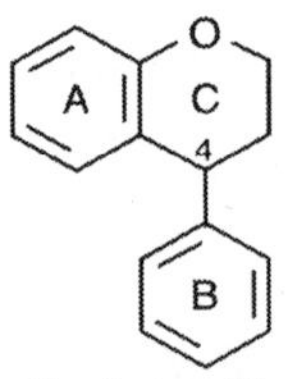

Neoflavonoid
(4-Benzopyran)

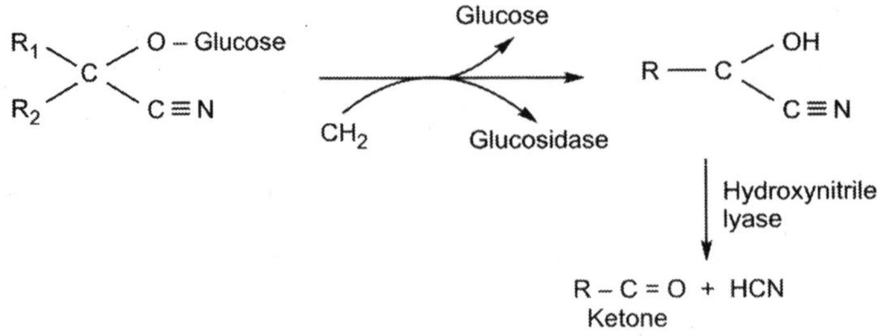

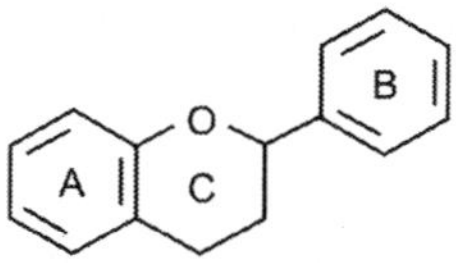

Flavan

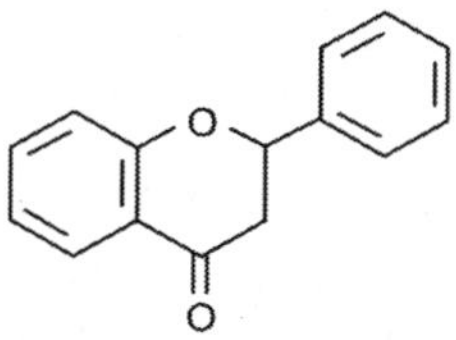

Flavanone

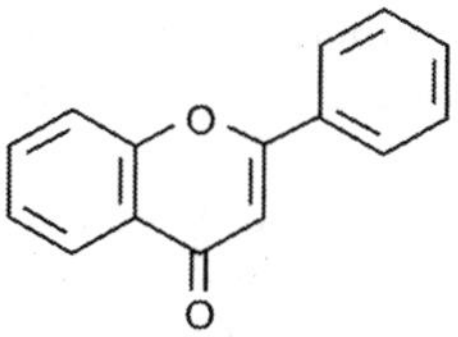

Flavone

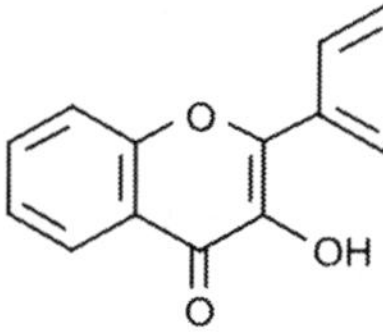

Flavonol

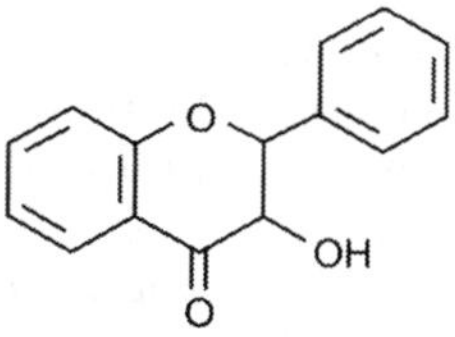

Dihydroflavonol

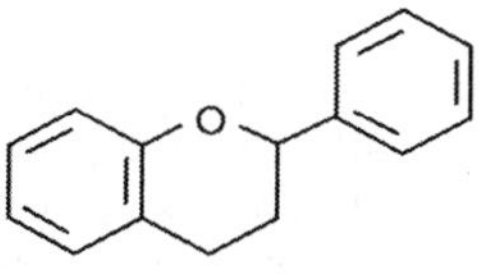

Flavan

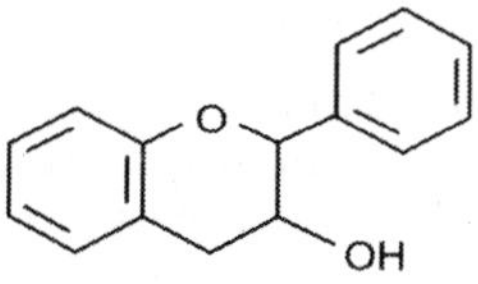

Flavan-3ol

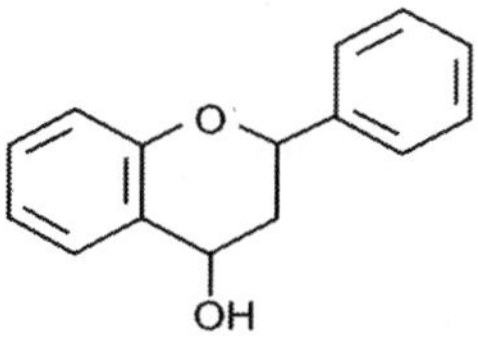

Flavan-4ol

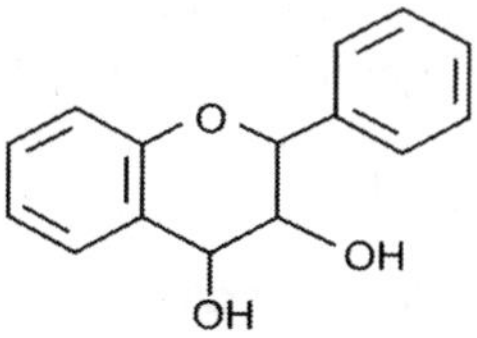

Flavan 3,4-diol

Isoflavonoid

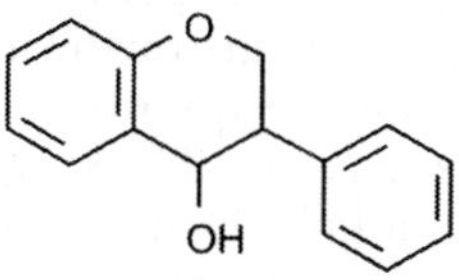

ISO-Flavanol

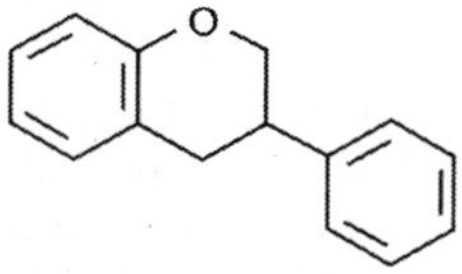

ISO-Flavan

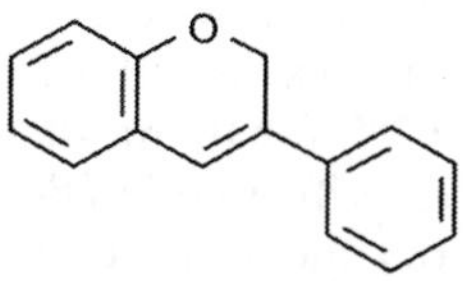

ISO-Flav-3ene

Aurone and chalcone: Chalcone and aurone also contain C_6-C_3-C_6 backbone. These groups include 2-hydroxy chalcone, 2-hydroxy dihydrochalcone, 2-OH retrochalcone, aurones (2-benzylidene coumaranone) and auronol.

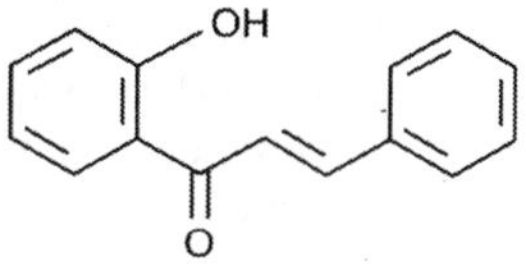

2′-OH chalcone

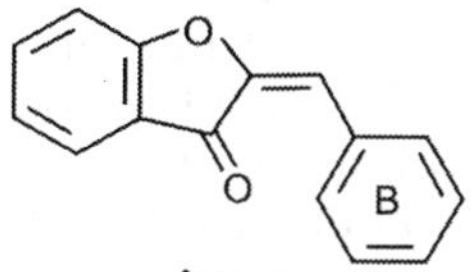

Aurone

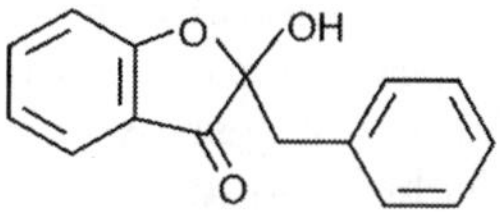

Auronol

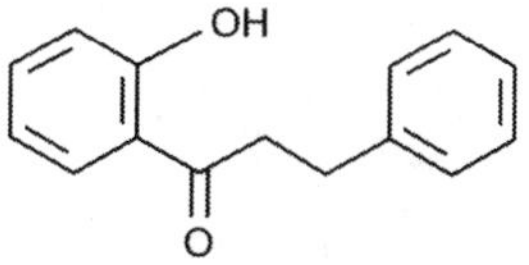

2-OH-dihydrochalcone

Physicochemical properties: Flavonoids are yellow coloured pigments, e.g. flavones, flavonoles, chalcones and aurones. But there are few which are **colourless**, e.g. flavans, flavanones, isoflavones.

On treatment with alkali some give blue coloration, e.g. anthocyanidins and in acidic media colour change to red.

Flavonoids are crystalline compounds soluble in water and alcohol but insoluble in organic solvents. **Aglycones** are soluble in ether and chloroform. Under ultraviolet light flavonoids give fluorescence of different colour. **Yellow → orange → brown → red.** Flavonoids on treatment with $AlCl_3$ give different colour in ultraviolet region. This property can be used for identification, e.g.

Flavone group—Green

Flavonol group—Yellow to yellowish green

Chlacone group—Brown-pink

Aurone group—Pale brown.

Qualitative Tests

Shinoda's test (cyanidin reaction): Four to five pieces of magnesium ribbons are added to alcoholic extract solution of flavonoids, followed by concentrated hydrochloric acid. Appearance of reddish colour indicates the positive test for flavonoids.

Alkaline reagent test: To the flavonoids extract add few drops of sodium hydroxide solution. Intense yellow colour indicates flavonoid or phenolic compounds but on addition of dilute acetic acid, yellow colour disappears which indicates the confirmation of flavonoids.

Wilson's reaction (Boric acid): On treatment with boric acid, flavonoids form complex between hydroxyl group and carbonyl group. Which is not destroyed by addition of citric acid alcoholic solution.

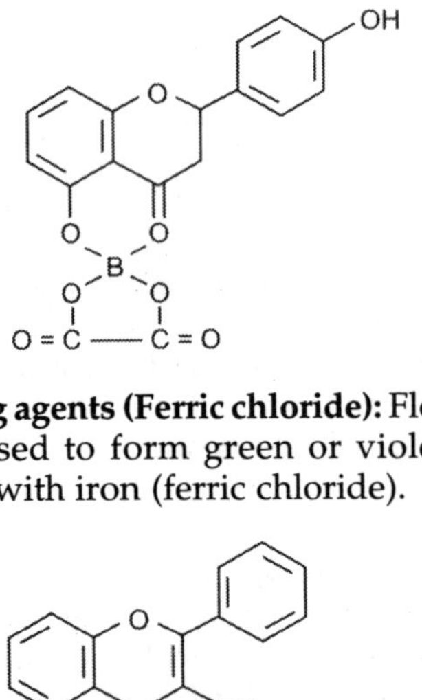

Oxidising agents (Ferric chloride): Flovonoids get oxidised to form green or violet colour complex with iron (ferric chloride).

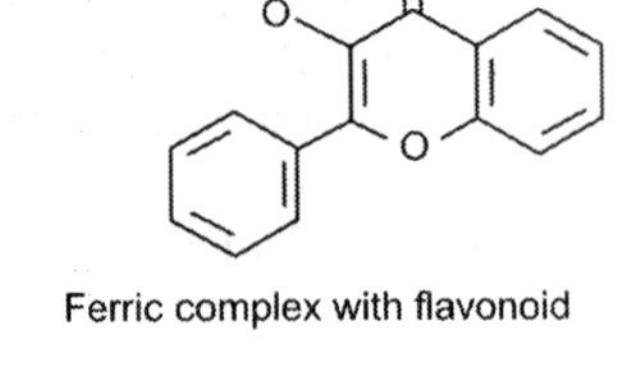

Ferric complex with flavonoid

Catechins on treatment with concentrated hydrochloric acid, catechin produce red colour.

Quantitative Analysis

i. Total phenolic contents: As the quantity of flavonoids present in vegetable or fruits drugs are usually low, data generally being recorded as total phenolic contents which can be most conveniently assessed by spectrophotometric method.

Colorimetric procedure for plant extract sample depends on the reaction of the flavonoid with one of a numbers of reagents of varying selectivity.

Folin-Ciocalteu reagent, which has been used before and after precipitation of flavonoid in acidic methanol and vanillin are the classic reagent.

Acid hydrolysis is done by refluxing the plant material with hydrochloric acid or formic acid, then aglycones are extracted with chloroform or ether.

Separation: Separation is done by liquid chromatography (LC). Usually reverse phase (RP) mode is best way on C_8 or C_{18} bounded silica columm in conjunction with binary mobile phase system such as acidified water, methanol and acetonitrile, less commonly tetrahydrofuran as organic modifier.

Formic, acetic and tetrafluoroacetic acid used.

Folin Ciocalteu

The reaction forms blue chromophore constituted by a phosphotungstic-phosphomolybdenum complex, where the maximum absorption of the chromophores depends on the alkaline solution and concentration of phenolic compound, hence the quantity of alkali should be in excess to check the cloudiness due to excess alkali, lithium salt added in the reagent which prevents turbidity.

Method: Take coarsely powdered drug sample about 1 g, extracted with 1 ml ethanol, centrifuged at 2°C for 10 minutes. Separate the aliquot, extract with 10 ml of 80% ethanol and centrifuge. Pool the aliquot and evaporate to dryness. Dissolve the residue and prepare dilute extract of different concentrations in a 10 ml test tube and total volume to 3 ml with distilled water, add 0.5 ml Folin-ciocalteu reagent (1 : 1 with water) and 2 ml sodium carbonate (20% w/v) solution heated on boiling water bath for 1 minute and measure absorbance at 650 nm (after cooling the reaction mixture) against the blank reagent. Standard curve to be drawn by using the standard phenolic campound (catechu).

ii. Total flavonoid contents: Aluminium chloride colorimetry method.

Aluminium chloride method: Aluminium chloride forms stable complex with C-4 keto group and either C-3 or C-4 hydroxy group of flavone and flavonol respectively. In addition, it also forms acid stable ortho-dihyroxyl group of A or B ring of flavonoid.

Method: 1 ml of known dilution of plant extract is used. Place in test tube, add methanol to make volume 2 ml, add 0.1 ml of aluminium chloride ($AlCl_3$) 10% w/v solution, then add 0.1 ml of sodium acetate and 2.8 ml distilled water. Keep the test tube for 30 minutes at room temperature, colour develops and absorbance measured at 415 nm by using spectrophotometer.

Standard curve prepared by using standard solution of quercetin.

Alternative Method by Zhishen et al (1999)

In this method known volume of plant extract (flavonoid fraction) transferred to 10 ml volumetric flask, add distilled water to make up the volume to 5 ml, then add 3 ml sodium nitrite ($NaNO_2$) (1: 20), then add 3 ml aluminium chloride ($AlCl_3$) (10% w/v). After 6 minutes add sodium hydroxide 2 ml (1 mol) solution and final volume made-up to 10 ml with more distilled water, mix well, the colour develops, measure the absorbance at 510 nm by means of spectrophotometer. Absorbance to be measured against blank solution.

COUMARIN AND THEIR GLYCOSIDES

Coumarins are benzo-α-pyrone derivatives. These are found in plants both in free state and as glycosides. It smells like **fresh hay** and

vanilla was originally used as flavouring agent but now its use has been banned by British Food Standards Agency, followed by Germany, China and other countries. They have made a law to forbid the usage of coumarin as food additive. It is found in Tonka beans (*Dipteryx odorata* family Fabaceae) and sweet woodruff (*Asperula odorata* family Rubiacea).

In ammoniacal solution, these compounds have a blue, blue-green or violet fluorescence. This property of coumarin is being used for qualitative test for coumarin containing plants such as umbelliferous resin present in asafoetida and galbanum.

2-pyrone   Coumarin

Bergapten
(Furanocoumarin)

Furanocoumarins are formed by fusion of furan ring to coumarin at either 6 and 7 position or 7 and 8 position and occur particularly in the families Rutaceae and Umbelliferae, e.g. celery fruits. Bergapten occurs in bergamot oil.

Coumarin found in 150 species belonging to over 30 different families.

Properties

Occurs as colourless, prismatic crystals.

Have characteristic fragrant odour and a bitter, aromatic, burning taste.

The glycosides are soluble in water and dilute alcohol.

In free state are soluble inorganic solvent, e.g. ether and chlorinated solvent.

Qualitative Evaluation

Spot test: They give blue or violet fluorescence in ammoniacal solution.

Presence of lactone: Place few drops of concentrated ether extract of the plant in a porcelain dish, add one drop of saturated solution of hydroxyl amine hydrochloride and one drop of saturated alcoholic potash. Heat the mixture on open flame till it starts bubbling, after cooling add 0.5 N HCl to acidify the mixture followed by drop of 1% ferric chloride solution. Appearance of violet colour indicates the positive test for lactone ring.

Quantitative Evaluation

Widely used method for quantitative estimation is based upon the conversion of **coumarin to coumaric acid** which in basic solution gives characteristic yellowish-green fluorescence on exposure to ultraviolet rays.

A known weight of drug to be analysed extracted with dilute alcohol by heating in a stoppered vessel on water bath, followed by addition of sodium hydroxide and heat it again, it will convert the coumarin to coumaric acid with the appearance of green fluorcesence which can be measured spectrophotometrically.

A freshly prepared coumarin standard, concentration of 0.1, 0.25, 0.50, 0.75 and 1.0% coumarin per mol, in 0.5 N NaOH, irradiated and read. The instrument used adjusted to read 100 with a fluorescence standard consisting 0.77% of quinine sulphate per ml in 0.1 N H_2SO_4. A curve to be plotted from the reading of the coumarin standards. Coumarin equivalence value for the sample to be read from the curve.

ANTHRAQUINONE GLYCOSIDES

Anthraquinone glycosides: These glycosides, upon hydrolysis, yield aglycones that are di-, tri-, or tetra-hydroxy anthraquinone or modification of these compounds, e.g. frangulin hydrolyzes to form emodin and rhamnose, examples of drugs are: e.g. Rhubarb, senna, aloe, cascara, etc.

Plant families:

Monocotyledons: Only in Liliaceae family. C-glycoside, e.g. barbaloin.

Dicotyledons family

Rubiaceae, Leguminaceae, Polygonaceae, Rhamnaceae, Ericaceae, Euphorbiaceae, Lythraceae, Saxifragaceae, Scrophulariaceae and Verbenaceae.

Absent in Bryophyta, Pteridophyta and Gymnosperms but occurs in fungi and lichens.

Pharmacologically, the drug containing anthraquinone glycosides are purgative in nature. The derivatives of anthraquinone responsible for purgative action are: Dihydroxyphenol, e.g. chrysophenol.

Trihydroxyphenol, e.g. emodin or

Tetrahydroxyphenol, e.g. carminic acid. Carmine natural red cochineal.

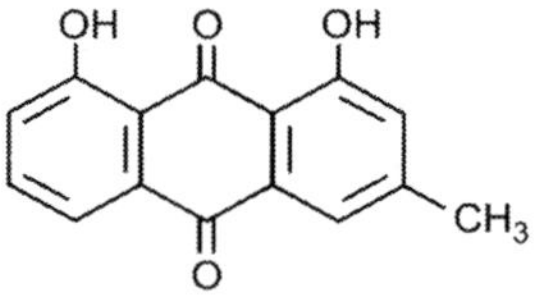

Chrysophenol

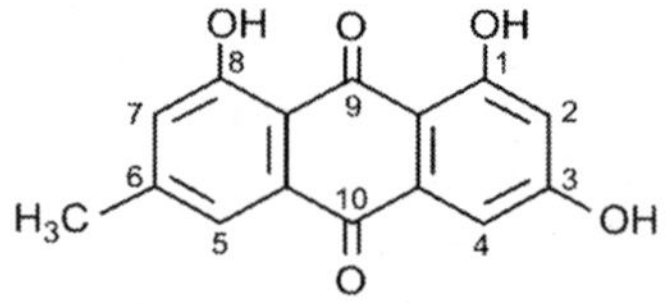

1.3,8-trihydroxy-6-methylanthracene-9,10-dione (Emodin)

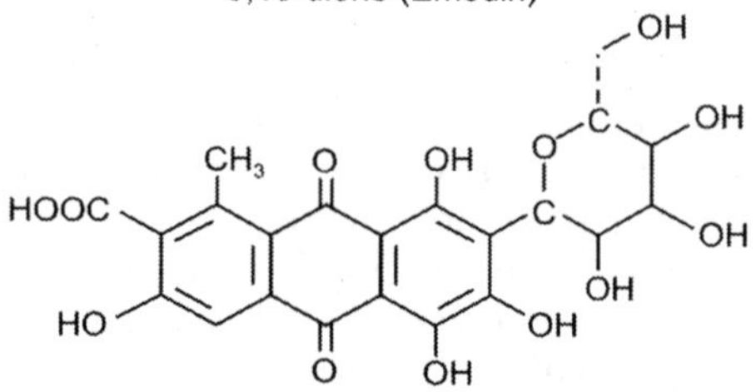

Carminic acid

Anthraquinone glycosides are present in drug as free state as well their derivatives. As

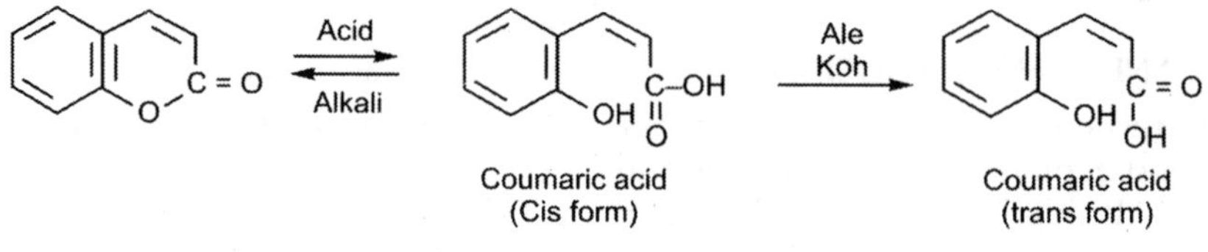

Coumaric acid (Cis form)

Coumaric acid (trans form)

it get easily hydrolysed, their derivatives often are found in plant as orange-red compound, e.g. medullary rays of rhubarb and cascara. As glycosides are soluble in hot water or dilute alcohol, while aglycones are soluble in organic solvents.

Test: Macerate the powdered drug with organic solvent (ether preferably) after filtration, filtrate is shaken with aqueous ammonia or caustic soda, appearance of pink red or violet colour in aqueous layer indicates the presence of anthraquinone derivatives.

Borntrager Test for Anthraquinone Glycosides

Hydrolyse the drug (powder form) with alcoholic potash or 2 M sulphuric acid by heating for 5 minutes, filter and on cooling extract with chloroform or dichloromethane, shake the oraganic layer with dilute solution of ammonia, red or pink colour in ammonia layer indicates the positive test.

Modified Borntrager's test: This test is being used for anthraquinone glycosides having C-C linkage, e.g. aloe-emodin. **Ferric chloride or dilute hydrochloric acid** are used for oxidative hydrolysis. The anthraquinone liberated is extracted with carbon tetrachloride. Add ammonical solution to the carbon tetrachloride layer, will produce rose red or pink violet

colour is positive test for anthraquinone glycosides.

Test for anthrone and anthranols: Anthrone and anthranol are the derivatives of anthraquinone, occur free or as their glycosides. They are isomeric to each other. Anthrone is pale yellow in colour, non-fluorescent and insoluble in alkali.

Anthranol is brownish yellow in colour and are strongly fluorescent in alkali solution.

Test: Give green fluorescence with borax or other alkaline solution. Anthranol on treatment with fuming nitric acid converted to anthraquinol which give violet colour on addition of ammonia.

Oxanthrone

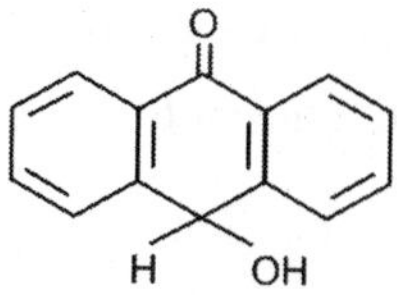

It is intermediate product between anthrone and anthranol. Oxanthrone gets oxidised to anthraquinone by heating the powder drug (cascara). Boil the powder drug with alcoholic potash (0.5 N) along with dil. hydrogen peroxide solution, after cooling add few drops of acetic acid, acidified mixture is extracted with benzene. Shake the benzene layer with

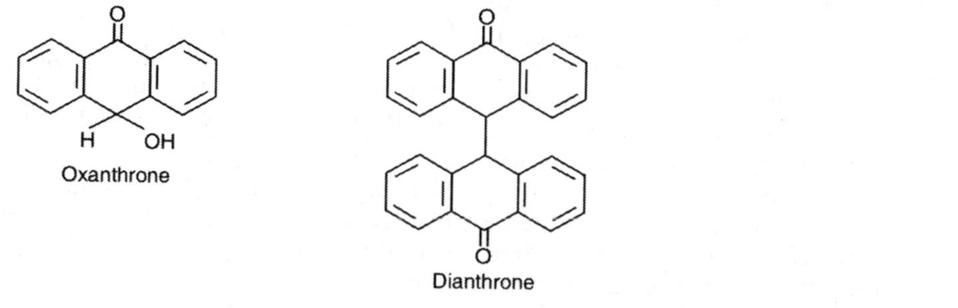

Anthraquinone

Anthrone

Anthranol

Oxanthrone

Dianthrone

ammonium hydroxide. It will give yellow colour in alkaline layer, indicates the positive test.

Dianthrone

Dianthrones are the compounds derived from two anthrone molecules, may be identical or different. They (aglycone) are present in cassia, rheum and rhamnus. The best known example is **sennoside A and B**.

Aloin type or C-glycoside

Aloin

This is strongly resistant to normal acid hydrolysis but may be oxidised with ferric chloride. In this compound sugar is linked directly with aglycone by C-C linkage.

Quantitation of Anthraquinone Glycoside

Anthraquinone produce colour with magnesium acetate or with potassium hydroxide that can be measured spectrophotometrically.

Since free anthraquinone in drug has no pharmacological important component, pharmacopoeias recommend the quantitation of anthraquinone in the combined form only.

General procedures include first extraction, oxidation followed by colour reaction and spectrophotometry analysis.

Extract the powder drug with water or hydroalcohol by heating at water bath. Filter, extract the filtrate with a polar organic solvent to remove the free anthraquinone. Then reflux the aqueous extract with ferric chloride followed by hydrochloric acid. The resultant aqueous layer extract with an **apolar organic solvent** (repeat the process three times), pool the organic layer, wash with water, dry over anhydrous sodium sulphate, evaporate to dryness, redissolve in methanolic solution of magnesium acetate, colour develops, measure the absorbance at 515 nm.

ESSENTIAL OILS (VOLATILE OILS)

Essential oils are liquid at ambient temperature also volatile in nature and almost completely volatilised without decomposition at room temperature leaving no spot on the paper. They are generally colourless, having density less than water exception clove, cinnamon and sassafras oil. The volatile oils have 'essence' or odour, hence also known as essential oils.

Chemically they are complex, highly variable mixture of alcohol, ketone, aldehyde, esters, phenols, terpenes, hydrocarbons, ethers, and degradation products of non-volatile constituents.

Essential oils are steam volatile hence can be isolated from drug containing volatile oil by steam distillation.

Only a few possess a single component in higher percentage, e.g. mustard volatile oil contains not less than 93% allylisothiocyanate; clove oil contains not less than 85% of phenolic substances chiefly eugenol.

Those volatile oils, which are obtained other than by distillation, e.g. lemon oil contain small proportion of non-volatile components/matter.

A few volatile oils, e.g. oil of anise are solid at 15–16°C, but melt to form liquid at slightly higher temperatures.

Common physical properties: All volatile oils possess a characteristic odour, high refractive indices (index), optically active and their specific rotation is valuable diagnostic character/property.

Solubility: Although the volatile oils are insoluble in water but they are sufficiently soluble to impart their odour and taste to water (Aromatic water).

They are soluble in ether, alcohol and most organic solvents.

Distribution in plant: Volatile oils are usually contained in some special secretory tissue, e.g. the **oil ducts** (Vitae) of Umbelliferous fruits; oil cells or **oil glands** present in the sub-epidermal tissue of lemon and orange and the **mesophyll** of eucalyptus leaves.

Few volatile oils do not pre-exist in plant but are formed by the **decomposition** of a glycoside, e.g. whole black mustard seeds are odourless but upon crushing the seeds and upon adding water a strong odour occur which is due to the decomposition of glycoside sinigrin by an enzyme myrosin. The enzyme and the glycoside exist into different cells of the seeds unable to react until the seeds are crushed.

Difference between Volatile oils and Fixed Oils

1. Volatile oils do not leave a grease spot on the paper or surface on evaporation. The fixed oil leaves permanent grease spot on a paper as they contain glycerol esters of fatty acids.
2. Volatile oil do not become rancid while the fixed oil gets rancid giving obnoxious odour.

   The volatile oil on exposure to light and air gets oxidized and resinified.

Methods of Obtaining Volatile Oils
Distillation

1. Three methods of distillation, i.e. water distillation, water and steam distillation, direct steam distillation. Selection of method depends upon the nature of the drug (plant/plant part or exudates, etc.).

   1.1. Water distillation:
   Dried plant material that is not subject to injury at the boiling temperature of water, e.g. turpentine oil.

   The crude turpentine exudates containing plant exudates, rainwater and wood chips, pine needles, etc. are put into distilling still along with water and heated to boiling till the oil along with water distilled out and condensed into the condensing chamber as a separate layer.

   1.2. Water and steam distillation
   Material: Dried or fresh plant material, which may be injured at boiling temperature, in the case of dried material (cinnamon, clove) drug is powdered and covered with layer of water and steam is passed (generated separately) though the pipe into the container containing the drug material. The steam along with oil drops is condensed into the condensing chamber, where the oily layer is separated from the aqueous layer.

   1.3. Direct steam distillation:
   This method is applicable to fresh plant material (peppermint, spearmint). The crop is cut in morning having moisture and placed directly into a metal distilling tank on a truck bed, the truck is driven into a distilling chamber where steam pipes are attached to the bottom of distilling tank. The steam is forced through the material. The steam will carry the oil drops along with water vapour to the condensing chamber. The oil layer will be separate from the aqueous layer.

2. **Expression method:** In this method plant material is crushed and treated with water followed by distillation.

   This method is applicable to volatile oil which does not pre-exit in plant but are produced by enzymatic hydrolysis, e.g. glycosidic volatile oil (mustard oil) the seeds are crushed, washed with water and distilled by distillation.

3. **Ecuelle method:** This method is applicable for the volatile oil present in oil glands (lemon oil, orange oil or citrus family).

   It involves the puncturing the oil glands by rolling over a trough lined with sharp projection long enough to penetrate the oil glands present in epidermis and could puncture the gland (piercing the oil glands). Water is sprayed in such a way that it washes away the oil from mashed peel, while juice is extracted through centered tube that crosses the fruit. The resulting oil/water emulsion is separated by centrifugation.

4. **Enfleurage method:** In this method, the odourless fixed oil or fat (melted) is spread over glass plates. The plant material especially delicate plant parts (flower petals) are placed on the fat/fixed oil for few hours. The volatile oil from the petals gets absorbed by the fat/fixed oil. After the fat has absorbed oil fragrance as much as possible, the absorbed oil is removed from the fatty matter by extraction with alcohol. This process of oil extraction is known as **enfleurage**; other methods of oil extraction are not commercially viable for the flowering petals, which is major source of fragrance in perfume industry (perfumery).

5. **Destructive distillation (dry distillation):** This method of distillation is applicable to woody part of the plant for obtaining **empyreumatic** oils (having an odour of burnt organic matter) from wood or resin of Pinaceae or Cupressaceae family plants. The destructive distillation is usually conducted in retorts. In this method wood is heated without access of air, decomposition takes place and volatile oil separates into two layers. An aqueous layer containing wood naphtha crude acetic acid and tar (depending on the type of wood) and the oily layer, e.g. volatile oils.

Evaluation of Volatile Oils

For qualitative evaluation; pharmacopoeias have prescribed tests to be performed as follows:

1. Miscibility with different organic solvents (ethanol, ether, etc.).
2. Physical measurements like refractive index, optical rotation, density, solidification, acid, ester and carbonyl value. Absence of any fatty oil; resnified materials and other residue on evaporation. Chromatographic (TLC, GC, HPLC) analysis for its purification/identification.

TLC (Thin Layer Chromatography)

Thin layer chromatography to be performed on silica gel plates, solvent systems to run the plate are toluene or benzene and chloroform; ethyl acetate or both in ration given in monograph.

Spray reagent: Detection of the separation profile (pattern) can be examined under ultraviolet region after spraying with sulphuric acid followed by vanillin and heating or can be sprayed with antimony trichloride.

Gas Chromatography (GC)

Volatile nature of the essential oils components, makes the gas chromatography method most suitable analytical technique for qualitative as well as quantitative analysis. It is fast, reliable, automatic and potential technique of analysis.

The use of gas chromatographic profile as references by pharmacopoeias and other standards are becoming more common means of standards for quantitation of the tested sample being representative and characteristic of an essential oil.

High Pressure Liquid Chromatography (HPLC)

HPLC is a liquid column chromatography system which employs relatively narrow coloumn about 5 mm diameter, operating at ambient temperature and even up to 200°C at pressure up to 200 atm.

This method is useful for analysing the non-volatile content of the essential oil, e.g. it is the efficient way to check the purity of citrus oils by analysing their non-volatile components. Citrus essential oil is widely used in food products for citrus flavours. Its relatively simple chemical composition and tremendous price difference among citrus species, the chances of adulteration are more and numbers of indistinguishable blends are available in market which are possible to analyse with conventional analysis GC, the reverse phase (RP). HPLC is the only method of analysis.

Electronic Noses (Artificial Nose)

It is designed in such a way that it mimics the mammalian nose. It contains different types of chemical gas sensors (organic polymers, metal oxide, quartz, etc.) which non-selectively interact with the odour molecules in response to which sensor produces signals recorded in computer which are designed to create data pattern for particular aroma.

This pattern recognition is used to identify the similarity between two samples. Once the fingerprint of an odour is integrated and stored in memory, it can be used as a reference for subsequent analyses. Hence, it is advance technology for measuring and characterising aroma released from the essential oils. It is helpful in the identification and classification of aroma mixture of foods and drugs.

In some cases one particular component or group of components can be used for creating electronic fingerprint, e.g. cineole in eucalyptus oil, eugenol in clove oil, carvone in caraway, etc.

TANNINS

Tannins are complex, organic, non-nitrogenous polyphenolic substance of high molecular weight (about 1000–5000) natural products, occurring in plants, confined to certain organs; such as leaves, fruits, barks or wood. They are found largely in unripe fruits and disappear on their ripening. They are amorphous substance soluble in water form colloidal, acidic aqueous solution with astringent and usually bitter taste.

The phenolic compounds, with relatively low molecular weight, e.g. gallic acid, catechin and chlorogenic acid are called 'pseudotannins'.

Classification

Tannins are classified into two main groups based on type of phenolic nuclei involved.

I Hydrolysable tannins (Pyro-gallol-tannins).

They are formed from several molecules of phenolic acids such as gallic acid hexahydro-xydiphenic acids, united by ester linkage to a central glucose molecule.

They may be hydrolysed by acids or by enzymes (Tannase), to yield phenolic acid such as gallic acid (gallotannins), ellagic acid (ellagitannins) and sugars, example of plants hamamelis leaf, chinese galls, oak bark and green tea.

II Condensed tannis (Phlobatannins) or nonhydrolysable tannins, contain only phenolic nuclei.

Most of the members of this group are derived from the dihydric phenol, catechol; and they do, contain sugar moiety. They are formed from the condensation of 2 or more flavn-3-ols such as catechin or flavan 3–4-diols, such as leucocyanidin.

Unlike hydrolysable tannins, these tannins do not hydrolysed readily to simpler molecule. When treated with hydrolytic agent, these tannins tend to polymerise, yielding insoluble, usually red coloured product known as **phlobaphenes** soluble in alcohol but practically insoluble in water example of drugs containing such tannins catechu, cinchona bark, cinnamon bark, krameri roots and wild cherry bark, acacia and male fern.

General Properties of Tannins

a. Tannins are soluble in water.
b. With iron salt they form dark blue or greenish black coloured (ink) soluble compound.
c. They are precipitated with all the other metallic salts such as copper, lead and tin.
d. They react with skin and hide to form leather and with gelatin protein form insoluble compound.
e. They react with alkaloids to form water insoluble tannate.

Gallic acid
R = OH

Ellagic acid

Hexahydroxy diphenic acid

Gallotannin

f. They form bulky precipitate with phenazone.

g. Many tannins are glycosides and hence on hydrolysis they give test for sugar.

Test for Identification

i. **Gelatin test:** About 0.5 to 1% w/v solution of tannins, precipitate 1% w/v solution of gelatin (containing 10% w/v sodium chloride), pseudotannins (concentrated solution) also precipitate the gelatin solution.

ii. **Goldbeater skin test:** Fix up the small piece of prepared gold-beater skin (OX intestine), flat on the hard paraffin, pour 1 ml of 2% hydrochloric acid solution and leave for 10 minutes, on the skin, washed the skin with distilled water and add 1 ml solution of tannin under test, leave for half an hour, wash and examine, the skin will be tanned or treat the tanned skin with 1% solution of ferrous sulphate. The colour of the skin will be brown or black.

Phenazone test: To about 5 ml of aqueous solution of tannins, add 0.5 g of sodium acid phosphate, heat on water bath, cool and filter, to the filterate add 2% solution of phenazone, bulky precipitate will be formed with tannins.

Matchstick test: Dip matchstick in tannins solution; dry and moisten with concentrated hydrochloric acid and heat near the flame, the wood will turn pink or red.

Iron tannate test: To about 5 ml of plant extract, add an equal volume of 0.25% solution of iron and ammonium citrate and 1–1.5 g of sodium acetate and boil. A violet or black precipitate of iron tannate will be formed.

Ferric chloride test: To about 5 ml of dilute solution of tannins (plant extract) add a few drops of ferric chloride solution. A black coloured precipitate will form.

Lead sub-acetate test: To about 5 ml of dilute solution of plant extract add 1 ml of concentrated solutions of lead subacetate, white coloured bulky precipitate will be formed indicate the positive test.

Extraction: Tannins are generally extracted with water and acetone mix (50–70%) by reflux/sonication/microwave extraction technique. However, microwave extraction technique is most safe (methanol to be avoided as it causes methanolysis of galloyl deposits).

Fresh leaves/plant tissues are preferable than the dried material (to avoid irreversible complex formation of polymers).

Eliminate the acetone by distillation, the aqueous layer left out to be extracted with dichloromethane or $CHCl_3$ to remove the lipid and pigments, followed by extraction with EToAc. It will separate the dimeric proanthocynidins and most of the gallotannins.

The polymeric proanthocynidins and high molecular weight gallotannins remain in the aqueous solutions.

For further purification, gel filtration to be done followed by reverse phase chromatography.

Mobile solvent system: Water, alcohol and acetone mixture.

Quantitative assay: The best mathods for tannins detection and quantitation is, to measure their specific ability to precipitate proteins:

I. **Hemolysed blood method basis:** Tannins form combination with hemoglobin and the non-precipitated hemoglobin can be estimated colorimetrically against a blank.

Standard (tannic acid) is used to determine the relative astringency, i.e. relative to that of standard.

II. **Alternative method:** In this very method haemoglobin is replaced with bovine serum albumin. The protein is solubilised at its isoelectric pH, then precipitated by the tannins present in the extract to be analysed.

The protein concentration of the precipitate is determined colorimetrically after alkaline hydrolysis and reaction with ninhydrin.

III. **Hide powder method (Traditional method):** First, an infusion (extract) of the drug is prepared, one aliquot is evaporated to determine the total soluble matter (S). In another aliquot the tannins are precipitated by the addition of hide powder. The precipitates are separated by centrifugation followed by decantation.

The supernatant is evaporated to dryness (residue N). The difference in weight between the two residues (S–N) is the weight of the tannins present in the aliquot.

Quantitative Analysis of Condensed Tannins

Proanthocyanidins can be estimated by measuring colour (absorbance) obtained upon conversion to anthocyanidins by boiling in n-butanol in the presence of HCl. Reaction can be accelerated and reproducibility is improved by addition of ferric chloride to the reaction medium (the absorbance at a given wavelength varies depending upon the structure of anthocyanidin).

Proanthocyanidins can also be quantitated as vanillin adition product in methanol in the presence of HCl.

Vanillin is an aldehyde, form adduct at 6-positon of the flavonoid unit, which are dihydroxylated at C-5 and C-7.

p-dimethylaminobenzaldehyde can be used instead, e.g. grape seeds tannins.

Quantitative Analysis of Hydrolysable Tannins

The gallotannins can be hydrolysed in the presence of H_2SO_4 following the reaction of the rhodamine gallic acid with rodamine. The absorbance of the product can be measured or reaction with potassium iodete can be used.

Determination of Hydrolysable Tannins (Gallotannins and Ellagitannin) After Reaction with KIO_3

Hydrolysable tannins are heated at 85°C for 20 h in methanol/H_2SO_4 to quantitatively release methyl gallate. Oxidation of methyl gallate by KIO_3 at pH 5.5, at 30°C forms chromophore with λ_{max} 525 nm which is determined spectrophotometrically. pH is to be adjusted with ethanol amine/H_2SO_4. The conventional quantitative procedure for ellagitannins involves a reaction with nitrous acid after sulphuric acid hydrolysis, form quinone oxime, which are measured colorimetrically.

Gallotannins Determination by Rhodamine Assay

Reagents

1. Rhodamine solution (0.667% w/v) in methanol. It is stable for at least 2 weeks stored in refrigerator.

2. KOH (0.5 N). Dissolve 2.8 g KOH in 100 ml D.W.

3. Sulphuric acid solution: Prepare 0.3, 0.4, 0.6, 22 and 26 N, H_2SO_4 solution by approximately diluting 98% commercially available H_2SO_4 (36 N).

Determination of free Gallic Acid

Pipette 200 ml supernatant (Ext) in four test tubes (160 × 12 mm), remove solvent (acetone) in vacuum oven at 40°C for 2 hours. or by flushing the nitrogen gas.

Gallic acid: Add to 200 µl of 0.2 N H_2SO_4 to the tubes containing dried supernatant. To three tubes add 300 µl of H_2SO_4 solution and to fourth tube add 300 µl methanol (blank). After 5 min. add 200 µl of 0.5 N KOH solution to all the tubes. Wait for 2.5 min. and then add 4.3 ml D.W. After 15 min. measure absorbance at 520 nm against proper blank.

Determination of gallic acid present in the free and gallotannin form: Pipette 3.34 ml of supernatant in duplicate in culture test tube. Remove acetone by flushing the tube with nitrogen gas. To 1 ml supernatant (or make to 1 ml with D.W.) add 0.1 ml of 22 N H_2SO_4 so that the final H_2SO_4 conc. is 2 N. Freeze the contents and remove the air by using vacuum pump. Keep these tubes at 100°C for 26 h to hydrolyse gallotannins to gallic acid. After hydrolysis, make-up the volume to 11 ml by adding 9.9 ml D.W. The H_2SO_4 conc. in this solution is 0.2 N. This solution is hydrolysed supernatant.

Now take 200 µl of the hydrolysed suspernatant and proceed further as above.

Total phenolic quantitation

Total phenolic contents from the extract are determined by **Folin-Ciocalteu's** reagent method. 0.5 ml of extract and 0.1 ml (0.5 N) **Folin-Ciocalteu's** reagent, mixed and to incubate the mixture at room tempterature for 15 min. Then **2.5 ml saturated sodium carbonate** solution to be added and further incubated for 30 min at room temperature and the absorbance measured at 725 nm. Gallic acid to be used as positive control. Total phenol contents to be expressed in terms of gallic acid equivalent (mg/g) of the extracted compound.

This procedure derived from **Folin-Denis method:** The phenolate ion formed by adding sodium carbonate is oxidised by a mixture of phosphotungstic and phosphomolybdic acid which is simultaneously reduced to give **blue** solution.

RESIN

See Chapter 1 (unorganised drugs).

FURTHER READING

1. Bandelin. The colorimetric determination of various alkaloids, Journal of American Pharmaceutical Association (Scientific ed.). 1950;18: 493–5.
2. Bruneton J. 1999. Pharmacognosy, Phytochemistry and Medicinal Plants, 2nd ed. Lavoisier Publication.
3. Evans WC. 2009. Trease and Evans Pharmacognosy, 16th ed., Elsevier; New York.
4. Francis Duric, et al. A colorimetric method for estimation of some tropine alkaloids, Journal of American Pharmaceutical Association (Scientific Ed.). 1950; 39:680–2.
5. Gunnar Samuelsson. Drugs of Natural Origin. A Textbook of Pharmacognosy, 4th Edition, Apotek Arsocieten, 1999; p. 307.
6. Harborne JB. Phytochemical methods, 1973, p. 185.
7. Mallick CP, Singh MB. Plant enzymology and plant histoenzymology, Kalaya. Pub., New Delhi, 1987:281–6.
8. Mervat MM, El Far, Hanan AA Taie. Australian J. Basic Applied Sc., 2009;3:3609–16.
9. Narasimhan Sreevidya and Shanta Mehrotra. Spectrophotometric method for estimation of alkaloid precipitate with Dragendorff's reagent in plant material. Journal of AOAC International. 2003;86(6).
10. Quantification of tannins in tree and shrub foliage. wwwspringer.com.
11. Quantitative Estimation, Wiley online library.
12. Rezaul Haque M, and Howard Bradbury J. Total cyanide determination of plants and foods using picrate and acid hydrolysis methods. Food Chemistry, 2002, 77:107114. Analytical nutritional and clinical methods section.
13. Tyler VE, Brady LR, Robbers JE. 1988. Pharmacognosy, 9th Edition-Leo and Fabiger. Philadelphia.
14. www.researchgate.net/publications 223138629 cyanogenic glycoside chapter by Roslyn Gleadow, Nanna Biarnholt, et al.
15. Zhishen J, Mengcheng T, Jinnamig W. The determination of flavonoid contents in mulberry and their scavenging effect on superoxide radicals. Food Chem., 1999;64:555–9.

Study of Biological Sources, Chemical Nature and Uses of Plant Products

8

Plant Products: Fibres— Cotton, Jute, Hemp

COTTON

Raw cotton: It consists of the epidermal trichomes of seeds of *Gossypium herbaceum* and other cultivated species of *Gossypium.*

Family: Malvaceae

Purified cotton (absorbent cotton): Purified cotton is free from adhering impurities, fatty matter, bleached and sterilised.

Chemical nature: Raw cotton consists of 90% cellulose, 7% moisture, and 3% wax, fat and remains of protoplasm.

Purified cotton consist of almost exclusively of cellulose, alpha, beta-linked linear glucopyranosyl polymer, free from wax, fat, alkali, acid and water soluble substances.

Description: Purified cotton occurs as white, soft, fine, filament like hairs that appear under microscope as hollow flattened and twisted band slightly thickened at the edges.

Hairs are unicellular, non-glandular from 2.5 to 44.5 cm long and 23 to 36 µ in diameter.

Odour: odourless and tasteless.

Chemical Test

Ignition test: On ignition cotton burns with flame without odour and fumes. It does not produce any beads, very little white ash, which differentiate it from wool, silk and rayon.

Iodine and sulphuric acid test: N/50 iodine solution soaked and dried cotton on treatment with 80% sulphuric acid—appearance of blue colour distinguish it from acetate rayon, alginate yarn, jute, hemp, silk and nylon.

Phloroglucinol and hydrochloric acid test: Cotton does not give red stain on treatment with phloroglucinol and hydrochloric acid, this distinguish it from jute and hemp.

Solubility test: Soluble in 80% (w/w) sulphuric acid. Insoluble in 5% (w/v) potassium hydroxide solution, distinguish it from oxidized cellulose also from wool and silk.

Also insoluble in 90% (v/v) formic acid and 90% (w/w) phenol distinguish from rayon.

Insoluble in acetone distinction from acetate rayon.

Cuoxan solution (ammoniacal copper oxide solution) test: Absorbent cotton dissolves completely with uniform swelling whereas raw cotton dissolves with ballooning leaving few fragments of cuticle.

Treatment with water

Absorbent cotton readily wetted and sink in water whereas raw cotton will not be wetted, but float.

Uses

Purified cotton used as a surgical dressing, to absorb blood, mucous or pus and to keep bacteria away from infecting wound thus providing mechanical protection.

Absorbent cotton is also source for the manufacturing absorbent gauze, microcrystalline cellulose, purified rayon and cellulose derivative, such as carboxycellulose, cellulose acetate phthalate, oxidised cellulose and pyroxylin used in pharmacy and in medicine (Fig. 8.1).

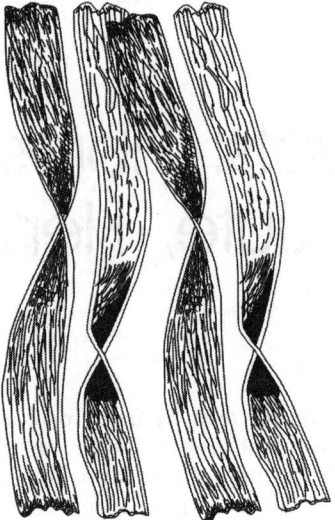

Fig. 8.1: Cotton

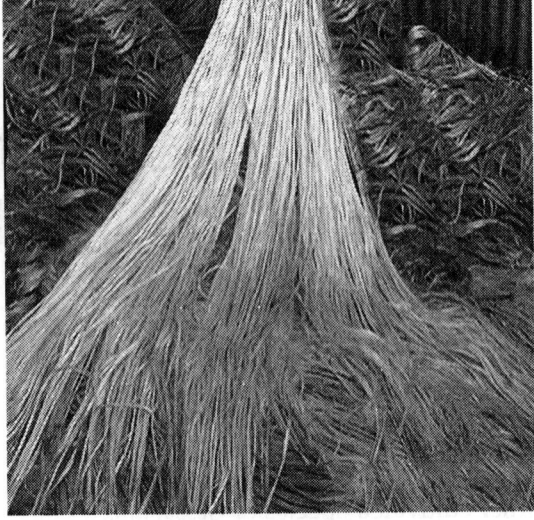

Fig. 8.2: Jute

JUTE

Botanical source: It is obtained from the phloem fibres strands of stem bark of *Corchorus capsularis*; *C. olitorius* and other species of *Corchorus*, family Tiliaceae.

It is obtained from the stem of annual plant (2 to 3 m) by rotting and scutching (mechanical beating and combing process) to get a mass of pale yellowish brown fibres up to 2 m in length. These strands are made into cheese rolls, constitute *tow* fibre bundles are then separated into individual fibres lengthwise.

Description

Fibres are yellowish brown or buff-coloured and free from adhering xylem tissue. Strands of fibre are 1 to 3 metre in length and 30 to 140 μm thick. These are brittle and dusty when dried but are hygroscopic and absorb moisture up to 25%.

Microscopic examination reveals that fibres are smooth free from any striation or transverse lines, the lumen or cavity is not uniform in diameter as at some point is narrow or even obliterated, apices are usually rounded but few are blunted. The length of fibre is 0.8 to 4 mm and 10 to 25 μ in diameter (Fig. 8.2).

Geographical source: Bengal, delta region of Ganga and Brahmaputra river Asom, Bihar and Odisha.

Chemistry: Chemically jute consists of lignocellulose bundle of phloem fibres, the middle lamina of which lignified. On disintegration with oxidising agent (nitric acid and potassium dichromate mixture) the bundle disintegrate into individual fibres.

Chemical Test

Test for cellulosic matrial: Digest the jute in N/50 iodine solution, remove the extra iodine solution then add the few drops of 80% w/v sulphuric acid, the fibres will stain with bluish-green colour which latter may become yellow, whereas the adherent phloem parenchyma will give full blue colour.

Test for Lignin: Digest the few strands of jute fibres in 1% alcoholic phloroglucinol subsequently add few drops of hydrochloric acid, the fibres will stained red.

Chlorzinc iodine solution test: On treatment with chlorzinc iodine solution the fibres will stain yellowish brown but the parenchyma present will stained blue to violet colour.

Aniline chloride solution test: The fibres get stained bright yellow.

Uses: It is also important vegetable fibres next to cotton used to make cloth for wrapping bales of raw cotton and to make sacks, carpets, chair covering, rugs and linoleums backing.

HEMP

It is vegetable fibre extracted from the pericylic fibres of the stem of *Cannabis sativa*, family Cannabinaceae.

The fibres are prepared by retting process as described under jute, from parenchyma fibres of a plant cultivated on rich soil in the temperate climate. These fibres are chiefly composed of cellulose (70%) but with some lignifications (8–10%).

Description: The average length of the fibre is 35 to 40 mm, diameter 16 to 50 μm, the apices of the fibres are mostly blunt and sometimes forked, surface with marked striations, large lumen, the transverse section shows roughly 3 to 6 sided, with rounded corners lumen cleft or branched (Fig. 8.3).

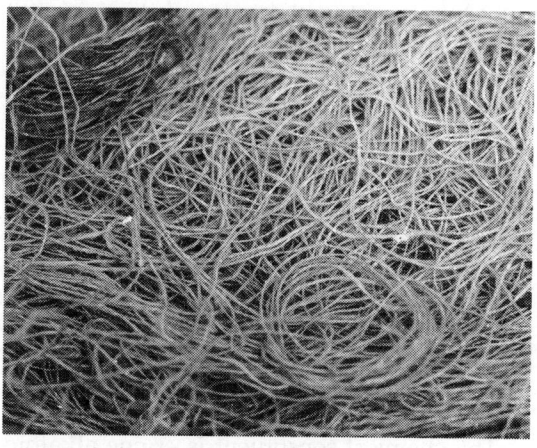

Fig. 8.3: Hemp fibres

Chemical test

Phloroglucinol and hydrochloric test: Stained slightly red.

Iodine and sulphuric acid test: Inner wall blue, middle lamella yellow.

Chlorzinc iodine solution test: Fibres stained purple to yellow colour.

Uses: It is used to make canvas, boat sails, cloth, papers, shiprigs, fish-nets and twine. It can block ultraviolet light (natural antibacterial).

FLAX FIBRE

It is prepared from the pericyclic fibre of the stem of *Linum usitatissimum*, family Linaceae.

The fibres are prepared by dew retting or water retting processes. The length of the fibre is 25 to 30 mm average but few of them are even 120 mm long and the average diameter is 12 to 30 μm. Lumen is narrow, walls are thick with cross lines (Fig. 8.4).

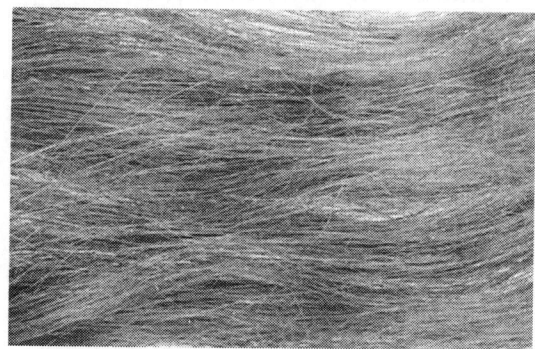

Fig. 8.4: Flax fibres

Chemistry: The fibres are non lignified except for the middle lamella.

Chemical test:

Iodine sulphuric acid staining test: Fibres get stained blue or violet colour.

Chlorzinc iodine staining test: Purple to yellow colour.

Phloroglucinol test: Remained colourless or slightly pink colour.

Uses: Coarse grade is used to manufacture twine, ropes, canvas and webbing equipment.

HALLUCINOGENS

A hallucinogens are psychoactive agents that causes distinct changes in perception, emotional state of mind, awareness of space and time. Medically defined as sensory delusions, synaethesia is another potential occurrence, where the senses become combined and individual feel that he can smell colour and see sound. The reported side effects are anomalies in perception and unusual deviations in thoughts, emotions and consciousness.

Within the plant kingdom the hallucinogens occur only among the evolutionary advanced flowering plants and in the more spore bearers fungi.

Most hallucinogens are alkaloids, a family of perhaps 5000 complex organic molecules. These active compounds may be found in various concentrations in different parts of the plants—roots, leaves, seeds, bark and flowers. They gets absorbed by the human body in the number of ways, by smoke or snuff, swallowing fresh or dried, by drinking decoction and infusions, or by topical application and also by enemas.

Following is the list of few well known hallucinatory plants in practice: *Peyote cactus, Datura* species, *Salvia divinorum* and morning glory species sach as *Turbina corymbosa.*

Psychoactive fungi with potent hallucinogenic compounds include—Red and white capped mushrooms *Amantia muscaria* and ergot (*Claviceps* species).

Peyote Cactus (*Lophophora williamsii*): Historically, Peyote plant was used as a medicinal plant to treat high fever, headache and other ailments. The religious and ceremonial use of Peyote still practiced among the Huichol Tarahumara and Yaqui people in North—Central-Mexico.

Chemistry: Psychoactive compound of the Peyote cactus is the alkaloids mescaline, a powerful vision—inducing intoxicant.

Formula

Mescaline

Uses: Members of Native American church can legally use peyote for **sacramental purposes**, otherwise the plant is protected under the Convention of International Trade in Endangered Species (CITES).

Ololiqui (*Turbina corymbosa*): It is a member of morning glory family, the vine like ololiqui is another new world ritual plant used by Hispenic culture. It is being used as psychoactive by the indigenous people of West Indies and North American Gulf Coast. The compound responsible for its psychoactive properties is alkaloid having closed relation to LSD.

Ebena (*Virola theiodora*): The snuff prepared From the **bark of Ebena** (Member of Nutmeg family) and leaves of *Justicia pectoralis* are used by Amazonian Shamans tribe.

Dimethyl trytamine (DMT): *Psilocybin* or *Psilocin* are hallucinogenic substances found in more than 180 species of mushrooms. They are mainly used for spiritual or recreational purposes and similar but distinct hallucinogenic experiences compared with LSD.

LSD (d-lysergic acid diethylamine): It is also known as acid, microdots, sugar cubes or window panes; is one of the most potent and perception altering hallucinogenic drug.

Description: It is white odourless water soluble material synthesised from lysergic acid derived from rye fungus. Its crystalline form known as microdot, thin gelatin square (window panes) blotter (LSD soaked paper punched into square).

Argyreia nervosa syn. *Argyreia speciosa*— elephant creeper: woolly morning glory, family Convolvulaceae.

The seeds of the plants are used mainly as hallucinogenic and have been used traditionally in a number of diseases in India as hypnotics and spasmolytic as well as anti-inflammatory.

In Hawaii used for religious and sacramental purposes.

The chemical constituent is ergine alkaloid (0.04% w/w) is the major component which is also used as a precursor to lysergic acid.

Psilocybin mushroom (*Psilocybe semilanceata*): Psilocybin (4-phosphoryloxy-N, N-dimethyl tryptamine) also known as a magic mushroom found in tropical and subtropical regions of South America, Mexico and United states. The biological genera containing psilocybin mushrooms include

Copelandia, gymnopilus, Inocybe, Mycena and psilocybin.

DMT (Dimethyl tryptamine): Also known as **Dimitri** a powerful hallucinogenic chemical obtained from Amazonia Plant spieces (*Ayahuasca*) also known as hoasca. Ayahuasca tea has traditionally been used for healing and for religious purposes.

Salvia divinorum (Diviner's sage) or magic-mint, family Labiateae.

It is a psychoactive plant common to Southren Mexico and central and south America

Fresh leaves are chewed or their juice is being used as hallucinogens. Dried leaves are also being smoked or inhaled for the purpose of hallucinogens.

INDIAN HEMP

Biological source: Dried flowering and fruiting tops of pistillate plants of *Cannabis sativa* and other species, *C. indica, C. ruderalis,* family Cannabinaceae.

Geographical source: India, Bangladesh and Pakistan.

Narcotic products of Cannabis: Ganja, bhang and charas or churus.

Ganja (Indian Hemp) IP1955: Ganja is the aerial part of the plant containing not more than 10% of the fruits, large foliage leaves and stem over 3 mm. It is also known as *Flat or Bombay-Ganja,* prepared by rolling the wilted tops between the hands.

Bhang (Hindustani) or Hashish (Arabic): It is the larger leaves and twigs of both male and female plant of *Cannabis sativa* or *Cannabis* species. It is used in India in the form of electuary for smoking alone or with tobacco, opium or datura.

Charas or Churus

It is a crude resin obtained by rubbing the tops of *Cannabis sativa* plant between hands or by beating on cloth or carpet or by worker wearing leather jacket walking among growing plants followed by collection of resin from the jacket by scrapping. It is used as narcotic purpose by mixing with other smoking material.

TERATOGENS

Teratogens are the substances (chemical, physical or biological) able to induce abnormalities in developing fetus leading to birth defect in the child. It came to known first time in 1962 with the occurrence of **Thalidomide disaster**, one of the darkest episode in the history of pharmaceutical research. The drug was marketed as a mild sleeping pill safe even for pregnant women, however it caused thousands of babies born worldwide with malformed limbs. Thalidomide is a synthetic drug for the treatment of Hansen's disease (leprosy).

Source of Naturally Occurring Teratogens

There are three source of naturally occurring teratogens **food, drugs** and **natural products**. The excessive use of plants and plant products by pregnant women can cause toxic effects on the foetus. Birth defect is one of the dangerous side effect of herbal drugs mainly due to misconcept that the herbal drugs are harmless being natural. Actually some plants are abortigenic, even endanger to maternal health in some cases. This is because of unawareness of the users as well as the prescribers about abortive effects of the plants. As these plants, do, not act during short period of gestation cycle, usually abnormalities appear in offspring, till that time causative plant source completely disappeared.

Following range of plant constituents are reported to have teratogenic effects in animals having given the larger doses at laboratory experiments: alkaloids, coumarins, lignans macrolides nitrites, terpenoids, toxic amino acid and other some unknown compounds.

Human Teratogens

Radiation (atomic weapons and radioiodine), infectious diseases caused by cytomegalovirus, herpes viruses, syphilis, Toxoplasma and Rubella virus.

Maternal metabolic factors: Alcoholism, diabetes, folic acid deficiencies and endemic cretinism.

Drugs: Aminopterin, busulfan, cocaine, coumarins, anticoagulants, cyclophosphamide, lithium, mercury, thalidomide and retinoic acid.

Herbal products containing one of the following plants: *Lupinus, Veratrum, Conium* and *Solanum* genus, *Trachymene* genus, *Sorghum* and *Senecio* genus. *Thermopsis cytisus, Sophora* and *Nictiana.*

Following is the list of some plants reported to have teratogenic effects: *Elaegnus angustifolia, Peganum harmala* Linn, *Carthamus tictorius* and Saffron all reported to have abortive effect.

Plants having teratogenics as a side effect: *Lavandula officinalis, Lawsonia inermis* and *Silybum marianum.*

Many poisonous plants common in the diet of domestic livestock poses teratogenic potential.

Some plants known to produce congenital deformities include *Lupinus, Astragalus, Veratrum, Leucaena, Lathyrus* and *Indigofera.*

Perovskia abrotanoides: This plant is being used in Iranian traditional medicine in the treatment of parasitic infection, but reported to have some abnormalities such as spine bifida, aglossia, tarsal extensor, gastroschisis and numerous skeletal abnormalities.

ALLERGENS

Allergens are inciting agents of allergy, i.e. the substances capable of sensitising the body in such a way that an unusual response occurs, in hypersensitive person. Allergen may be of biologic, chemical or of synthetic origin. It is common to speak about the substances such as pollens, danders, dust, etc. as natural allergens. Although the chemical identity of allergen is unknown but most known **allergens are protein or glycoprotein** and do not have much difference from other immunogens except perhaps being somewhat smaller in size (mol wt. 10,000–70,000). Most allergenic substances are mixture in composition. Allergens from related sources often are similar chemically and cross allergenic.

A number of low molecular weight chemicals (**allergenic haptens**) are partial immunogens and induce allergy after combining covalently with a suitable protein carrier, viz. drug allergy.

WHAT IS ALLERGY?

The allergy (**hypersensitivity**) may be defined as a specific **immunologic reaction** to an immunogen, a normally harmless substance (allergen). It was first defined in 1906 by **Clemens von Pirquet** who described **allergy as changed or altered reaction in the body of an individual, in response to a substance or condition that is harmless to others**.

Sneezing is always considered to be a symptom of a cold but sometimes it is an allergic reaction to something in the air. According to reports available approximately 30% population suffers from some sort of allergic syndromes. However, few persons develop symptoms that are sufficiently severe to require the services of allergist or physician. The occurrence of allergic disease is determined by the characteristics of the individual as well as those of the allergen and even the condition of exposure.

Disease occurs only in those individuals who are previously sensitised by exposure to the allergen and becomes more sensitised on subsequent exposure but sometimes it is genetically determined in children of allergic parents who are more likely to develop allergies to the particular allergen even on first exposure, even if only one parent is allergic. Sensitisation may also vary with the age of the individual, nature of the allergens, route and degree of exposure and many other factors.

The immunological processes involved in allergy results in tissue damage which otherwise do not differ fundamentally from those seen in the normal immune response.

Normally, the immune system functions as the body's defence against invading agents, such as bacteria and viruses. When an allergic person first comes into contact with an allergens, the immune system treats the allergens as an invader and mobilises to attack. The immune system does this by generating large amount of a type of **antibody** (a disease fighting protein) called **immunoglobin E** or **IgE**. Each **IgE** antibody is specific for one particular allergenic (allergy producing) substance. In the case of pollen allergy, the antibody is specific for each type of pollen. One type of antibody may be produced to react against oak pollens and another against ragweed pollens. Thus, antibodies are considered to be specific and because allergenic substances do produce specific antibodies, each type of allergy is constitutionally different from other types. Allergy can be classified into **four types** on the basis of immune effectors, mediators and cell involved in the reaction (Table 8.1).

Most of the environmental allergens produce Type I allergies. Type II and Type III allergies are produced due to autoimmune and in alloimmune diseases.

The IgE molecules are special because IgE is the only class of antibody that attached to the body's mast cells (Tissue, cells and to basophils). When the body is first subjected to the allergen (antigens) the condition is referred to as the primary exposure. Because no antibodies have been formed previously, hence no symptoms of the allergy are produced during primary exposure, however on subsequent exposure its specific IgE attach the allergens and **antigen antibody reaction**

occurs; with the liberation of powerful inflammatory chemicals like histamine, cytokines, leukotrienes or SRS (slow-reacting substance) and bradykinin. These chemicals act on tissues in various parts of the body, such as the respiratory system and causes the symptoms of allergy.

Some people may develop asthma with allergy the symptoms of asthma include coughing, wheezing and shortness of breath due to narrowing of bronchial passages in the lungs, production of excess mucus and inflammation. It can be fatal and requires immediate medical attention.

Following are predisposing factors which make the person hypersensitive to allergens:

  i. Hereditary tendency to allergic response.
 ii. Dysfunction of the endocrine glands.
iii. Increased excitability of sympathetic and parasympathetic nervous systems.
 iv. Absorption of metabolic and catabolic substances.
  v. Hepatic dysfunction.
 vi. Psychic influences.

Table 8.1: Allergy manifestations and their mechanisms of action

Basis	Type I (Immediate Reagin-mediated)	Type II (Cytotoxic)	Type III (Immune complex Arthus type)	Type IV (Delayed: Cellular-mediated Tuberculin-type)
Immune effectors	IgE	IgG; IgM	IgG (IgM)	Effector T cells
Cells involved in inflammation	Mast cells Basophils	Macrophages (cell-mediated lysis)	Neutrophils	Macrophages Lymphocytes
Mediators	Histamine Leukotrienes	Complement (C′-mediated lysis)	Lysosomal enzymes	Lymphokines
Time of onset in sensitised individuals	0–30 min	Immediate but may not be apparent for some time	2–24 hr	6–24 hr
Manifestations	Rhinitis Urticaria Angioedema Asthma Anaphylaxis	Hemolytic anemia Neutropenia Thrombocytopenia	Serum sickness Vasculitis Glomerulonephritis Extrinsic alveolitis	Contact dermatitis Allergy of many infections

TYPES OF ALLERGENS

The allergens can be classified on the basis of types of symptoms, which depend on the shock organs affected by the particular allergens and its route of entry into the body;

• Inhalant allergens
• Ingestant allergens
• Injectant allergens
• Contactant allergens
• Infectant allergens
• Infestant allergens

Inhalant Allergens

Inhalant allergens are airborne substances as chemicals, causing respiratory disease, inflammation in the nose and lungs. Inflammation in the nose is manifested by sneezing, lacrimation, itching and swelling of nose and eyes. The condition is known as **Sinusitis or hay fever**. The odour emanating from new mown hay is often responsible for the 'fever' or stuffiness of the nasal passages. Inflammation of lungs is often expressed as **asthma**. Air pollution, both in-door and out-door, play a significant role in the aggravation of airway disease in the asthmatics and may contribute to the overall increase in asthma morbidity.

Symptoms of allergies to airborne substances are:

• Sneezing often accompanied by a runny or clogged nose.
• Coughing and postnasal drip
• Itching eyes, nose and throat.
• Allergic shines (dark circles under the eyes caused by increased blood flow near the sinuses).
• The 'allergic salute' (in a child persistent upward rubbing of the nose that causes mark on the nose).
• Watering eyes, conjunctivitis (an inflammation of the membrane that lines the eyelids causing red-rimmed, swollen eyes and crusting the eyelids).

As soon as the allergens land on mucous membrane, an inside lining of the nose, a chain reaction occurs that leads the **mast cells** in these tissue to release histamine and other chemicals. These powerful chemical contract certain cells of some small blood vessels in the nose, that allow fluid to escape, which causes the nasal passage to swell resulting in nasal congestions.

The allergens that can cause airborne allergies (**inhalant allergens**) include pollens, dust, mites, mold spores and animal allergy (epidermis or dander).

The type of allergen can be identified from the symptoms which occurs in the patient.

Pollen Allergen's Symptoms

• Symptoms intensify in the morning and worsen on windy days.
• Symptoms flares on days with high pollen counts. Eyes may itch or swell.

Mold Allergen's Symptoms

• Symptoms intensify, during evening especially as the day cools off when humidity is present.
• Symptoms intensify when mowing grass, and raking leaves.
• Symptoms intensify with exposure to moldy foods such as blue cheese, mushrooms, etc.

House Dust/Dust Mite Allergen's Symptoms

Symptoms are worse inside a dusty building or house. Symptoms flare within 30 minutes after going to bed.

Itching of eyes is more in comparison to skin itching.

Pollen Allergens

Pollens are the tiny, egg shaped, round, angular, square, rectangular or otherwise shaped male cells (organ) of flowering plants. These microscopic, powdery granules are necessary for plant fertilisation. The average pollen particle size is less than the width of an average human hair.

Most pollen grains are single entities but some may be 2-compound, 3-compound, tetrad, or so forth. They may either have no germinal apertures as such (**acolpate**) or have many pores (**multicolpate**) or range in between (**dicolpate, tricolpate, tetracolpate**). The surface appearance of outer wall (**exine**) is characteristic, it may range from smooth (**psilate**) to spiny (**echinate**) with various intervening gradations (reticulate granulate, lophate).

These pollens can be further classified into two types:

1. Anemophilous (wind pollinated).
2. Entomophilous (insect pollinated).

Anemophilous

Anemophilous pollens are usually small 15–45 µ in diameter, light, non-adhesive and relatively smooth and are produced by plain looking plants, e.g. **Trees** (oak, walnut); **grasses** (bermuda grass and timothy) and weeds (ragweed, plantain).

Entomophilous

Entomophilous pollens are usually larger in size (up to 200 µ in diameter), heavier, adhesive and may be somewhat spiny. Plants are scented, with coloured flowers such as clover, hollyhock, honey suckle and rose.

Most common allergic reactions are produced by wind pollinated (anemophilous) pollens, because of their lightweight and the dry nature these pollen grains are carried for long distances. It is difficult to get rid of an area from pollens, as the pollens can drift in from many miles away. In addition, most allergic pollen comes from plants that produce them in huge quantities. A single ragweed plant can generate a million of pollen grains a day.

The chemical composition of pollen is the basic factor that determines its likelihood cause hay fever. For example, pine tree pollen is produced in large amount by common tree, which makes it a good candidate for causing allergy. However, the chemical composition of pine pollen, appears to make it less allergic than other type; moreover, pine pollen is heavy, it tends to fall straight down and does not scatter, therefore they rarely reaches human noses.

The plants responsible for seasonal pollinosis have the following criteria:

1. The pollen must contain an excitant of hay fever.
2. The pollen must be anemophilous or wind born, with regards to its mode of pollination.
3. The pollen must be produced in sufficiently large quantity.
4. The pollen must be sufficiently buoyant to be carried to considerable distances.
5. The plant producing pollen must be widely and abundantly distributed.

Early Spring Pollinating Trees

Ulmus americana L. (American elm)	*Acer Saccharinum* (silver maple)
Ulmus rubra muohlenb (slippery elm)	*Acer rubrum* (red maple)

List of plant or tree producing pollens (allergens):

Alfalfa	Eucalyptus
Almond	Gladiolus
Apple, Acacia	Hazelnut
Barley	Juniper
Blue grass	Mulberry
Canary grass	Mustard
Cherry	Lemon and related species of citrus

Grasses

The following is the list of grasses that shed allergenic pollens:
- *Cynodon dactylon* (Linn.) Pers (Bermuda grass)
- *Sorghum halepense* (Linn.) (Johnson grass)
- *Dactylis glomerata* Linn. (Lockshoot) (Orchard grass)
- *Phleum Pratensis* Linn. (Timothy)
- *Poa pratensis* Linn. (Kentucky bluegrass)
- *Agrostis alba* Linn. (Red top)

- *Anthoxanthum odoratum* Linn.
  (Sweet vernal grass)
- *Lolium perenne*
  (Perennial rye)

The grasses pollinate throughout the year and no particular season is apparent.

Weeds

The weeds belonging to the family Chenopodiaceae, Polygonaceae, Plantiginaceae, Amaranthaceae and Compositae are responsible for shedding allergenic pollens.

Some weed plants pollinate in the beginning of summer while others pollinate later in the summer depending upon their geographical location extending into late fall. *Plantago major* L. (Common plantain) and *Plantago lanceolata* L. (English plantain) are cause to widespread early summer weed pollinosis.

Following are other hay fever weeds that shed allergenic pollens:

- *Rumex crispus* Linn.
  (Yellow dock)
- *Rumex acetosella* Linn.
  (Sheep sorrel)
- *Chenopodium album* Linn.
  (Lamb's quarters)
- *Chenopodium ambrosioides* Linn.
  (Mexican tea)
- *Amaranthus palmeri* wats
  (Palmer's amaranth)
- *Amaranthus retroflexus* Linn.
  (Pigweed)
- *Acnida tamariscina* (Nutt) wood
  (Western water hemp.)
- *Salsola kali* Linn. var. *tenuifolia* Mey
  (Russian thistle)
- *Iva xanthifolia* Nutt
  (Marsh elder)
- *Franseria tomentosa* Gray
  (False ragweed)
- *Artemisia ludoviciana* Nutt
  (Western mugwort)
- *Artemisia tridentata* Nutt
  (Sagebrush)

- *Ambrosia species*
  (Ragweed)
- *Kochia scoparia* L.
  (Burning bush)

The genus *Ambrosia* is responsible for approximately 90% of the pollinosis in the United States. The two species that may be found in greatest abundance are the **gaint or great ragweed** (*Ambrosia trifida* L) and the dwarf or **Common ragweed** (*Ambrosia artemisiifolia* Linn.). Although these vary considerably in the height, leaf structure and general habit, their pollens are practically indistinguishable. They range in size from 18–21 μ, are uniformly rounded, are tricolpate and have somewhat spiny exine.

Mold Allergy

Along with pollens from trees, grasses and weeds, molds are an important cause of seasonal rhinitis or non-seasonal hay fever. Mold season often peaks from July to late summer. Unlike pollens, molds may persist after the first killing frost, some can grow at subfreezing temperatures, but most become dormant. After the spring thaw, molds thrive on the vegetation that has been killed by the winter cold in the warmest areas, however, molds thrive all year and can cause year-round (perennial) allergic problems. In addition, molds growing indoors can cause perennial allergic rhinitis even in the coldest climate.

Microscopic fungal spores or sometimes, fragments of fungi may cause **allergic rhinitis** (hay fever). Because they are so small, they (mold spore) may evade the protective mechanisms of the nose and upper respiratory tract to reach the lungs. In some people, symptoms of mold allergy may be brought on or worsened by eating certain foods, such as cheeses, processed with fungi. Occasionally, mushrooms, dried fruits and foods containing yeast, soya, sauce or vinegar, will produce allergic symptoms.

Allergenic molds: Like pollens mold spores are also important airborne allergens, only if they are abundant, easily carried by air currents. Found almost everywhere, mold spore areas are numerous in number ever more than the pollens in the air.

The most common mold genera are *Alternaria*, Macrosporing, *Helminthosporium*, Hormodendrum (*cladusporium*), *Aspergillus*, *Penicillium mucor*, *Rhizopus*, *Syncephalastrum*, *Curvularia*, *Brachysporium* and *Pullularia*. *Alternaria* and *Cladosporium* (Hormodendrum) are the molds most commonly found both indoors and outdoors throughout the United States and in India.

House Dust and Dandruff Allergens

Dust is almost indefinable because it differs from one place to the next; but commonly it composed of mold spores; cotton linters, or fragments of cotton fibres that are light enough to float in the air, animal danders (epithelial scales), cat, dog, guniea pigs, chicken, rabbit, human hair and dandruff, chicken excreta, mice dandruff and house mites, cockroach excreta, odours and perfumes, etc. In-house dust, common allergens are particularly the acarine mite, dermatophagoides and specifically its species *D. pteronyssinus*. About 30% of patients with symptoms of asthma or hay fever are sensitive to disintegrating bits of insect, dust inhaled from air and soil; hence it is not possible to diagnose the sensitivity to dust.

House dust sensitivity differs from pollen allergy in several respects and suspected particularly when the patient's history includes one or more of the following factors:

Perennial symptoms that worsen when the patient remains indoor, increased nocturnal symptoms increased symptoms when performing household chores and increased symptoms associated with turning on/off heating or air conditioning systems.

Dust Mite Allergy

Dust mite allergy is an allergy to a microscopic organism that lives in the dust and is found in all dwellings and work places. Dust mite is perhaps the most common cause of **perennial allergic rhinitis**. It produces symptoms similar to pollen allergy and can produce asthma.

The dust mites appear to be distributed universally and usually found in furnishings stuffed with vegetable fibres (e.g. cotton). It is generally believed that mite allergens are responsible for most dust allergy but there are some peoples who are allergic to dust but not the dust mites as it is not found in some dusts.

Ingestant Allergens

Allergens which are present in foodstuff and swallowed are termed **ingestant** (food allergy). **A food allergy is an immune system response to a food.** Once the immune system decides that a particular food is harmful it creates specific antibody to it.

The gastrointestinal symptoms are mainly effected by the food allergens but they also causes skin rash, puffed lips and tongue, migraine, rhinitis or other symptoms like severe eczema of hand and feet. The effects of food allergens are not localised to one organ or area of the body, but it may transferred to other organs by the blood. Thus, an **atopic dermatitis**, such as tomato rash, strawberry rash, or that caused by eating oranges, chocolate or shellfish, is developed by patients.

Some most common food allergens ingested by patients are:

Milk, egg, peanut, tree nut (walnut, cashew nut, etc.), fish, shellfish, soy, wheat, orange juice, cod liver oil or other vitamins—containing fish liver oils. In addition to the above-mentioned normal food there are food additive, which also could be allergic to any individual, *viz.* mannitol, sorbitol, polysorbates, maltdextrins, citrus, bioflavonoids, artificial preservatives, artificial colours, citrus pectin, talc, soy lecithin, gluten, soy flour, rice flour, alfalfa, potato starch and gum acacia.

Most satisfactory method of combating food allergens is elimination of the offending substance from the diet. Dairy milk allergy is a specific immunologic antibody-antigen reaction due to a lacto-albumin, because heating and boiling alter this protein. Milk allergy may result in severe dermatitis, recurrent rhinorrhea, bronchitis and asthma.

Its antigenicity can be avoided by the use of commercial milk substitutes that are prepared from soya bean isolates.

Injectant Allergens

Injectant allergens causes symptoms similar to those of the antibiotics, e.g. Penicillin, cephalosporin and semi-synthetic penicillin, etc. Itching of the palms of the hands and the soles of the feet, erythema and peeling of the skin are characteristic. In severe cases anaphylactic shock may occur.

OH

OH

R = C-15 aliphatic side chain (Poison oak)
R = C-17 aliphatic side chain
R = May possess 0, 1, 2 or 3 double bands

R

Urushiol

The natural sources of injectable allergens are produced by the sting of bees, hornets and wasps. The allergens injected by the stings of such insects can induce severe local and constitutional reactions sometimes causing death.

In addition to penicillin products, other injectable that may cause allergies are liver extract, antitoxins and the glandular products.

Contactant Allergens

A number of plants and their products have been identified as the causes of contact allergies. The plant most responsible for contact dermatitis in North America belong to the Ancardiaceae family, primarily the genus *Toxicodendron* (Rhus) and include **poison ivy**, **oak** and **sumac**. The allergen component of these plants, called **urushiols** (a phenolic compound) are found in the oleoresin fraction and are derivatives of pentadecylcatechol or heptadecylcatechol. Many plants of Compositae family, which include the ragweeds also cause contact dermatitis and the allergens responsible had been identified as **Sesquiterpenoids lactone**.

Allergen plants are responsible for considerable hazard in USA where **poison ivy** are widespread as a woody vine lacquer used for producing oriental type finish on furniture. Its use causes industrial hazard for the craftsman. Similar type of compounds have been isolated from fruit pulp of *Ginkgo biloba* and from the glandular trichomes of annual *Phacelia* spp. (*Hydro-phyllaceae*) of the Californian Mojave desert. **The dermatitic action of these compound is due to the oxidation of the allergen to quinone, which then bind with protein nucleophiles giving an antigenic complex.**

Another class of chemical compound, **Sesquiterpene lactone** isolated from plants of compositae, lauraceae and magnoliaceae and from Liverwort Frullania (*Jubulaceae*), causes allergic contact dermatitis in the hypersensitive individuals. **The α-methylene group exocyclic to the γ-lactone is the principle immunochemical responsible for the allergic reaction.** Such compound (Pseudoguaianolide) is obtained from the plant *Parthenium hysterophorus*, an aggressive weed causing public health problems in parts of India.

Other plants species, which can give rise to contact allergic reactions are *Ruta graveolens*, asparagus, ornamental "dumb cane" (*Dieffenbachia seguine*), buck wheat, butter cups, catalpa leaves, chrysanthemums, ginkgo leaves, lobelia, marigolds, may-apple, osage orange, flowering spurge, snow on the mountains and smart weeds.

Aeroallergens, such as the various pollen grains containing oils, trichomes from various leaves, flowers and small fragments of plant tissues carried by smoke originating from brush fires, grass fires and burning leaves are also cause for contact (allergens) dermatitis.

A number of plant products used as additives in cosmetics and perfumes are irritants and cause skin allergy to some hypersensitive individuals. These types of allergens are termed **Hypoallergenic Cosmetics**, to denote this fact, the cosmetic manufacturer add the brand names of Ar-ex, Allercreme, Almay and Marcelle are example of hypoallergenic cosmetics.

Certain natural products added to cosmetics such as talcum and perfume are chief source of contact allergy such as orris root, an ingredient to talcum powder.

Dibromofluorescein, commonly used in lipsticks.

Wool fat (lanolin) in cosmetics, soap and soap powders, plain detergents and enzyme detergents, nail polishes, hair dye and hair spray are also included among the major causes of contact dermatitis.

Infectant Allergens

Allergy caused by the metabolic products of living microorganism in the human body. The continual presence of certain types of bacteria, protozoas, molds, helminths and other parasites in the body of human being are responsible for chronic infection for which patients are not aware but metabolic product of their growth causes some patient sensitised and the patient may exhibit allergic symptoms, which does not response positively to routine skin test for inhalant allergens. In such patient bacterial metabolic waste are considered to be infectant allergens.

The continuous presence of growth products and metabolic waste of parasitic organism such as hookworms, tapeworms, pinworms, threadworms and dermatophytes are referred as **infectant allergens**.

ALLERGENIC EXTRACTS

Allergenic extracts are concentrated solutions or suspensions of allergens used for the diagnosis and therapeutic purposes. Extracts are **aqueous** (0.9% Sodium chloride used as diluent) or glycerinated (50% glycerin as diluent). Most preparations are buffered at pH 8 and contain phenol (<0.4%) as an antimicrobial preservative. They are sterilised by aseptic filtration and used as injectable products administered in the physician's office and for many years were prepared by the individual users. Commercial extracts have gradually replaced extemporaneous preparations as number of small speciality companies marketing allergenic extracts several decades ago have today disappeared with merger into larger. Pharmaceutical companies and the several other manufacturers of allergenic extracts are multinational corporations.

The manufacturing of allergenic extracts intended for international export or import must be carried out in licensed laboratories as per the terms and condition laid down by section 351 of the Public Health Services Act.

Preparation

The preparation of allergenic extracts required same general procedure and precautions required with all parenteral products. In addition to the general aseptic condition the extraction process should be carried out in a cold room. The extracts are thermolabile and must be sterilised by aseptic filtration. Sterility test for both aerobic and anaerobic microorganism must be performed in guinea pigs particularly for autogenous extracts where unknown toxic constituents may be present.

In addition to general procedure used for the preparations of other extractives the following is the unique procedure for most allergenic extracts.

Materials

The allergenic substances to be extracted are obtained from commercial suppliers and only the most reliable sources are selected. It should be free from adulteration and should not contain more than 1% of extraneous foreign matter, prompt and proper dehydration is important to prevent alteration of the allergens and prevent microbial contamination.

Grinding

The material to be extracted must be ground or subdivided for the efficient extraction of the allergens. Materials such as hair, feathers and textiles should be divided finely with shears.

Defatting

Many allergenic substances, including all pollens should be defatted before final extraction, ether and petroleum ether are most commonly used for this purpose. It provides clear final extract free from irritants (cotton seed, pepper, mustard and ginger, etc.). This defatted extract can be used in the preparation of some patch testing substances.

Extraction

The extraction procedures are based upon the assumption that allergens are water soluble proteins or glycoproteins. Extraction is carried out normally for 24–72 hours in cold room using sterile, pyrogen free buffered saline, coca's solution or similar aqueous menstrum of pH 8.

Buffered saline

Sodium chloride	5.00 g
Monobasic potassium phosphate	0.36 g
Dibasic sodium phosphate anhydrous	7.00 g
Phenol crystals	4.00 g
Water for injection USP to make 1000 ml	

Cocoa Solution

Sodium chloride	5.0 g
Phenol crystals	5.0 g
Sodium bicarbonate	2.5 g
Water for injection USP to make 1000 ml	

After extraction, mixture is clarified by coarse filtration. Some extracts are dialysed against saline or running tap water to remove irritants or colouring matter (e.g. house dust, mustard, potato, spinach, beets). The processed extract is sterilised by filtration through cellulose membrane filter.

Freeze-dried pollen extracts: These are prepared with the same procedure except water rather than electrolyte solution is used as extracting medium.

Standardisation

Most allergenic extracts carry the statement 'No US standard of potency'. The two most common measures of allergenic potency are weight/volume (w/v) and the Protein Nitrogen Unit (PNU), unit of potency for allergenic extracts. 1 mg protein nitrogen equal 1,00,000 PNU (Table 8.2).

Stability and Storage

The potency of allergenic extracts start reducing within a matter of week or months after their preparation, very dilute solution tend to reduce potency by absorption to the surfaces of containers used for packing but the inclusion of TWEEN 80, TWEEN 20 or human serum albumin reduce this absorption.

Table 8.2: Units of potency for allergenic extracts

Unit	Description	Used
Weight/volume (w/v)	Allergen (g) per volume (mL) of extracting fluid	Worldwide
Protein Nitrogen Unit (PNU)	1 mg protein N = 100,000 PNU	Worldwide
Allergy Unit (AU)	Skin testing to end point	US
Biological Unit (BU)	Skin testing relative to histamine	Europe

All the allergenic extracts should be refrigerated at 2–8°C and freezing should be avoided.

Expiry Date

Aqueous extract	18 months
Glycerinated scratch test and bulk extract	3 years
Lyophilised products	4 year
After reconstitutions	18 month

Pollen extracts

Pollens are the most common cause of atopic disease in most parts of the country, but allergens vary somewhat with the region. Therefore allergen extracts prepared from some of the common pollens (e.g. ragweed, several grasses and tree) have been among the most widely studied and it has been reported that these products are reliable for both diagnosis and in several cases for therapeutic use when properly prepared (Table 8.3).

Dust Extracts

The allergens in house dust are not related to the inorganic dirt from outside but to the products of aging and decompositing materials in and around the house. The dust for commercial extracts generally is obtained from house cleaning or rug cleaning firms and is pooled to get some homogencity.

Dust mites are of more concern, as mites are more responsible for most dust allergy. Standardised extract of Dermatophagoides species are available. The dust mite is

Table 8.3: Pollen extracts

TREES

Acacia	Elderberry	Osage orange
Alder, grey	Elm, American	Palo verde
Almond	Eucalyptus	Peach
Apple	Hackberry	Pear
Apricot	Hazelnut	Pecan
Arbor vitae	Hemlock	Pepper tree
Ash	Hickory	Pine
Bayberry	Hop-hornbeam	Plum
Beech	Ironwood	Poplar
Birch, spring	Juniper	Privet
Birch, white	Locust	Redwood
Bottle brush	Maple	Russian olive
Box elder	Melaleuca	Spruce
Carob tree	Mesquite	Sweet gum
Cedar	Mock orange	Sycamore
Cherry	Mulberry	Tamarack
Chestnut	Oak, white	Tree of heaven
Cottonwood	Olive	Walnut
Cypress	Orange	Willow

GRASSES

Bahia	Corn	Redtop
Barley	Fescue, meadow	Rye grass, perennial
Beach	Grama	Salt
Bent	Johnson	Sorghum
Bermuda grass	June grass	Sudan
Bluegrass, Kentucky	Koeler's	Sweet vernal grass
Brome	Oats	Timothy grass
Bunch	Orchard grass	Velvetgrass
Canarygrass	Quack	Wheat
Chess		Wheatgrass

WEEDS AND GARDEN PLANTS

Alfalfa	Fireweed	Poppy
Amaranth	Gladiolus	Povrtyweed
Aster	Goldenrod	Quailbush
Balsam root	Greasewood	Ragweed, giant
Bassia	Hemp	Ragweed, short
Beach bur	Honeysuckle	Ragweed, western
Broomweed	Hops	Rose
Burrow brush	Iodine Bush	Russian thistle

(Con...)

Table 8.3: Pollen extracts (Con...)

Careless weed	Jerusalem oak	Sagebrush
Castor bean	Kochia	Saltbrush
Chamise	Lamb's quarters	Scale
Clover	Lily	Scotch broom
Cocklebur	Marigold	Sea blight
Coreopsis	Marshelder	Sheep sorrel
Cosmos	Mexican tea	Snapdragon
Daffodil	Mugwort	Sugar beet
Dahlia	Mustard	Sunflower
Daisy	Nettle	Western waterhemp
Dandelion	Pickleweed	Winter fat
Dock	Pigweed	Wormseed
Dog fennel	Plantain, English	Wormwood

distributed universally and is usually found in furnishing stuffed with vegetable fibres (e.g. cotton) (Table 8.4).

Table 8.4: Dust extracts

House dusts	Dust mites
• House	• *D. farniae*
• Mattress	• *D. pteronyssinus*
• Upholstery	• Mite mix
	• Cedar and red cedar
	• Cotton gin
	• Oak
	• Grain elevator
	• Padauk
	• Wood dusts

Fungal Extracts

Fungi are omni present and may be found in the home on textiles, leather goods, upholstered furniture, food and plants. Therapy should include efforts to create mold and fungi free environment. The allergenic extracts are prepared variously from mycellium, medium or both but little know how is available of fungal allergenic extracts preparation method. Some of the fungal and mold allergen extracts available are given in the Table 8.5.

Table 8.5: Fungal extracts

Alternaria	Mucor
Aspergillus	Mycogone
Botrytis	Nigraspora
Cephalosporium	Penicillium
Cephalothecium	Pullularia
Cladosporium	Rhodotorula
Curvularia	Rusts
Epidermophyton	Saccharomyces
Fusarium	Spomdylocladium
Gliocladium	Trichoderma
Helminthosporium	Trichophyton
Hormodendrum	Verticillium
Microsporium	

Insect Extracts

Sensitivity testing and immunotherapy are commonly recommended and employed for the stinging insects. The venom extracts have been shown to be highly effective when properly employed. The list of the standardised extract is given in Table 8.6.

Table 8.6: Standardised extract

INSECT EXTRACTS

Stinging insect: Whole body

- Ant black
- Ant red
- Ant carpenter
- Ant mix (black/red)
- Ant fire

Stinging insect: Venom protein

- Honeybee
- Yellow hornet
- Wasp
- White faced hornet
- Mixed verpid

INHALANT ALLERGY TO INSECT

Blackfly	Horsefly	Spider
Butterfly	Housefly	Sow bugs
Cockroach	Mosquito	Waterfly
Daphnia	Moth	
Fruitfly	Mushroomfly	

Miscellaneous Inhalant Extracts

Miscellaneous allergens are those other than pollen, dust and molds that cause atopic allergies, these includes epidermal from domestic animals (cat, dog and horse). The number of other inhalant allergens is remarkable (Table 8.7).

Table 8.7: Miscellaneous inhalant extracts

MAMMALIAN EPIDERMAL/FEATHERS

Camel	Chicken	Pigeon
Cat hair	Dog	Goose
Cat pelt	Goat	Duck
Deer	Guinea pig	Parakeet
Canary	Hog	

MISCELLANEOUS INHALANT

Acacia	Hemp fibre	Orris root
Algae	Henna	Silk
Cartor bean	Guar gum	Sisal
Cotton seed	Jute	Tobacco leaf
Derris root	Leather	Tragacanth
Grain dust	Lycopodium	Wood dust

FURTHER READING

1. Hallucinogenic Plants: A Golden Guide (pdf) June 15, 2010 https://anthrome.wordpress.com› 2010/06/15›hallucinogenic-plants-a-g.
2. Hallucinogenic Plants: A Golden Guide by Richard Evans Schultes, Elmer W. Smith (Illustrator).
3. Kalia AN. Textbook of Industrial Pharmacogonsy. (2005). CBS Publishers and Distributors, New Delhi.
4. Richard F Keelar. Effects of Natural Teratogens in poisonous plant on Fetal Development in Domestic Animals. Drugs and Fetal Development. 1970:107–25.
5. Schultes RE. 1976. Hallucinogenic plants. Golden Press.
6. Tyler VE, Brady LR, Robbers JE. 1988. Pharmacognosy, 9th Edition-Leo and Fabiger. Philadelphia.
7. Evans WC. 2009. Trease and Evans Pharmacognosy, 16th ed., Elsevier; New York.

Chapter

9

Primary Metabolites

INTRODUCTION

Plants produce two types of metabolites, primary and secondary metabolites.

Primary metabolites involved directly in growth and metabolism, and they are produced by each and every plant irrespective of their genera and family, e.g. carbohydrates, lipids and proteins, etc.

The secondary metabolites are the end products of the primary metabolism not involved in metabolic activity of plants, they are toxic but defensive for the plants. Secondary metabolites are gene specific and not common for all plants, e.g. alkaloids, glycosides, phenolics, steroids and essential oils.

CARBOHYDRATES

Carbohydrtes are the primary plant products biosynthesised by photosynthesis, from water and carbon dioxide in the presence of sunlight. They can be grouped into sugars and polysaccharides.

Sugars

Sugars are water soluble and more or less sweet in taste. They are monosaccharide or oligosaccharides.

Monosaccharide are sugars containing from three to nine carbon atoms, but sugars with five or six carbon atoms (pentose, $C_5H_{10}O_5$ and Hexoses, $C_6H_{12}O_6$) are accumulated in large quantity in plants, e.g. glucose, fructose or oligosaccharides.

Oligosaccharides

Saccharides containing from two to ten units. They are derived from two, three, four to ten monosaccharides molecules, respectively with the elimination of two, three, four to ten molecules of water respectively. They can also be known as di-, tri-, tetra-saccharide or pentasaccharides depending on the numbers of monosaccharides involved in formation. One of the commonest plant di-saccharides is sucrose.

The monosaccharides units in oligosaccharides may be different or same.

Polysaccharides

These are high molecular weight polymers formed by condensation of large number of monosaccharides molecules in a exactly similar manner to the formation of di-, tri- or tetra-saccharides. Each sugar is linked with its neighbour sugar through a glycosidic linkage formed by the theoretical elimination of water molecule between the hemiacetal hydroxyl group C-1 of one sugar molecule with any of the hydroxyl group of other sugar molecule. The hydrolysis of polysaccharide, by enzyme or reagents, breakdown into pentose, hexose or their derivatives.

They are responsible for the rigidity of cell wall in higher plants (cellulose) or the flexibility of the thallus of lower plant (Algae) or as energy storage forms (starch in plants and glycogen in animals). Other substances also occur along with cellulose (primary cell wall) are the hemicelluloses which are also of high molecular weight polysaccharides but are more soluble and easily hydrolysable than cellulose. Closely related to **hemicelluloses** are **gums** and **mucilages**, which are also important group of drugs and pharmaceuticals. **Pectin** is also an another form of polysaccharide associated with cellulose, having pharmaceutical importance.

Chemistry: Chemically carbohydrates are polyhydroxy aldehydes or ketone containing carbon, hydrogen and oxygen. The proportion of hydrogen and oxygen is the same as that is in of water (H_2O). The general formula $(C_nH_{2n}O)_n$ or CH_2O.

The oxidation product is the corresponding carboxylic acid –$COOH$, i.e. oxidation product of glucose is uronic acid and of galactose is galacturonic acid.

Sugars and starch are important product in the economy of mankind. They are used as food and pharmaceuticals.

Identification Test

Molisch test: All the carbohydrates give purple colouration on treatment with molisch reagent (1% alcoholic solution of α naphthol) along with sulphuric acid, poured down on the side of test-tube: in the case of soluble carbohydrates a deep violet colouration is produced where the liquids meet, in the case of insoluble carbohydrates (cellulose) colour will appears on shaking the test mixture.

Sulphuric acid test: Heat small quantity (0.2 g) of carbohydrates with 1 ml of concentrated sulphuric acid (H_2SO_4)on a small flame, immediate blackening will take place.

Action with sodium hydroxide: Boil a small quantity of (0.2 g) of carbohydrates with about 5 ml of 10% (w/v) sodium hydroxide solution (NaOH); the solution turns yellow, then brown and emits the caramel smell with soluble carbohydrates but insoluble carbohydrates will not give colouration.

Fehling solution test: Add 5 ml of carbohydrate solution to 5 ml of freshly prepared fehling solution (Fehling solution A & B in equal quantity) and boil. Reduction will take place with the formation of red colour precipitate of cuperous oxide with reducing sugars. while non reducing carbohydrates (sucrose and polysaccharides) will appear on hydrolysis as on hydrolysis non-reducing sugar will be converted into reducing sugars but precaution to be taken to neutralise the any acid used for hydrolysis before adding fehling solution.

Resorcinol test for ketones: Carbohydrates solution with equal volume of concentrated sulphuric acid heated on water bath in the presence of resorcinol crystal. Appearance of rose-red colour show the presence of ketones, e.g. fructose and honey.

Test for pentose: Solution of carbohydrate with equal volume of hydrochloric acid and phloro-glucinol is heated on water bath, appearance of red colour indicate the pentose sugar, e.g. D-ribose, D-arabinose, D-xylose and xylulose.

ACACIA GUM

Source: Dried gummy exudates obtained from the stem and branches of *Acacia senegal* Linn; and other species of *Acacia*, family Leguminosae.

It is commonly known as gum Arabic.

Geographical source: Sudan, central and west Africa (chiefly Senegal) and Nigeria.

Method of preparation: Most of the official drug comes from cultivated tree in Kordofan (Sudan).

Collection: Gum is collected from 6 to 7 year old tree after the rainy season till the next year rains. Lower branches from the tree are removed at the time of leaves wilting and falling down. The trees are trapped by making transverse cut in the bark with sharp axe, avoiding damage to the cambium and xylem. A strip about 1.5 to 2.5 feet long and 2 to 3 inches in breadth is removed. Gum start exudating immediately in hot weather while in cold weather it is slow in exudation. On exudation gum solidify in the form of tears and remained adhere to the tree. The tears are removed after 2 to 3 weeks of trapping, sbsequently transferred to grading house where they are graded, cleaned and bleached.

Cleaning means picking by hand and removal of adherent fragments of bark followed by shifting of tears.

Bleaching: The tears are spread in thin layers on canvas and exposed to sunlight for two to three weeks; during this process small cracks developed on the outer surface of the tears and make them opaque in appearance. Whereas, the unbleached tears are glassy in appearance and termed **natural** ungraded gum containing all sorts of tears and fragments is called **sorts**. Graded tears are packed in jute bags and marketed.

Chemistry: Raw gum contain 10 to 15% water, some tannins (in coloured gum only), oxidase enzyme but no starch. The chief constituents of gum acacia mainly consists of arabin (Acidic polysaccharide) which is complex mixture of calcium, and to less extent, of magnesium and potassium salt of arabic acid. Which on hydrolysis with dilute sulphuric acid gives sugars [l-rhamnose (18%), d-galactose (32%), l-arabinose (38%)] and d-glucuronic acid. The uronic acid residue represent about 18% of the gum. Peroxidase and carboxydase (oxidase enzymes) are also present.

Evaluation: The **good** quality gum is almost colourless translucent and striated. The medium grade has marked pinkish tingue, while lower grade of gums are dark and having few fragments of bark.

B.P. requirement include limit of insoluble matter and loss on drying not more than 15%. It should be free from tragacanth and starch.

Ash value between 2.7 and 4%. **Taste**—blanded. **Fracture**—Freshly fractured surface is glassy and odourless, otherwise tears are opaque or pale-yellow colour.

Chemical test: Solubility test: It is almost completely soluble in equal weight of water the solution is slightly viscous and mucilaginous, pH slightly acidic in cold water solution but in hot water acidity increases, on dilution with water no sedimentation on standing. Solution is levorotatory.

Test for the **absence of tragacanth** and **agar:** Aqueous solution (10% w/v), of gum acacia do not give precipitation with dilute solution of lead acetate.

Test for the absence of starch and dextrin: Ten percent aqueous solution of gum acacia do not give blue or red colour with weak iodine solution.

Peroxidase enzyme: Blue colour with benzidine solution.

Sucrose and fructose: Aqueous solution (10% w/v) do not give any colour with chlorohydric resorcinol (resorcinol-hydrochloric acid).

Absence of tannins: No blue colour with ferric chloride solution.

Uses: It is used as suspending agents and binding agent in pharmaceutical formulations. It is compatible with other plants hydrocolloids.

Indian Gum or Ghati Gum

It is used as a substitute of gum acacia. It is obtained from *Anogeissus latifolia* Wall, family Combretaceae.

This gum is viscous exudates of wild forest tree of India and Sri Lanka. Its tears are vermiform and show fewer cracks even less than gum acacia.

It is a complex polysaccharide which contains d-mannose, d-galactose, l-arabinose, d-xylose, d-glucuronic acid. It very often contains tannins

Water produce more viscous solution hence used as emulsifier and stabiliser.

Solubility—Approximately 90% of the product is water soluble.

Purity Tests

Borax test: Aqueous solution of gum acacia (10 g in 15 ml of water) should be translucent but not glairy. To 5 ml this solution add 0.1 g of borax (in solution form) stiff translucent mass will form with acacia gum and Indian gum but not with tragacanth.

Lead sub-acetate test: To dilute solution of mucilage (1 : 4 dilution) add few drops of lead sub-acetate solution.

Acacia gum will give thick precipitate; Indian gum and Tragacanth mucilage will yield only slight precipitate.

Test for oxidase enzyme: To 5 ml of mucilage add few drops of 1% solution of guaiacum resin in alcohol.

Acacia gum mucilage will show blue colour, similar colour develop in Indian gum mucilage however no colouration in tragacanth mucilage.

TRAGACANTH

Biological source: It is dried gummy exudates obtained by incision from the trunk and branches of *Astragalus gumifer* Lbill, family Fabaceae (Leguminoseae) and other species of Asiatic *Astragalus*; *A. kurdicus* Bioss, *A. gossypius* and more. The better grade tragacanth known as Persian Tragacanth.

Geographical source: More than 2000 species are known but gum produce from thorny subshrub found at the height of 2000 to 3000 M in the mountaneous district of Anatolia, Syria, Iran, Iraq and USSR.

Peparation: A transverse incision is given at the base of the stem of a two years, old plant with sharp knife having a thin cutting edge; a wedge-shaped wooden piece inserted into the injured trunk to keep the wound open, after 24 hours wooden piece is removed gum start exuding with force (gum produced by gummosis process).

Fresh gum is white in colour but on exposure to air, water gets evaporated and it gradually harden and change in colour, the shape of the gum depends upon the incision, The gum exuding from the natural injury is of worm like and twisted into coil known as Vermiform tragacanth of ¾ inch in length.

To increase the yield of exudates, in some countries, plant are burnt at the top after having injury/incision, the quantity of the yield may be increased but quality of the product is poor therefore this process is not followed by many of the countries.

Description: The official Persian Tragacanth is odourless, tasteless, flattened white ribbon-shaped, about 25 mm long and 12 mm wide and 1 mm thick, horny with transverse striation on the surface (indicate the stoppage of flow). Microscopically, the powder dug shows the presence of rounded starch granules (4.5 to 10 μm) with central hilum.

Commercially tragacanth is available in number of grades; No. 1: colourless flate ribbons; No. 2 White flat ribbons; No. 3 Light cream curly ribbons; No. 4 Cream coloured flat ribbons; No. 5 Pinkish coloured ribbons. As the colour darkens grade No. increases, as ambered-coloured are graded as No. 28 whereas reddish brown coloured ribbons are graded No. 55, etc. the good quality form the official drug while the lower grades are used as food, laxative and for industrial purposes.

Chemistry: Gum tragacanth is cosidered to be a mixture of two polysaccharides (**tragacanthin** and **bassorin**), starch (3%) and about 3 to 4% minerals but does not contain oxidases enzymes. **Tragacanthin** is neutral and soluble in water and alcohol mixture and dissolve in water to form colloidal solution. The **bassorin** part is acidic, incompatible with ethyl alcohol but swells in the presence of water to form gel (60 to 70%).

Tragacanthin is a demethoxylated bassorin; about 30% of the gum is an arabinogalactan and have galactose backbone; the **bassorin** (tragacanthic acid) on the other hand cemically is partially methylated glycano galacturonan built from four monosaccharides: D-galacturonic acid, D-galactose, D-xylose and l-fucose. The central backbone of the molecule is chain of 1,4-linked galacturonic acid; the chain is substituted by disaccharides (fructoxylose or galactoxylose).

The Persian Tragacanth contains traces of starch while the unofficial grade contain more starch and give blue colour with weak iodine solution. Tragacanth hydrocolloid is resistant to acid hydrolysis hence preffered for use in highly acidic conditions.

BP limit foreign matter to 1.0% and microbial limit test.

Storage: To be stored in cool and dark room, protected from microbial contamination.

Uses: In pharmaceutical formulation as suspending agent. In cosmetics as a demulscent and an emollient. Dilute solution (0.5 to 1.5%) of tragacanth is very viscous and stable in acid pH and heat, compatible with most plant hydrocolloids, and easy to conserve hence good stabiliser for suspension and as emulsion. It is also used in textile industry in cloth printing and in confectionary.

Identification Tests for Tragacanth

Solubility test: Tragacanth is partially soluble in water (distinction from acacia and agar).

Mucilage formation: It forms mucilage with water (1 : 20 H_2O) on boiling.

Iodine solution test: On boiling with strong solution of iodine tragacanth develops green colour.

Ferric chloride solution test (10 %w/v): Deep yellow colour precipitate will appear.

Lead acetate solution test: Tragacanth solution will give heavy precipitate with strong solution of lead acetate.

Alcoholic potash solution test: On warming the solution of tragacanth with alcoholic potash solution will produce canary yellow colour.

Ruthenium red solution test (0.1% w/v): No pink stain will be developed with the ruthenium red solution.

Test for reducing sugar: Hydrolyse the tragacanth solution (4 ml) with hydrochloric acid (1 ml), on heating at water bath for an half hour. Divide the hydrolysed mixture into two portion.

To one portion add 1.5 ml of sodium hydroxide (NaOH) to neutralise solution, followed by the addition of Fehling solution 3 ml and heated on water bath—appearance of red coloured precipitate indicate the presence of sugar.

The second portion add a few ml of barium chloride solution—no precipitate formation distinct it from Agar.

AGAR

Agar is the dried gelatinous substances obtained from decoction concentrates of *Gelidium cartilagineum* (Linn) Gaillon, family Gelidiaceae and other species of Gelidiaceae.

It is also refered to as Japanese isinglass obtained from *Gelidium amansii* spp. and related red algae (class Rhodophyceae).

Geographical Source: Most of the commercial supply comes from Korea, South Africa, both Atlantic and Pacific coasts of USA, Spain, Mexico and New Zealand.

Method of preparation

Method of preparation is divided into four steps:
1. Collection of algae (seaweeds)
2. Cleaning of seaweeds
3. Bleaching
4. Conversion to strips.

Collection of algae (seaweed): Collection is done from two sources; cultivated and natural source, grown on rocks in shallow water. Cultivation carried out in special areas by planting poles in the sea as support for the development of seaweed, poles being withdrawn and algae stripped off.

From the shallow water algae is collected by using small boats either by diving or by using long handeled rackes, collection is done in summer.

Cleaning: The collected algae is taken to sea-beach, dried in sun, shaken to remove dust, sand and shell, etc. adhered; bleached partially by washing and exposure to sun.

Bleaching: Partially bleached algae spread on loosely made bamboo tray or plateform, and exposed to sun, during the process it is being washed from time to time during exposure until it is almost colourless.

Extraction

Extraction of algae is obtained by decoction process. It is carried on in winter season in two steps.

First step decoction is done by boiling the bleached algae in acidified water (1 : 60) in kettles for several hours to get viscid product, while it is hot passed through coarse strainer to remove the undissolved material and then by reheating, it is passed through Linen bags into trays, allowed to cool and set to form jelly followed by cutting into bars.

Strips formation: The bars (jelly) are then forced through wire netting to form strips, which are subsequently dried by freezing, thawing and drying at 35°C.

Description: It occurs usually as bundles consisting of thin membranous agglutinated strips or as a coarse granulated powder or flakes. Indian agar occurs as thin transparent membranous pieces or as yellowish white powder.

Colour—yellowish white to greyish to colourless. **Solubility**—swell in cold water but spairingly soluble in water. It is soluble in hot water (1 : 60) and on cooling form stiff jelly. **Taste** is mucilaginous; **odour**—odourless to slightly odourous.

Fracture: It is tough when damp, brittle when dry.

Chemistry: It consists chiefly of calcium salt of sulphuric acid, mixture of complex carbohydrate and the magnesium salt may also be present. The primary carbohydrate consist of alternating 1,3-linked d-galactopyranosyl and 3,6-anhydro-l-galactopyranosyl. The carbohydrate consists of long chain of d-galactopyranose which on acid hydrolysis (dilute hydrochloric acid) produce galactose and sulphate ion and thus reduce the fehling solution; the sulphate ion gives white precipitate with barium chloride solution.

This complex polysaccharide consist of two major fractions **agarose** and **agropectin**. The agarose is responsible for gel strength of agar while **agropectin** is responsible for the viscosity of solution.

Uses: As a laxative, a culture media for bio-technology experiment, a pharmaceutical aids in the form of emulsifying, suspending and gelating agent. It is also used as a surgical lubricant, in food processing and other industrial processing.

Identification tests

1. Agar is non-nitrogenous hence show negative test for gelatin and ammonia:
   a. 0.2% aqueous solution of agar do not give precipitate with tannic acid
   b. On heating with soda lime no ammonia evolved.

2. Fehling solution reduction test.
3. Test for starch.
   Moisten the powdered drug with weak solution (N/50) of iodine, deep crimson colour is produced which distinguish agar from acacia and tragacanth.
4. *Test for sulphate ion*: To about 5 ml of 0.5% aqueous solution of agar add 0.5 ml of hydrochloric acid and heat on water bath for 30 minutes, on cooling add few drops of barium chloride solution, a slight white coloured precipitate produced. This test differentiate agar from tragacanth.
5. *Test for the presence of sponge spicules*: Boil about 1 g of agar with 10 ml of acidified (hydrochloric acid) water for 10 minutes. Cool and centrifuge the mixture, decant and observe the deposit under microscope, sand particles, diatom and **sponge spicules** will appear.
6. *Acid soluble ash*: Ash treated with dilute hydrochloric acid, observe under micro-scope for **diatoms**.

HONEY

It is saccharine secretion of flower nectar, deposited in honeycomb by worker bees (*Apis melifera* Linn), family Apidae.

Geographical source: Honey is produced in England but main suppliers are West Indies, New Zealand, California, and various parts of Africa and Australia.

Method of preparation: The worker bee collect the nectar from the surrounding flowers which contains mainly sucrose, store into honey sac where it is converted into invert sugar by invertase enzyme present in saliva of honeybee; on reaching to hive the bee bring back the contents of the sac into storage cell of honeycomb.

Honey is removed from the comb by first removing the wax cap followed by pressing or by centrifuging, however the best quality of honey is obtained by draining.

Purification: The collected honey is heated on water bath; the layer of wax and other impurities rises to the surface; which are skimmed off from the surface and the purified honey is strained. International standard for strainer is mesh size not smaller than 0.2 mm which will keep pollen in the honey but will remove all the other impurities.

Moisture contents

Water content less than 20 g/100 g. The European Union accept maximum limit of water 21 g/100 g.

Acidity: 50 milliequivalent/kg.

Proline contents: 180 mg/kg is the indicator of ripen honey and for sugar adulteration.

Invertase activity: This is the indicator of freshness as the fresh and unheated honey should have invertase number more than 10.

Specific sugar contents: The general standard of minimum contents of sum of fructose and glucose is 60 g/100 g for all blossom honey (nectar honey), and 45 g/100 g for all honey-dew honey but the sucrose content is 5 g/100 g.

Hydroxymethyl furfural contents (HMF)

HMF contents icreases on storage in warm climate the European standard (EU) demand for maximum 40 mg HMF/kg.

Diastase activity: It is also indicator of freshness as activity decreases on storage as per EU standard is 8.

Water insoluble solid contents: EU standard is 0.005 to 0.5 g/100 g.

Chemistry: Honey mainly consists of invert sugar, water and other components in small quantities are sucrose, dextrin, formic acid, protein, volatile oil, pollen grains and waxes.

The protein content of floral honey is about 1–1.5%, while in honeydew honey is about 3%. The amount of amino acid is 1% and proline is the major component, about 50–85%.

Description: Fresh honey is a clear syrupy liquid pale-yellow to reddish-brown colour, the odour depends upon source of nectar; on storage it tends to crystallise and appearance of granular mass.

Uses: Honey is used as nutrient and sweetener traditionally being used as demulscent in cough preparation. It is also used in many folklore remedies.

Adulterants: Synthetic invert sugar.

Commercially, it is prepared by the treatment of mineral acid with sucrose.

Sucrose added in the form of syrup.

Identification test—fehling solution test for reducing sugar: Dissolve 0.5 g of honey in 10 ml of water, add Fehling solution (A & B) heated on water-bath. Reddish-brown precipitate indicates the presence of reducing sugar.

Presence of invert sugar: To 10 ml of honey add 5 ml of ether and mix by sterring, allowed to separate ether layer, pour the ether to porcelain and evaporated to dryness, to the leftover residue add 1% solution of resorcinol in hydrochloric acid. A faint pinkish colour, fading within seconds but not persistant cherry reddish colour. This red colour is due to the presence of methoxyfurfuraldehyde. This test is known as **Fiehe's test**.

PROTEINS AND ENZYMES

GELATIN

Biological source: Gelatin is gel-forming protein obtained from partial hydrolysis of collagen derived from skin, bones and connective tissue of animals.

Commercial gelatin is obtained from suitable by-products of slaughtered cattles, sheep and hog (cowhide, cattle bones pork skin and scales).

Method of preparation: It is prepared by boiling the animal tissues (skin, collagen and bones) with water and filter but preliminary stage varies with nature of raw material.

Bones as raw material: Bones are made free from fatty materials by treating with organic solvent followed by decalcification by treating with hydrochloric acid; the material is then extracted with boiling water and steam under pressure until the collagen is partially hydrolysed and converted to gelatin in solution. The solution is decolourised and filter by electro-osmosis, concentrated under reduced pressure to 45% gelatin contents, allowed to gel and dry over metting or in shallow trays in current of warm air (40–60°C).

Description: Gelatin occurs as flakes, sheets, shreds or as a coarse or fine powder. It is colourless to faint yellow or ambered coloured, translucent having characteristic odour and taste. It is insoluble in cold water but gradually swell and soften by absorbing 5–10 times its weight of water. It dissolves on heating and 2% solution form jelly on cooling.

It is stable when dried but its gelling power is reduced on prolonged heating.

Evaluation: Quality of gelatin evaluated by its jelling strength which can be measured by an instrument known as Bloom Gelometer (BP).

Types: Commercially gelatin is of two types, A and B. Both have different isoelectric point. **Type A** has pH between 7 and 9. Therefore, it is incompatible with tragacanth and agar.

Type B exhibits isoelectric point pH between 4.7 to 5 and is compatible with anionic compounds hence useful in such mixtures.

The principle nitrogenous compound responsible for swelling in cold water but do not dissolve is known as **glutin** (protein) and hence gives the test of protein.

Chemistry: Gelatin consists of number of amino acids including high proportion of lysine but do not contain tryptophan, therefore, it is incomplete nutritional protein.

The gelatin prepared from cartilages contain **chondrin**, the gelatinising power of chondrin less than that of gelatin and the jelly prepared is less tenacious, therefore, the official gelatin should not contain chondrin.

Uses: Gelatin is a pharmaceutical aid as suspending, encapsulating, tablet binder and coating and in pastilles and sponge. High grade gelatin (with blooming strength) is used for making capsule body and also for bacteriological medium. Zinc gelatin is used as topical protectant, it is also being used in many food products.

Chemical test for identification: Gelatin solution is prepared by dissolving 0.2 g of gelatin in 40 ml of hot water to perform the following chemical test:

Tannic acid test: Take 2 to 3 ml of gelatin solution, add few drops of 10% solution of tannic acid white to pale yellow to pale buff coloured precipitate appear, which do not dissolve on warming.

Millon's reagent test: Add few drops of Millon's reagent to the 5 ml of gelatin solution, white precipitate forms which turn red on heating (protein).

Trinitrophenol test: To 5 ml of gelatin solution add trinitrophenol saturated solution in excess yellow-coloured precipitate formed—this test differentiate gelatin from agar.

Ammonia test: Heat the gelatin powder in a dry test tube with soda lime, ammonia vapour will evolve with the decomposition of gelatin.

Absence of chondrin: Heat the gelatin with acetic acid, gelatin powder will be completely soluble excluding chondrin if present.

Standard: As per British pharmacopeia gelatin should pass the limit test for arsenic, copper, lead, zinc, sulphur oxide ash and loss on drying. Blooming strength (150–250 g).

CASEIN

Caseins are the primary group of milk protein. Casein from bovine milk is a phosphoprotein. There are four types of caseins which makes up approximately 80% of total protein in bovine milk, S1 casein, S2 casein, β-casein and K-casein, all these different types are distinct molecule but similar in structure.

All other protein of the milk are grouped together under the name of whey proteins. The major **whey** protein in cow milk are β-lactoglobulin and β-lactoalbumin.

Casein and other major proteins are biosynthesised by mammary glands.

Casein is composed of several amino acids, important for the growth and development of the nursing young. This high quality protein in cow milk is one of the major reasons for an important human food.

It is a mixture of several similar proteins in the form of casein micelle. These micelles in addition to casein molecules also contain water, calcium and phosphorus salts and some enzymes.

The micelle structure of casein makes the casein digestible in stomach and intestine and best for milk products.

The individual molecule of caseine is insoluble in aqueous media, therefore if the micelle structure is disturbed the caseine will be precipitated forming gelatinous mass of curd and cheese.

Preparation: The milk is made free from fat (removal of cream) by low speed centrifugation (5000 to 10000 g) resulting the separation of cream at the top, the aqueous supernatant is decanted off carefully form the debris and then subjected to ultracentrifugation (usually about 50,000 g or greater) resulting in pelleting of casein and supernatant whey protein, (serum plasma). Thereafter the casein is separated leaving behind whey protein.

Or milk is to be acidified with hydrochloric acid (0.1 N) to pH 4.6 at 20°C, the casein will gradually form precipitate, whereas, the whey protein remains soluble at pH 4.6 after the precipitation of casein.

Cow milk contains approximately 82% casein as milk protein (36%) and remaining 18% is plasma.

Cow milk contain about 5% casein

Buffalo contain about 3.8% casein

Goat milk contain about 3.25% casein

Uses: Protein supplement, sustained supply of amino acids, and is an ideal protein supplement to sustain long periods of an anabolic environment to muscle growth.

PROTEOLYTIC ENZYMES

Enzymes are organic catalyst synthesised by living organism. They are protein in nature, having molecular weight range from 13000 to 840,000. They have different chemical structure but have several common properties.

1. They are colloid and soluble in water and dilute alcohol but are precipitated by concentrated alcohol.
2. They all are active at temperature between 35°C and 40°C, but at higher temperature (65°C and above) in the presence of moisture they completely decomposed.

3. They are very much sensitive to pH.
4. Their activity is retarded by heavy metals, formaldehyde, and iodine.

Classification: They are classified into six major classes on the basis of their action.

a. **Oxidoreductases:** Catalyse oxidoreductions reaction between two substances.

b. **Hydrolases:** Catalyse hydrolysis of ester, ether, peptide, glycosyl acid C—C, C—halide, and P—N bonds.

c. **Transferases:** Catalyses the transfer of a groups other than hydrogen between pairs of substances.

d. **Lyases:** Catalyse the removal of group from substances by mechanism other than hydrolysis, leaving double bonds.

e. **Isomerases:** Catalyses the interconversion of optic, geometric and positional isomer.

f. **Ligases:** Catalyses the linkage of two compounds coupled to the breaking pyrophosphate bond in ATP.

Another nomenclature which is uniform for enzyme is based on the name of substrate and the termination 'ase' the classes of enzyme were named similarly, e.g. 'esterase' which include lipase which hydrolyse fats.

Esterase: Include lipase, phospholipase and acetylcholinesterase.

Carbohydrases: Include diastase, lactase, maltase, invertase, cellulase, etc.

Nucleases: Ribonuclease, deoxyribonuclease, nucleophosphatase.

Nuclein deaminase: Include adenase, adenosine, deaminase and others such as amidases arginase, urease, etc.

Proteolytic enzymes examples: Pepsin, trypsin, chymotrypsine, papain, fibrinolysin, streptokinase, urokinase, etc. These enzymes act on peptide linkage thus hydrolysing the C-N linkage.

Papain

It is dried and purified latex obtained from the unripe fruit of *Carica papaya* Linn, family Caricaceae.

Geographical source: Papaya tree is indigenous to tropical America and cultivated in Sri Lanka, Tanzania, Hawaii and Florida.

Preparation: Fully grown healthy unripe fruits are selected, all the four sides of the epicarp of the fruit are incised, white coloured latex start flowing freely for few seconds and gets coagulated very soon after exuding, after one week interval the lumps of coagulated latex is collected, are shredded and dried in artificial heat at 40–60°C known as crude papain.

Purification of crude papain: Crude papain is dissolved in water and precipitated with alcohol, filtered and dried known as **vegetable pepsin** because it also contain enzyme similar to pepsin but the enzyme papain can work in acid, neutral or alkaline media.

Character: It is white to light brown, amorphous or slightly granular powder with characteristic odour; sparingly soluble in water and insoluble in alcohol, chloroform and ether.

Chemsitry: It is mixture of enzymes but the major one is peptidase (proteolytic) able to breakdown protein into peptides (di- and poly-peptides) and to digest, other enzymes are renin-like; casein coagulating enzyme and enzyme similar to pectase (Amylolytic enzyme) and an enzyme that has feeble activity on fat.

Papain can digest about 35 times of its own weight of lean meat because of this properties it is being used as meat tenderiser; it can also digest egg albumin to about 300 times its own weight.

Storage: To be kept stored in air tight light resistant container in cool and dry place.

Uses: Used as a protein digestant, in meat packing industry; therapeutically to relieve the symptom of episiotomy.

Standard: It should be free from *Escherichia coli* (*E. coli*), and Salmonellae. Loss on drying should not be more than 7%, on drying 1 g of papain in hot air oven at 60°C.

Assay I.P. 1996.

Weigh accurately about 0.5 g of papain, triturate with 10 ml of cysteine hydrochloride solution and dilute to 100 ml with water, Pour 30 ml each of this solution to two flask separately followed by the addition of 15 ml casein solution and maintained at 60°C over water bath. To the first flask add 5 ml of solution to be tested and in the second flask same amount of the same solution but previously boiled for 2 minutes and cooled. Maintain the solution at 60°C for 30 minutes and cool rapidly at room temperature and add to each flask 0.75 ml of phenolphthalein and 10 ml formaldehyde solution previously neutralised to phenolphthalein solution, titrate with 0.1 M sodium hydroxide to similar definite pink colour, the difference between the two titration is not less than 4.5 ml.

Bromelain

It is protein digesting and milk-clotting proteolytic enzyme obtained from the juice of pineapple *Ananas comosus* Linn Family Bromeliaceae.

Brief history: Bromelain was first isolated from pineapple juice in 1891 and introduced as therapeutic supplement in 1957, the active ingredient, bromelain is found in juice and stem of the pineapple but stem contain more bromelain than the fruit.

Preparation: First step healthy pineapple fruits are collected, cleaned by washing with water to make it free from debris, crushed into pieces and prepare the paste with sodium acetate buffer, separate the extract by filtration followed by centrifugation at 600 rpm for 10 minutes; decant the supernatant (crude extract).

Purification: Purification of the extract is done by means of precipitation with ammonium sulphate, to 1000 ml of the crude extract add 4.4 g of ammonium sulphate at 4°C for 45 minutes to one hour, then kept at 4°C for overnight incubation. Next day centrifuge the extract at 10,000 rpm for 10 minutes. Discard the supernatant and to the residue add 10 ml tris hydrochloric acid followed by further purification by dialysis or by ion-exchange chromatography.

Preparation of bromelain from fruit peel: Cleaned peel of the fruit is crushed and ground in a juicer with water or buffer, filter and centrifuge at 8000 g at 4°C for 30 minutes. The supernatant cooled at 4°C and precipitated the protein with ammonium sulphate (40 to 80%) saturated solution, the solution to be added slowly with constant agitation; after the complete addition of salt continue the stirring at 4°C for half an hour, allow to stand for overnight, centrifuge at 8000 g at 4°C for 15 minutes, then discard the supernatant and dissolve the precipitate in minimum volume of 25 nm[1] potassium sulphate buffer at pH 7, it is to be desalted on gel-filteration column, frozen in liquid nitrogen and lyophilised. Purification to be done by ion exchange chromatography.

Uses: Used as analgesic in arthritis patient and reduce the swelling. Anticoagulant, to reduce the clumping of platelets in arteries, brain, and thus help in the treatment of cardiovascular disease.

Antiasthmatic: By reducing the mucous formation and in hay fever.

Analgesic: Reduce the painful symptoms of varicose vein.

Anticlotting: It is employed in the production of protein hydrolysates.

Meat tenderiser and in leather industry.

Pepsin

Pepsin is bio-synthesised and secreated in the gastric membrane in an inactive form called **pepsinogen** (PG) molecular weight 40 K Da. It contain about 44 amino acids and stable in neutral and weak alkaline environments. On exposure to hydrochloric acid (pH 1.5 to 2.0) the 44 amino acids are proteolytically removed in an autocatalytic way to activate it to pepsin.

Main role in protein protolysis is to cleave aromatic amino acid (phenylalanine and tyrosine) from the N-terminus of protein.

Pepsin is an important **acidic protease**, widly applied in the hydrolysis of protein.

It has been isolated from various mammals including human, Japanese Monkey, bovine, goat, rat and rabbit. It can also be removed from fish waste especially fish viscera constituting 5% of fish waste.

Official source: Pepsin is obtained from the grandular layer of fresh stomach of the hog; *Sus scrofa* Linn Var. *domestica* Gray.

Family: Suidae

Preparation: Prepared stomach is minced and digested with Tris hydrochloric acid, cleaned by centrifugation at 40°C, partially evaporated, dialysed, concentrated or poured on glass plate to dry.

Characters: It is available as scales or granular powder or spongy mass. **Colour**—cream coloured amorphous powder or light yellow to light brown colour powder or translucent scales; **Odour**—odourless; **Taste**—slightly acidic.

Uses: Industrial application of pepsin:
 Collagen extraction
 Medical research
 Cheese making
 Fish processing
 Fish silage.

Collagen extraction: Conventionally collagen is extracted by an acid solubilisation process (acetic acid), since pepsin can breakdown cross linkage in the telopeptide region of collagen without harming the secondary structure, thus enhance the yield of collagen from 5.30 to 8.40% from skin.

Medical research: Pepsin is used in the regulation of digestion, as a dental antiseptic and in the treatment of **dyspepsia, gastralgia. Obstinate vomiting, infantile diarrhoea,** apepsia and in some cancer.

Pepsin hydrochloride combination in the form of tablet and capsules are used in digestion improvement as well as appetiser. Pepsine from porcine stomach along with bismuth complex are used to heal stomach ulcer. In animal feed to enhance the digestibility of protein.

Cheese making: Tuna pepsin is effective as rennet in cheese production at pH range from 5.5 to 6.5.

Fish processing: Cod pepsin is used in de skinning of herring and used to descale hake and haddock under weak acidic conditions.

Fish silage (liquified product of minced fish): Pepsin play major role among all enzymes in preparation of silage.

Streptokinase (Fibrinolytic Enzyme)

Fibrinolytic enzymes are one of the largest group of proteolytic enzymes involved in number of regulatory process related to fibrinolytic action.

It is an extracellular protein (fibrinolytic enzyme), extracted from strains of β- haemolytic *Streptococcus*. It is non-protease plasminogen activator that activate plasminogen to plasmin enzyme which degrade the fibrin clots, through its specific lysine binding site.

Bacillus **genus** is well known producer of potent fibrinolytic enzymes like **streptokinase, urokinase, nattokinase,** etc. oral administration of **urokinase** and **nattokinase** can enhance fibrinolytic activity in plasma and the production of plasminogen activator type tissues.

Streptokinase has molecular mass 47 KDa and is made-up off 414 amino acids residue; protein exhibit maximum activity at pH 7.5 and isoelectric pH is 4.7. It is produced by different group of **streptococci.**

Note: *All streptokinase producing streptococci are pathogenic hence special attention is required for biosafety.*

Preparation

Culture media used for the growth of bacteria should be maintained at pH 7.0 during the incubation at 37°C for 8 hours by adding 4% glucose and 5 N NaOH. The crude enzyme produced on incubation at 37°C for 24 hours is separated. Secreted enzyme is separated by centrifugation at 8000 to 10,000 g rpm for 10 to 15 minutes. The supernatant containing crude enzyme is purified by precipitation with ammonium sulphate salt. After complete precipitation the clear solution of upper layer is discarded and lower layer precipitate (colloidal solution) re-centrifuged for another 10 to 15 minutes followed by removal of clear supernatant and pellet to be suspended in 0.1 M tris hydrochloric acid (HCl) buffer (pH 7.0).

Purification: The precipitate are desalted by dialysis followed by standard protocol, further purification is done by column chromatography using sephadex-G100 as adsorbent and 0.1 M tris HCl buffer as a solvent.

Standardisation: Analysis is done for the thrombolytic activity by means of streptokinase enzyme assay method.

Uses: It is used as a therapeutic agent in the treatment of thromboembolic blockage including coronary thrombosis.

Storage: To be stored at cool place at 4°C in a dark place away from light.

Urokinase

Urokinase is a **serine protease,** which specifically cleaves the proenzyme/zymogen plasminogen to form active enzyme plasmin which degrade (breakdown) the fibrin polymers of blood clots.

Source: Commercial scale source of urokinase enzyme is human urine produced by kidney cells but it is very difficult to isolate and purify from human urine being present in traces (10 to 15 µg/ml therefore in these days produced by *in vitro* cultivation by using kidney cells culture. This enzyme is of glycoprotein in nature and is a mixture of A and B enzymes having different molucular weight.

Preparation: Human kidney cell line HT1080 are available from NCCS, Pune, India.

Human kidney cells are cultured in DMEM containing 10%. Newborn calf serum (NBCS), Dulbecco's modified eagle media (DMEM), the enzyme produced is separated by centrifugation and purification done by precipitation with ammonium sulphate salt method and further purification being done by chromatography (ion-exchange chromatography method).

Standardisation: Standardisation is done by means of enzyme assay method to determine the amidolytic activity.

Isolation and Purification of Urokinase from Human Urine

Step 1: Prepare slurry of human male urine at pH 3.0 to 6.0 with non-reactive insoluble mineral adsorbent (bentonite, silicon dioxide, kaolin and titanium dioxide) having high surface area.

Step 2: The urokinase adsorbate is separated by centrifugation and extracted with hdroxy methyl amino methane buffer solution which will contain 99% of urokinase in urine. The pH of buffer is between 6.50 and 9.60 at temperature 50°C.

Recovery of urokinase: Add saturated solution of ammonium sulphate (40–50% saturation) with continuous stirring and allowed to stand over night at 4–5°C temperature followed by separation of urokinase precipitate by centrifugation, dissolve the precipitate in tris hydrochloric acid buffer (pH 10.40) in ice cold solution, followed by cold centrifugation to remove the insoluble portion.

Purification: The supernatant acid solution is then purified by dialysis, and ion exchange chromatography to achieve the final purity of the urokinase enzyme.

Serratiopeptidase

Serratiopeptidase or serrapeptase or serralysin is the proteolytic enzyme produced by the bacterium *Serratia marcescens* as extracellular secretion in submerged and solid state fermentation product. Family Enterobacteriaceae.

Brief history: Isolated initially from the enterobacteria *Serratia marcescens* strain E-15 found in the gut of Japanese silk worm *Bombyx mori*.

It selectively dissolve the dead protein but do not affect the healthy tissue in the body; moreover it inhibits the attachment of protein in healthy tissue. It is an immunological active enzyme and it is anti-oedemic, analgesic, anti-inflammatotry, solubilise non-living tissue such as mucous, plaques and blood clots; therefore it is named fibrinolytic/thrombolytic enzyme.

Production: Bacteria *Serratia marcescens*

Culture media: Trypticase soy broth

Composition of media: Carbon source maltose; Organic nitrogen source peptone; Inorganic nitrogen source—ammonium sulphate; Inorganic salt dihydrogen phosphate, sodium bicarbonate, sodium acetate, glycerin and ascorbic acid. Yield – 27.36 µl/ml.

Second media: Tryptic soy broth (TSB-SM) (30 g/L) and skim milk (5% w/v).

The enzyme produced is filtered using filter paper and stored at 4°C till further use. Maximum production is observed in 48 hours.

Other bacteria used are *Streptomyces hydrogenans*, *Bacillus licheniformis*.

pH of the medium 7.50.

Purification: 1. Ammonium sulphate precipitation; 2. Dialysis; 3. Ultrafiltration (Aqueous two-phase system) HPLC.

Or ultrasound assisted three phase portioning method.

Evaluation of enzyme: Reverse phase HPLC method, Radioimmunoassay, and Lowry assay.

Proteolytic activity:

1. **Skim milk agar plate method**
   Clear-zone formation indicate the proteolytic activity of the enzyme.
2. **Well-diffusion method**
   Culture filtrate is added in wells in agar medium followed by staining and destaining to visualise the clear zone around the well.

LIPIDS (FIXED OIL, FATS AND WAXES)

Lipids (fixed oils, fats and waxes) are esters of long-chain fatty acids and alcohols.

The chief difference between these substances is the type of alcohol.

Waxes: The alcohol has higher molecular weight, e.g. cetyl alcohol.

The term **fixed or fatty oil** is applied to those which are liquid at 15.5°C and **fat** to those which are solid or semisolid at that temperature.

The British Pharmacopoeia has used the terms oil uniformly to all oils obtained from vegetable origin even when **semisolid**, e.g. hydnocarpus or **solid**, e.g. oil of theobroma at room temperature.

Source: The fixed oil and fats are obtained from either plant (e.g. olive and peanut oils) and animals (e.g. lard). Their important function is food storage (energy).

Fixed oil, fats: The glycerol combine with fatty acids.

Fixed oil and fats cannot be distilled without undergoing decomposition.

Solubility: Fixed oils are insoluble in water but are freely soluble in organic solvents (ether, light petroleum, benzene and chloroform). They are slightly soluble in alcohol.

Physical properties: They are more or less viscid, non-volatile, their specific gravity is less than 1. They possess characteristic odour. Most of the oils and fats develop rancid odour on exposure to air, moisture and light for a long period.

Types of fixed oils: Drying and non-drying oil.

Drying oil: The oil which on exposure to air in a thin film absorbs oxygen and forms a hard film on drying, e.g. linseed oil.

The oils like olive oil, almond oil and certain other oils do not form hard film on exposure to air hence they are known as **non-drying oil**. **Third category** oil is which dry partially or very slowly, e.g. cotton seed oil.

Extraction: Most of the oils are derived either from seeds or fruits by **expression**. It is of two types—Hot and Cold expression.

Following are the general steps before the expression:

1. Remove the dust, dirt and other fragments if any, by sifting. etc.
2. Removal of husk (seed coat) having no nutritive value but increase the percentage yield of the oil. Seed coats are removed by slightly crushing followed by winnowing.
3. Rupture the cells of decorticated or un-decorticated seeds to free the oils by grounding.

Hot expression: In this method the ground material is subjected to heating in a steam trough (cooking). This step will help to increase the yield by two ways:

a. The oil contained in cell becomes mobile.
b. The protein gets coagulated and remains fixed up in tissue. The hot material is then subjected to pressure, the separated oil is purified by centrifugation or by solvent extraction.

Cold expression: In this process grounded material is not cooked but is pressed at room temperature only. This cold expression method is preferably used for medical and edible purpose oil.

Initial treatment before extraction depends on the botanical source of the material, e.g. cotton seed require delinting, castor seed and groundnut seeds require decorticating.

Extraction by solvents: This process is applicable to both the fresh intact seeds as well as to partially extracted with expression. The solvent hexane (65°C) or light petroleum ether (40°C) are used, followed by removal of the solvent at reduced pressure.

Refining the crude oil: The oil obtained by the above process contain moisture, free fatty acids, lecithins, resins, pigments, sterol and substance which give different odours, therefore the refining of the crude oil is required. Following are the steps to refine the crude oils:

Removal of lecithin, mucilages and proteins: The oil is heated and hydrated, all these impurities will form gell or colloids which will be removed by filteration.

Neutralisation: The crude oil is treated with dilute sodium hydroxide or sodium carbonate or ammonium hydroxide. The soap will be form which will adsorb the impurities like colouring pigments, phenols, sterols, waxes, ester and other substances, and removed by decanting.

Bleaching: This is being achieved by passing the oil through activated charcoal or diatomaceous earth.

Deodouring: The unpleasant odour of aldehyde or ketone of crude oil is removed by passing steam through hot oil under pressure.

Animals oil is obtained by rendering the tissue with steam, with or without pressure.

Chemical tests: The United States pharmacopoeia includes several tests for the identification and purity of fixed oils.

Acid value or acid number: The number of milligram of potassium hydroxide required to neutralise free fatty acid present in 1 g of the oil. This test indicates the amount of free acid present in the oils.

Saponification value: The number of milligrams of potassium hydroxide to neutralise the free acid and saponify the ester contained in 1 g of the substance, under the conditions specified.

Ester value: It is the difference between the saponification and acid values.

Iodine value: Number of grams of iodine absorbed under prescribed conditions by 100 g of the substance. It indicates the unsaturation of the oil. Drying and semidrying oil have high iodine values (e.g. linseed oil).

Volatile acidity: This test is useful for animal fat such as butter. As the lower fatty acid such as butyric acid are volatile in steam. This can be measured by gas chromatography, HPLC or by enzymatic method.

Unsaponifiable matter: The compounds which are not volatile at 100 to 105°C, are obtained by extraction with organic solvents after saponification of the substances; or the compounds (sterol) which remains after saponification of the acylglycerol and removal of the glycerol and soaps by means of organic solvents.

Acetyl value: It is the number of potassium hydroxide needed to neutralise the acetic acid freed by hydrolysis of the acetylated fat or other substances.

CASTOR OIL

It is fixed oil obtained from ripened seeds of *Ricinus communis,* family Euphorbiaceae.

Geographical source: Its origin is in India but nowadays cultivated in all tropical and sub-tropical countries, the main producing countries are India, Brazil, Soviet Union, China and Thailand.

Preparation: The testa of castor seeds is hard hence for the production of oil the seeds are decortified by pressing through a decorticator and is separated from endosperm and embryo, by sieves and compressed air, the kernels are then expressed at room temperature in hydraulic press. The yield of cold expressed oil (medicinal oil) is about 45 to 60%. The colour of the oil is light coloured, (high grade) and the remainder of oil obtained by other methods is of lower grade (solvent extraction) or by expression at higher temperature.

The oil is refined by steaming (to destroy the albumin and to denature the ricin if present), filteration and bleaching.

Description of the medicinal oil: The oil is pale yellow to colourless, transparent, viscid liquid having faint mild odour and a bland characteristic acidic taste. The acid value increase with the age.

Solubility: Partially soluble in hexane but give clear liquid with equal volume of alcohol.

Specific gravity: 0.957 to 0.961.

Free fatty acids: 10 g require 3.5 ml of 0.10 N sodium hydroxide.

Hydroxyl value: 160 to 168; **iodine value:** 83 to 88; **saponification value:** 176 to 182.

Chemistry of castor oil: The medicinal oil (virgin oil) consists of the glycoside of ricinoleic, isoricinoleic, stearic and dihydroxy stearic acid. The main component (75%) of castor oil is triglyceride of ricinoleic acid (an unsaturated hydroxylated fatly acid).

$$CH_2(CH_2)_5-CHOH-CH_2-CH =$$
$$CH-(CH_2)_7COOH$$

The remainder consists of diricinoleo glycerides with third acyl group; representing either oleic, linoleic, dihydroxystearic or a saturated (palmitic or stearic acid).

The purgative action of the oil is due to free ricinoleic acid and its stereoisomer which are produced by the hydrolysis by enzyme lipases in the duodenum, to release ricinoleic (12-hydroxy-octadec-9-enoic) acid which exert cathartic effect. This acid causes local irritation, leading to increased intestinal motility.

Use: Stimulant cathartic.

Polyethoxylated castor oil used as non-ionic surfactant in intravenous preparations of the drugs with aqueous solubility.

Pharmaceutical preparations: Flexible collodion, beauty product like hair lotion, etc. Ricinoleic acid is an ingredient (0.5 to 0.7%) in vaginal jellies for restoration and maintenance of vaginal acidity.

Commercial use: In the manufacture of soaps, paints, varnishes and as a lubricant for the internal combustion engine and also in manufacture of Turkey red oil.

Chemical test for the detection of adulterant

1. **Solubility in alcohol:** Fixed oils are slightly soluble in 90% alcohol whereas castor oil gives a clear solution with equal volume of dehydrated alcohol and glacial acetic acid.

2. **Partial solubility in light petroleum:** Most of the fixed oils mixed in all proportion with light petroleum, whereas the castor oil gives clear solution with its half volume of light petroleum, but on addition of more light petroleum the solution becomes turbid and separates into two layers on standing.

3. **Optical rotation:** Fixed oils are optically inactive but castor oil is active (+3.5). This is because of asymmetric carbon atom of ricinoleic acid.

CHAULMOOGRA OIL

Botanical name: *Hydnocarpus laurifolia* Slumer.

Synonyms: *Hydnocarpus wightiana* Blume

Hydnocarpus inebrian wall

Hydnocarpus pentandra Linn

Family: Flacourcaceae

Source: It is fixed oil obtained from *Hydnocarpus wightiana* Blume and *Hydnocarpus anthelmintica* and other species of *Hydnocarpus* by cold expression of the fresh ripe seeds.

Geographical source: Plant is found in India wildly in Western Ghats at the height of 650 **m** and in Burma and Siam of Indochina.

Method of preparation: Obtained from fresh seeds by **cold expression** by means of hydraulic press at room temperature.

Other methods of extraction are **solvent extraction** with petroleum ether and hot expression. But the cold expression method is widely used and is official in IP and BP.

Characters: Cold expressed oil is yellow to brownish yellow in colour.

Taste: Acrid taste

Odour: Slight characteristic

Optical rotation: Oil is optically active and generally dextrorotatory.

Melting point: 22–23°C

D_{25} – 0.958, $[\alpha]_D$: + 57.7°C (Chloroform)

Acid number: 3.8

Saponification number: 207

Iodine number: 113.4

Chemical constituents: Fixed oil contains the following acids—hydnocarpic acid, chaulmoogric acid palmitic acid and cyclopentene fatty acids present as glyceride.

The unusual monosaturated cyclopentenyl fatty acid (CFA) are the characteristic component of chaulmoogra oils. These acids constitutes about 80% of total fatty acid constituents of the oil.

H. wightiana oil: The major constituents are: Chaulmoogric acid (35.0%), hydnocarpic acid (33.9%), gorlic (12.8%), and palmitic (5.6%).

Formula

Hydnocarpic $C_{16}H_{28}O_2$

Chaulmoogric $C_{18}H_{32}O_2$

Gorlic $C_{18}H_{30}O_2$

Hydnocarpic acid

Chaulmoogric acid

Gorlic acid
(Cyclopentenyl fatty acids)

Uses: Chaulmoogra oil has a prominent place in the history of medicinal plants in the treatment of leprosy. It is also used in number of skin ointments, i.e. eczema, leucoderma and dermatitis.

Biological activities: Astringent, anti-inflammatory, anodyne, antirheumatic, bitter, carminative, emetic, purgative and vermifuge.

For parenteral use modified oil as iodised oil, ethyl esters and sodium salt are prepared and administered subcutaneously and found to be more effective and less irritant.

Storage: Oil and its derivatives turn rancid on storage and causes pain and irritation.

Preservation: Cresote 0.1 to 0.2% or hydroquinone (0.02%) inhibit the oxidation and improve shelf life.

Note: Hydnocarpic acid and its homologous is the active compound in Chaulmoogra oil.

ALMOND OIL

Source: It is fixed oil, obtained by expression from the kernels of *Prunus amygdalus* var. *dulcis* (sweet almond) or *P. amygdalus* var. *amara* (bitter almond), family Rosaceae.

Geographical source: The oil is mainly produced from almonds grown in the countries bordering the Mediterranean (Italy, France, Spain and North Africa).

Methods of preparation: The kernels are grinded and expressed in canvas bags kept heated by keeping the bag between slightly heated iron plates. The collected oil is purified by sedimentation followed by filtration.

Description: It is a pale yellow liquid with characteristic odour and nutty taste.

Constituents: It consists of glycosides of oleic (77%), linoleic (17%), palmitic (5%) and myristic (1%) acid. It also contains considerable amount of olein.

Uses: Expressed oil is used as an emollient. As a vehicle for oily injection. It is used in the preparation of cosmetic and to many toilet preparations.

Olive Oil (Salad Oil, Sweet Oil)

Source: It is fixed oil, expressed from the ripened fruits of *Olea europaea*, family Oleaceae.

Geographical source: Mostly all the Mediterranean countries and California.

Method of preparation: Edible or medicated oil (Virgin oil).

Virgin Oil

Oil is obtained by gently pressing the peeled pulp free from endocarp.

It is obtained from the handpicked fruits, collected before fully matured. Fruits are crushed in a mill without breaking the endocarp. Turbid oil flows from the fruits is allowed to stand and then filtered. Prolonged contact with water or tissue contents is avoided to prevent the hydrolysis.

The acid value of official edible oil should not exceed 2. High grade edible oil is obtained by pressing the above marc by hydraulic press. The pressure released followed by adding cold water on the marc and pressure is again applied (water is usually added to the turbid liquid to wash the oil) and mixture is immediately filtered and sold as edible or salad oil.

For technical oil: The marc obtained after the edible oil is removed from the press, mixed with hot water and again expressed pressed once or twice.

Technical oil can also be obtained by solvent extraction or by pressing the fermented fruits.

Description: Olive oil is a pale yellow or light greenish yellow oily liquid.

Odour: Slight but characteristic.

Taste: Bland to faintly acrid.

Solubility: Miscible with ether, carbon disulfide and chloroform but slightly soluble in alcohol.

Specific gravity: 0.910 to 0.915 at 25°C on cooling tends to become cloudy. At 0°C a whitish granular mass in formed.

Constituents: BP specifies the following limit of the standard olive oil.

Oleic acid: 56–85%.
Linoleic acid: 3.5–20%.
Palmitic and stearic acid: 8–23.5%.

Uses: Oilve oil used as pharmaceutical aids and in the preparation of soaps, plasters, etc. It is widely used as a salad oil, being nutrient. It is demulcent, emollient and laxative.

COD LIVER OIL

Source: Medicinal cod liver oil is fixed oil obtained from fresh liver of *Gadus morhua* Linn and other species of family Gadidae containing a due proportion of vitamins.

Geographical source: The main fishing grounds are located from New England, North Dakota to Nova Scotia, with small amount coming from Norway.

Collection and extraction: In early days the fish were cleaned on shipboard. The edible fish was salted and separated livers were thrown into barrels, where through the process of rolling, the liver tissue disintegrated and the oil rose to the top and separated. These days, fish are brought to fish houses just few hours after their trapping. The livers are removed with care and gallbladder completely separated and transferred to steamer or steamed in closed vessel (kettles), where the oil (crude) released, separated and stored at a low temperature in carbon dioxide atmospheres it is then delivered to the refinery for further processing.

Processing at refinery

1. Separation of impurities
2. Drying
3. Removal of solid stearin
4. Deodourisation
5. Standardisation

Separation of impurities: Nowadays this whole process of purification is being done in refinery under air-free atmosphere to prevent oxidation. It is carried out in continuous automatic, hermetic refining plant. It removes the impurities as well as further dissolution of the liver tissue, if any there, the oil and water are removed in hermetic separator and automatically purified oil is collected.

Drying: It is made free from any water traces in vacuum drying tower.

Removal of solid stearin: All the medicinal and veterinary oil are cooled to about 0°C. The solid stearin is removed by cold filtration.

Deodourisation: Deodourisation means to remove the aldehyde and ketone impurities by steaming.

Standardisation: Finally oil is adjusted to a definite vitamin content by admixture of higher or lower vitamin value oils.

Storage: Store in well-fitted air tight containers protected from light and stored in a cool place.

Description: Medicinal cod liver oil is a thin oily pale yellow liquid, having slightly fishy but not rancid odour and taste.

It is slightly soluble in alcohol and freely soluble in ether, chloroform, carbon disulphide and ethyl acetate.

Acid value: <1.2 (not more than 1.2).

Constituents: The oil consists of glyceryl esters of unsaturated (about 85%) and saturated (about 15%) fatty acid. The medicinal properties of cod liver oil is due to vitamin A (growth promoting vitamin) and vitamin D (anti-rachitic vitamin).

Uses: It is mainly used for the prevention and cure of rickets. Nowadays it is used as food supplement for the nutritional requirement as it is being reported to have cholesterol lowering property.

LARD

Source: It is purified internal fat (abdomen and other parts) of the hog, *Sus scrofa* Linn. order Ungulate, family Suidae.

Preparation: For medicinal purpose lard is prepared from the abdominal fat of the pig, called flares. These consist of fat enclosed in membranous vesicles enveloped in membrane. The fat is separated by first removing the external membrane and then minced the material to free from the enclosed fat. The minced material is heated at a temperature not exceeding 57°C (for commercial variety higher temperature is used to ensure complete separation of the fat).

Description: Prepared lard is a soft, white fat with non-rancid odour.

   Acid value: <1.2

   Melting point: 34–41°C

   Iodine value: 52–66

   Saponification value: 192–198

Adulterant: Beef fat, sesame seed and cotton seed oils.

Constituents: Lard mainly consist of triglycerides composed of three fatty acids, oleic (46%), stearic (12–14%), myristic and palmitic acids (25–28%), and solid glycerides (about 40%), e.g. myristin, stearin and palmitin and about 40% liquid glycerides such as olein.

Following are chief grades of lard:

1. Neutral lard No. 1, prepared from the 'leaf' (the fat adjacent to kidneys and bowels) by rendering between 50 and 60°C.
2. Neutral lard No. 2, prepared from the fat of the back (kidneys and bowels).

Leaf lard: This is prepared from the leftover material of neutral lard No.1. The material is steam heated and pressed.

Lower grade: It contains not only free fatty acids but also contains excessive portion of olein and too low melting point (33–41°C).

Uses: Ointment base.

Suet

It is purified internal fat of the abdomen and other parts of the sheep *Ovis aries*. This fat contains about 50 to 60% solid glycerides, fatty acid (palmitic and stearic acid), about 70% and oleic acid.

Uses: Ointment base.

Wool Fat (Hydrous Wool Fat) or Lanolin

Source: It is purified anhydrous fat-like substance obtained from the wool of the sheep *Ovis aries* Linn, family Bovidae.

Hydrous wool fat: Wool fat containing 25 to 30% of water is known as hydrous wool fat.

Preparation: Wool fat is secreted by sweat glands in the skin of sheep and exudes onto the hairs of the fleece.

Extraction or preparation of wool fat has two steps:

1. Raw wool grease
2. Purification

   Raw wool grease is obtained by acid cracking process.

First stage: Washing the clipped wool with detergents, such as soap, sulfonated alcohol and oil or alkali to give oil in water emulsion of wool fat (wool greese).

   Oil in water emulsion is then cracked by treating with sulphuric acid; with the result grease will separate as a separate layer over the aqueous (soapy) solution. This is known as raw wool greese.

Purification: Raw wool greese is then boiled with sufficient quantity of alkali (equivalent to the quantity of free acid content) in the presence of organic solvent (benzene or ethylene dichloride). The mixture is allowed to stand and separate into two layers – upper benzene layer containing wool fat and lower aqueous layer. Upper layer is removed and distilled off the organic solvent leaving behind the residue of neutral 'wool wax'. It is further purified by bleaching with sodium peroxide, sodium hypochloride or hydrogen peroxide by centrifuging with water and with bleaching agent.

   Raw wool greese can also be obtained by centrifuging the emulsion or by direct solvent extraction from wool.

Description: Wool fat is a yellowish white ointment like mass with a faint but characteristic odour. When heated over steam bath it separates into two layer.

   It is soluble in water and high proportion of water can be incorporated by melting at 15°C.

   Melting point: 36–42°C

   Specific gravity at 15°C: 0.94–0.97

   Refractive index (40°C): 1.48

   Free acid content: 4–10%

   Free alcohol content: 1–3%

   Proportion of fatty acid: 50–55%

Soluble in ether, chloroform. It can be saponified with alcoholic alkali but not with aqueous potash.

Saponification value: 94–106

Iodine value: 18–32

Acid value: <1

Constituents: The chief constituents are cholesterol and isocholesterol. Esters of lanopalmitic, lanoceric, carnaubic, oleic, myristic and other fatty acids. It also contains aliphatic alcohols such as cetyl, ceryl and carnaubyl alcohols.

Uses: It is used as a water absorbable ointment base. It is an ingredient of many skin creams and cosmetics.

WAXES

Waxes may be defined as esters of higher molecular weight, straight chain acids and high molecular weight primary straight chain alcohols or it may also be defined as mixtures of different molecular weight acids and alcohols. Although sometimes applied to the hydrocarbons mixture **hard paraffin**.

Difference between fats and waxes: Fats may be saponified by means of either aqueous or alcoholic alkali but waxes can only be saponified by alcoholic alkali.

Sources: Both plant and animals are the source of waxes.

Plants: In plants waxes are present in the outer cell walls of epidermis of leaves and fruits. They protect the penetration or loss of water, e.g. **Carnauba wax.**

Animal waxes: The insects secrete waxes, e.g. beeswax and lac, wax Spermaceti.

Uses: In pharmaceutical preparations waxes are used to harden ointments and cosmetics. In industry waxes are used as protective coating.

Carnauba Wax (Palm Wax)

It is derived from the leaves of *Copernicia prunifera* H.E. Moore, family Palmae. Plant grows from northern Brazil to Argentina.

Preparation: The leaves of carnauba palm are collected, dried and beaten to loosen the wax, collected by shaking them followed by purification and bleaching. In the pure form usually come in the form of hard yellow brown, moderately coarse powder or irregular lump.

Taste: Tasteless, free from rancidity.

Composition

Myricyl cerotate (80%) (aliphatic ester)

Free monohydric alcohol 10%; diesters of 4-hydroxycinnamic acid 21% w/w; ester of W-hydroxy carboxyl acids.

Lactone, resin and other minor components.

Acid value less than 12

Saponification value 75–95.

Iodine value 7–14.

$$C_{30}H_{61} - O - \overset{\overset{\textstyle O}{\|}}{C} - C_{15}H_{31}$$

Mericyl cerotate

Uses: In the manufacture of candles, wax varnishes, leather and furniture polishes and substitute of beeswax.

In pharmacy: Tablet coating agent.

Spermaceti: It is solid wax obtained from the oil, derived from the head of the sperm whale *Physeter macrocephalus* Linn, family Physeteridae order Cetaceae and also from *Hyperoodon rostratus* (bottlenose whale).

Geographical source: Pacific, Indian and Atlantic Oceans.

Note: This sperm whale is an endangered species and has been protected by international agreement, hence it is no more source for spermaceti. It has led to the use of synthetic spermaceti of Jojoba oil.

Synthetic spermaceti: It is mixture consisting of esters of saturated fatty acid and saturated fatty alcohols (C14 to C18) (cetyl ester wax).

Jojoba oil: It is liquid wax derived from seeds of *Simmondsia chinensis* Scheider, family Buxaceae.

Method of extraction: Expression method.

The seeds contain about 45 to 55% of an ester mixture, liquid at ambient temperature.

Constituents of the oil: The oil contains 35% eicosenoic acid (C_{20} unsaturated acid), 22% eicosenol (C_{20} unsaturated alcohol) and 21% of docosenol.

Hydrogenation of the oil yields crystalline wax, which in appearance and properties looks like spermaceti.

Uses: Used as emollient in pharmaceuticals.

Bees Wax

Yellow bees wax and white bees wax. Yellow bees wax is the purified wax obtained by melting and purifying the honeycomb of the bee *Apis mellifera* Linn, family Apidae.

Wax is present in four segments of abdomen on the ventral surface of honeybee. It passes out through the pores in chitinous plates and is used by the young worker honeybees for the formation of comb.

Geographical source: East Africa, West Africa, Chile, Morocco, India, Jamaica, France and Italy.

Preparation: After the removal of honey the honeycomb is melted by boiling in water, cooled, separated as solid cake, strained and allowed to harden in moulds.

Characters: It is solid mass, having colour from yellow to grayish brown with characteristic odour of honey. **Taste**—faint characteristic. When cold, it is brittle, dull, granular non-crystalline fracture.

Solubility: Insoluble in water, sparingly soluble in alcohol but dissolves in chloroform and warm fixed and volatile oils.

Composition: It consists of mostly 80% alkyl esters of fatty and wax acids chiefly myricyl palmitate 72% (myricin) and small proportion of myricyl stearate (10–15%), free wax acid (about 14 to 15%) especially cerotic acid. Other components are aromatic substances, hydrocarbon (10%) and other constituents in traces are: moisture, pollens and propolis (bee glue) responsible for the colour of wax.

Uses: Stiffening agent in the topical preparation. Commercially, it is component of polishes.

White Bees Wax

It is bleached purified wax obtained from honeycomb of honeybee *Apis mellifera* Linn, family Apidae.

Method of preparation: The melted wax is poured slowly over revolving wetted cylinder. Thin ribbon-like layers are formed which are removed and exposed to sunlight and air till they are bleached. The bleached wax is then melted and transferred into moulds to give the shape of cakes of various sizes.

Adulteration can be detected by saponification test. As waxes cannot be saponified with aqueous alkali whereas all the fats can be saponified by means of either alcoholic or aqueous alkali.

Uses: Used pharmaceutically in ointments and cold creams.

FURTHER READING

1. Ajitkumar DS, et al. Production, purification and characterization of streptokinase using Baccillus licheniformis under solid state Fermentation Journal of Global Biosciences, 2015;4(7):2703–12.

2. Braz. Arch. Boil.Technol.vol56 No 6 Cuirtiba Nov./Dec 2013.

3. David C, et al. Purification & characterization of single chain urokinase type Plasminogen activator from human cell culture; The journal of biological chemistry, 1986;261(3):1274–8.

4. Dubey R, et al. Asian journal of chemistry. Extraction and purification of Bromelain. 2012; 24(4);1435–8.

5. Encyclopedia.com

6. Honey quality and international Regulatory Standard (1999).

7. Journal of dairy science.

8. Kalia AN. Textbook of Industrial Pharmacogonsy. 2005. CBS Publishers and Distributors, New Delhi.

9. Pharmacognosy 8th edition by Varro E. Tyler Lynn R. Brady James E. Robbers, 1981, p 291–2.

10. Ramesh KB, Hisham A, Latha PG . Chemistry and theraupeutic potential of chaulmoogra oil chapter in www.research gate.net publication.

11. Selvarjan Ethiraj, Shreya Gopinath. Production, purification characterization immunolization and application of Serrapeptase A Review:Front Biol.2017,12 (5):333–48.

12. Trease and Evans. Pharmacognosy. (16ed), 2009.

13. US37755083 patent. Method of isolation and purification of urokinase from human urine.

14. Visha Bansal, et al. Urokinase separation from the cell culture broth of human kidney cell line; Int. j.Biol sci.2007; 3(1):64–70.

Chapter

10

Marine Pharmacognosy (Novel Medicinal Agents from Marine Source)

INTRODUCTION

Marine pharmacognosy is a sub-branch of pharmacognosy, which is mainly concerned with the naturally occurring substances of medicinal value from marine. It is not a new area for pharmacognosy, even the early civilisations of Greece, Japan, China and India have explored marine life as a source of drugs. In the western medicine **agar, alginic acid, carrageenan, protamine sulphate, spermaceti and cod, and halibut** liver oils are the marine medicinal established products.

The oceans cover more than 70% of the earth's surface and contain over 200,000 invertebrates and algae species.

Macroalgae or seaweeds have been used as crude drugs in the treatment of iodine deficiency states such as goitre, etc. Some seaweeds have also been utilised as sources of additional vitamins and in the treatment of anaemia during pregnancy. Marine products have also been used for the treatment of various intestinal disorders as vermifuges, hypocholesterolaemic and hypoglycaemic agent, e.g. *Cystoseira barbata; Sargassum confusum* and *Jania rubens*.

Seaweeds have also been employed as dressing materials, ointments and in gynae-cology. For example, *Porphyra atropurpurea* have been used in Hawaii to dress wounds and burns; and *Durvillaea antarctica* to treat scabies in New Zealand. Prepared, sterilised stripes of *Laminaria digitata* in conjunction with prostaglandins have been used to dilate the cervix, as the strips swell up to

several times to their original diameter when moistened.

During the last 30–40 years numerous novel compounds have been isolated from marine organisms having biological activities, such as antibacterial, antiviral, antitumour, anti-parasitic, anticoagulants, antimicrobial, anti-inflammatory and cardiovascular active products.

Marine flora and funa play significant role as a source of new molecular entity. The oceans of the world contain over 5 million species in about 30 phyla. Because of the diversities of marine organism and habitats, marine natural products enclose a wide variety of chemical classes, including **terpenes, shikimates, polyketides, acetogenins, peptides, alkaloids** of varying structures and a multitude of compounds of mixed biosynthesis.

While terrestrial sources have yielded numerous drugs, marine natural products represent a relatively untapped resources for new drug development. The marine environment may contain over 80% of the world's plant and animal species. During the past 30–40 years, numerous novel compounds have been isolated from marine organisms and many of these have been reported to have bio-logical activities, some of which are of interest from the point of view of potential drug development. On the other hand some of the compounds pose potential risk to human health. In this latter category are the **paralytic or diarrhetic and amnesic shellfish toxins**. The former can be fatal, but the latter, although producing very unpleasant effects, are not fatal. Both paralytic and diarrhetic shellfish toxins are produced by dinoflagellates, while amnesic shellfish, poisoning result from the ingestion of shellfish contaminated with diatoms. The ingestion of other marine organisms which can also lead to serious poisoning, include the potent neurotoxin, tetrodotoxin, resulting from eating pufferfish and ciguatoxin, associated with ingestion of tropical fish which have fed on the dinoflagellate, *Gambierdiscus toxicus*.

MARINE ORGANISM AS POTENTIAL SOURCE OF DRUGS

Knowledge of biological activities and/or chemical constituents of marine organisms is important not only for the discovery of new therapeutic agents but such informations may also be of immense value in exploring, new sources of economic materials, precursors for the synthesis of complex chemical substances and compounds of novel chemical structure, thereby prompting the chemist for the synthesis of a series of modified compounds of therapeutical importance. Thus, in recent years, considerable importance is attached to the discovery of new biodynamic agents from marine source to search new source of drugs from sea.

A survey of literature indicated that extracts from marine organisms had been evaluated for various biological activities. This has led to the isolation of substances possessing antimicrobial, antibiotic, antiviral, anticancer, cardioactive, anti-inflammatory, anthelmintic, anticoagulant neurophysiological and insecticidal activities.

Although, numerous compounds have been isolated from marine organisms and the biological activities attributed to many of them; but still very few of them have been marketed or are under development. There are number of reasons that is why more number of compounds originating from marine plants and animals have not been developed. There is no doubt that much of the work undertaken in the 1960s, 1970s and probably the early 1980s was driven by an interest in the chemistry of new compounds rather than in their biological activities. The earlier studies on chemistry of marine natural products were limited to the isolation, structure elucidation and phylogenetic relationship of specific substances, such as quinonoid pigments and sterols. Now, this field attracted the attention of not only the natural product chemists but also those of marine biologist, biochemist, pharmacologist, etc. The invention of the aqualung and the advent of new technology in the past few decades led to the awareness that the oceans may be a new frontier of biomedical research, as it has a vast resources for the discovery of marine derived medicine. Increasing sophistication of the tools available to explore the deep sea has expanded the habitats, which can be sampled; and has greatly improved the opportunities for discovery of novel metabolites.

Much of the earlier work limited the biological testing to antimicrobial activity, but this was often extended later to testing for cytotoxic properties, which may provide useful leads for anticancer drugs. This latter area is one that most of the compounds in various stages of clinical trials are located. Screening for other activities has of course, also been undertaken, e.g. for antiviral, anti-inflammatory, anticoagulant, antiparasitic and prostaglandins.

Many of the marine compounds have shown promising biological properties but have complicated chemical structures, the synthesis of which would be hard and expensive. These organisms are valuable as source of new biologically active chemical structures, but unless either the compounds or a derivative of them can be readily synthesised they are of little commercial interest to the pharmaceutical industry.

CONOTOXIN

Conotoxin (Conus venom) present in marine are used to develop new moiety drugs for producing receptor mediated effects without much side effects, e.g. CNS drugs, anti-hypertensive, anti-asthamatic and neurovascular blocking agents.

The active principle site of action of these toxins are peptide with disulphide linkage. About four conotoxins are of therapeutically importance.

Marine Algae

Four types of marine algae reported:

1. Cyanophyceae (blue green algae)
2. Chlorophyceae (green algae)
3. Phaecophyceae (brown algae)
4. Rhodophyceae (red algae)

These algae are of significant importance in therapy. They are being used as CNS drugs, antimicrobial agents, antifouling, antiviral, anticoagulant, hypotensive, diuretic and hypoglycaemic agents.

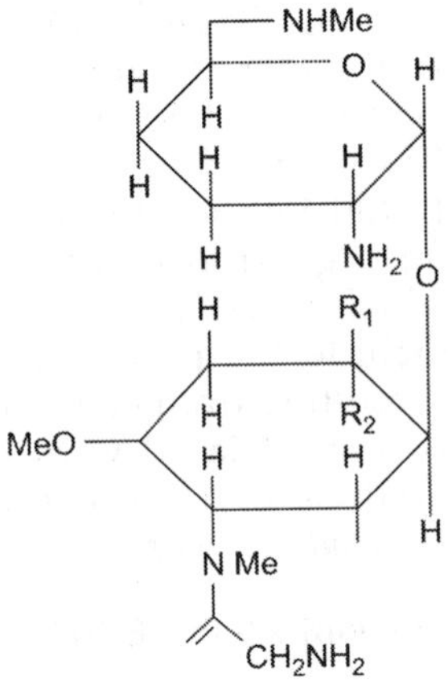

ANTIMICROBIAL COMPOUNDS

Cephalosporins: Discovered in the 50's from a marine fungus, *Cephalosporium acremonium* **Cephalosporin C** (Fig. 10.1) was isolated. The modification of the original cephalosporin (cephelothin sodium), has been widely used as an antibiotic drug active against microbes insensitive to penicillin and ampicillins.

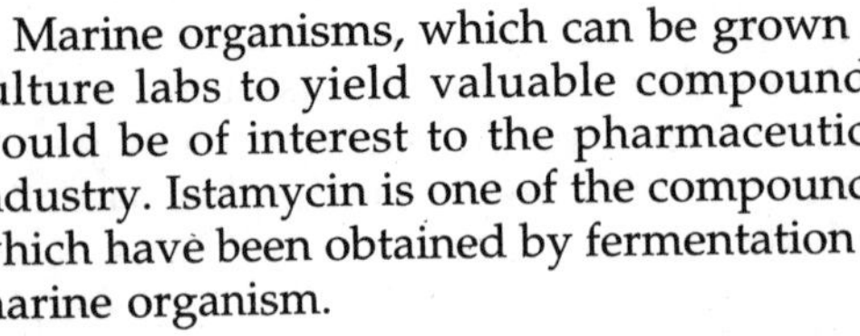

Fig. 10.1: Cephalosporin C

Marine organisms, which can be grown in culture labs to yield valuable compounds, would be of interest to the pharmaceutical industry. Istamycin is one of the compounds, which have been obtained by fermentation of marine organism.

Istamycins (Fig. 10.2): These are the fermentation products of marine microoganism, *Streptomyces lenjimariensis* SS-939. These compounds are reported to have *in vitro* activity against both gram-negative and gram-positive bacteria, including those with known resistance to the aminoglycoside antibiotics.

Istamycin A $R_1 = H$, $R_2 = NH_2$
Istamycin B $R_1 = NH_2$, $R_2 = H$

Fig. 10.2: Istamycin

Marine sponges are colourful and have resistance for bacterial decomposition; they can be the potential source of novel antimicrobial agent. On screening the sponges, it was observed that sponges of family Verongidae contain a series of antimicrobials and closely related compounds.

A list of few antibacterial or antimicrobial, agents isolated from sponges given in Table 10.1.

Novel series of **sesquiterpenes** have also been isolated from sponges such as **nitenin** and **furospongin** from *Spongia nitens* and *Spongia officinalis* respectively.

Antimicrobial agents are obtained from *Gorgonian corals* belonging to phylum Cnidaria.

Eunicin (Fig. 10.3)—a macrocyclic cembrenoid compound has been isolated from gorgonian *Eunicia mammosa* with antibacterial activity.

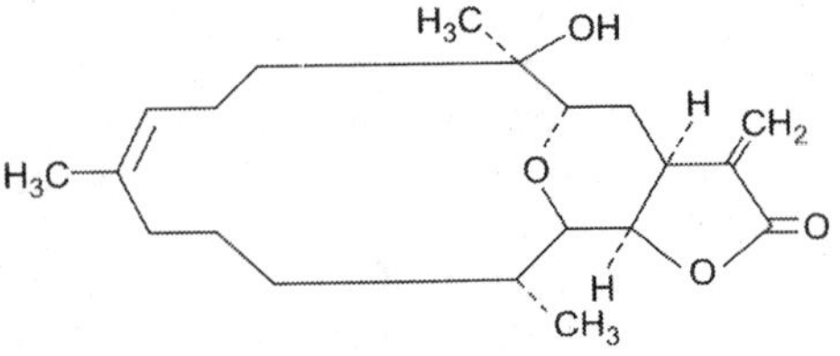

Fig. 10.3: Eunicin

Table 10.1: Antibacterial, antimicrobial and antibiotic agents isolated from marine sponges

Name	Structure (see page 208 and from no. 1 to 14)	Source	Biological Activity
3,5, dibromo-1-hydroxy-4-oxo-2, 5-cyclo-hexadiene-1 acetamide	(1)	*Verongia cauliformis, V. fistularis, V. aerophoba, V. thiona*	Antibiotic
3,5-dibromo-1-hydroxy-4, 4-dimethoxy 2, 5 cyclo-hexadiene-1-acetamide	(2)	*V. cauliformis*	Antibacterial
Aeroplysinin-1 (+)	(3)	*Verongia aerophoba*	Antimicrobial
Aeroplysinin-1 (–)	(4)	*Lanthella aridis*	Antimicrobial
2-cyano-4,5 dibromopyrrole	(5)	*Agelas oroides*	Antimicrobial
5,6-dibromo-1-H-indole-3-ethanamine	(6)	*Polyfibrospongia maynardii*	Antibacterial
5,6-dibromo-1-H-indole-3 (N-methyl ethanamine)	(7)	*Polyfibrospongia maynardii*	Antibacterial
3-Bromo-2-(4-bromophenoxy)-phenol	(8)	*Dysidea herbacea*	Antibacterial
Monobromo and Dibromophakellin	(9)	*Phakellia flabellata*	Antimicrobial
Acanthellin-1	(10)	*Acanthella acuta*	Antibacterial
Nitenin (sesquiterpene)	(11)	*Spongia nitens*	Antibacterial
Furospongin-1	(12)	*Spongia officinalis*	Antibacterial
Ircinin-1	(13)	*Iricinia oros.*	Antibacterial
Variabilin	(14)	*Iricinia variabilis*	Antibacterial

Antimicrobial and Antibiotic Activity from Algae

Zonarol and isozonarol (Fig. 10.4) obtained from brown algae *Dictyopteris zonariodes* have fungicidal properties.

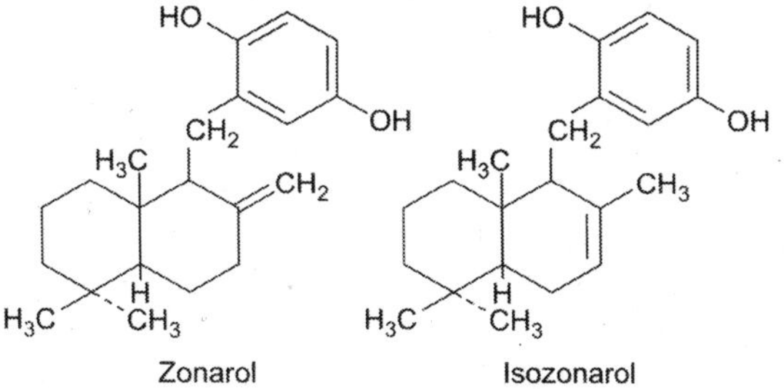

Fig. 10.4: Zonarol and Isozonarol

Tetrabromoheptanone (Fig. 10.5) has shown antimicrobial properties against large number of microorganisms. It is obtained from red algae *Bonnemaisonia hemifera*.

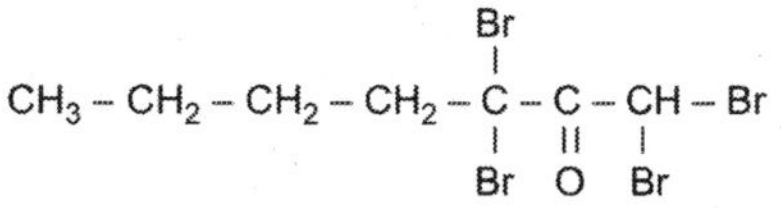

Fig. 10.5: Tetrabromo heptanone

Polyhalo-acetones (Fig. 10.6) and its isomers and four *polyhalo-3-butene-2-one* obtained from red algae *Asparagopsis taxiformis*, possess antimicrobial properties.

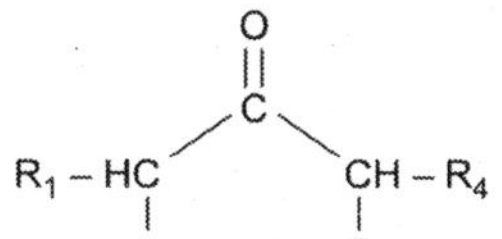

	R_1	R_2	R_3	R_4
a	Cl	Br	Br	Br
b	Br	Br	Br	Br
c	Cl	H	Br	Br
d	Cl	Br	H	Br

Fig. 10.6: Polyhalo-acetone

Sargassum species (brown algae) contain brominated polyphenol, which is used as antimicrobial agent as well as antifouling agents.

Structures of compounds in Table 10.1

Antibacterial, antimicrobial and antibiotic agents from marine sponges

ANTIVIRAL COMPOUNDS

Many marine microorganisms have been screened for antiviral activity and wide range of active compounds have been reported, but only few compounds are reported to have significant therapeutic activity and these are:

Antiviral and Anti HIV agents: Laminaran species from brown algae are reported to have antiviral, anti HIV and anticoagulant activity.

Ara-A (Fig. 10.7): It is a semi-synthetic compound based on the arabinosyl nucleosides isolated from the sponge *Tectitethya crypta*.

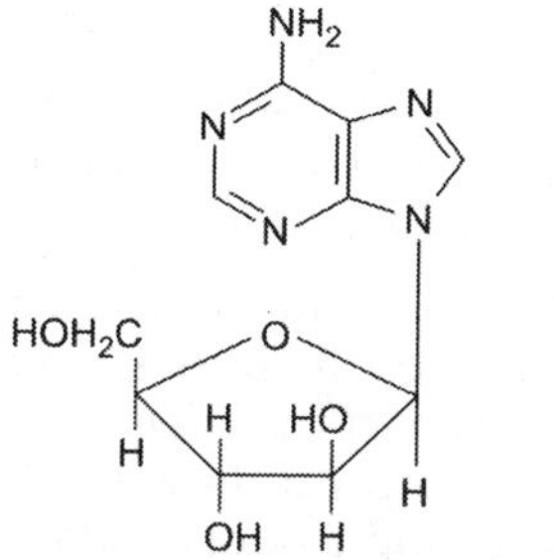

Fig. 10.7: Ara-A (vidrabine)

Avarol and Avarone (Fig. 10.8): These compounds (sesquiterpene hydroquinone) are isolated from a sponge, *Dysidea avara* schmidt. These compounds inhibit the immunodeficiency virus, have high therapeutic indices and the ability to cross blood–brain barrier.

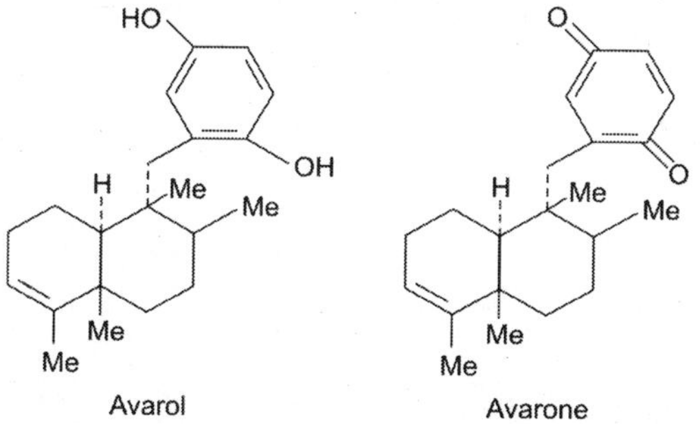

Fig. 10.8: Avarol and avarone

Didemnins: These are cyclic depsipeptides isolated from tunicate, *Tectitethya crypta*.

Eudistomin A (Fig. 10.9) *and β-Carbolines:* This is also isolated from tunicate, *Eudistoma olivaceum*.

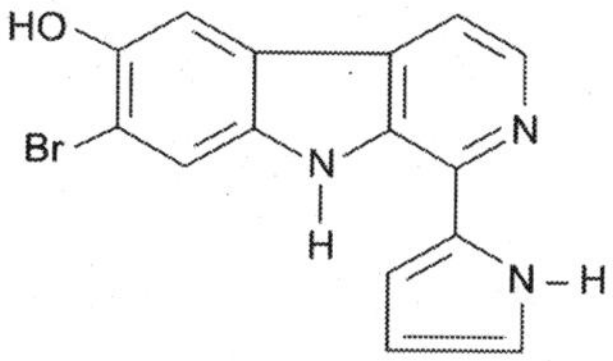

Fig. 10.9: Eudistomin A

Laurenterol (Fig. 10.10) possessing antibacterial activity against gram-positive bacteria obtained from *Laurencia* spp. (*Ophioderma variegatum*) and from the sea hare *Aplysia californica*.

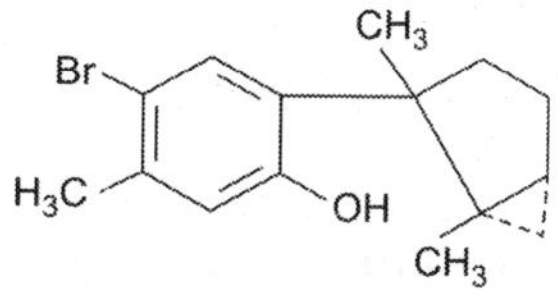

Fig. 10.10: Laurenterol

Oppositol (Fig. 10.10a) antibacterial agent from *Laurencia suboppostia*; against *Staphylococcus aureus*.

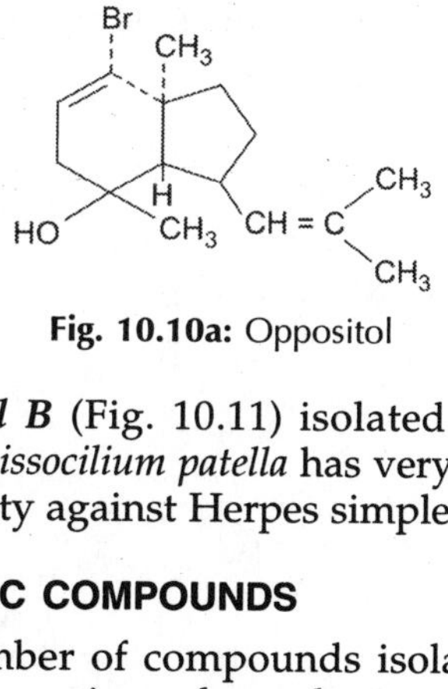

Fig. 10.10a: Oppositol

Patellazol B (Fig. 10.11) isolated from the tunicate, *Lissocilium patella* has very potent *in vitro* activity against Herpes simplex viruses.

CYTOTOXIC COMPOUNDS

Large number of compounds isolated from marine organisms have been tested for cytotoxicity in the search for drugs active against cancer. Among all, the best known novel compounds with high potential as anticancer drugs are found to be macrolides, known as **bryostatins** isolated primarily from the **bryozoan**, *Bugula neritina* and later some have been extracted from sponges and tunicates.

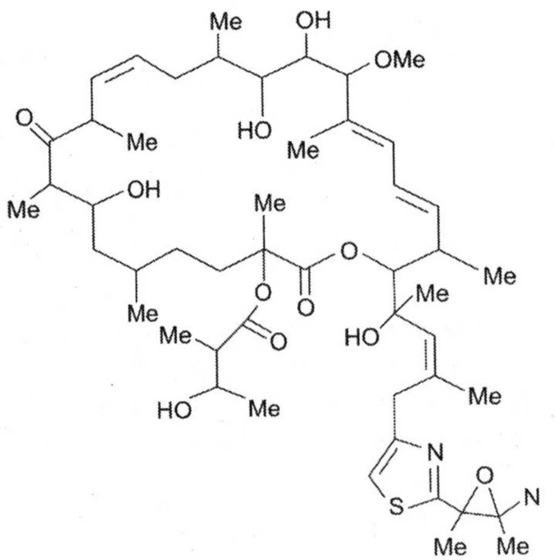

Fig. 10.11: Patellazol B

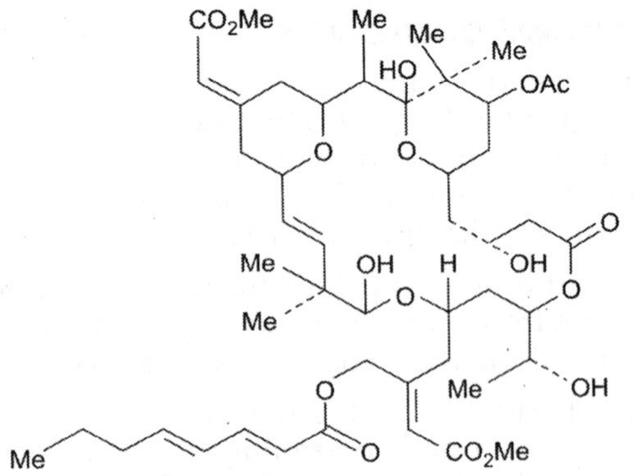

Fig. 10.12: Bryostatin-I

acid metabolite release. Both Bryostatin 1 and 2 enhance the efficiency of interleukin-2, in initiating the development of *in vivo* primed cytotoxic T-lymphocytes.

Many Bryostatins (1–18) are reported to have antileukaemic activity but only Bryostatin-1 and Bryostatin-2 have undergone phase 2 clinical trials.

Bryostatin (Fig. 10.12) triggers activation and differentiation of peripheral blood cells from lymphocytic leukemia patients. It also causes activation of protein kinase C and arachidonic

Dolastatins is a family of cyclic and linear peptides and depsipeptides; isolated from the sea hare, *Dolabella auricularia*. The highly cytotoxic compounds are Dolastatin 10, Dolastatin-H and Isodolastatin-H (Fig. 10.13).

In addition to the peptides, the polypropionate, Antipyrone A and B have also been extracted from *D. auricularia*.

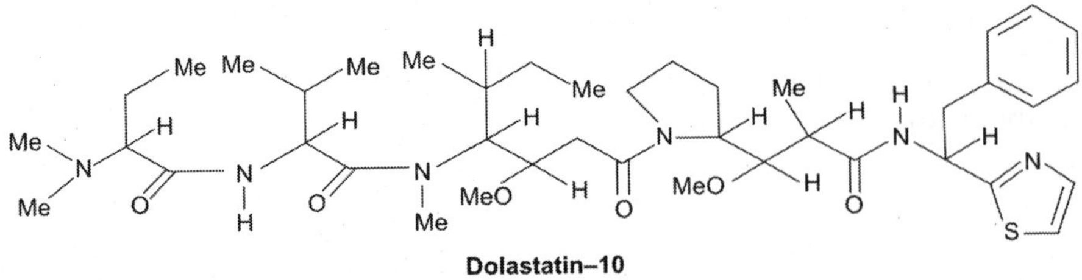

Dolastatin–10

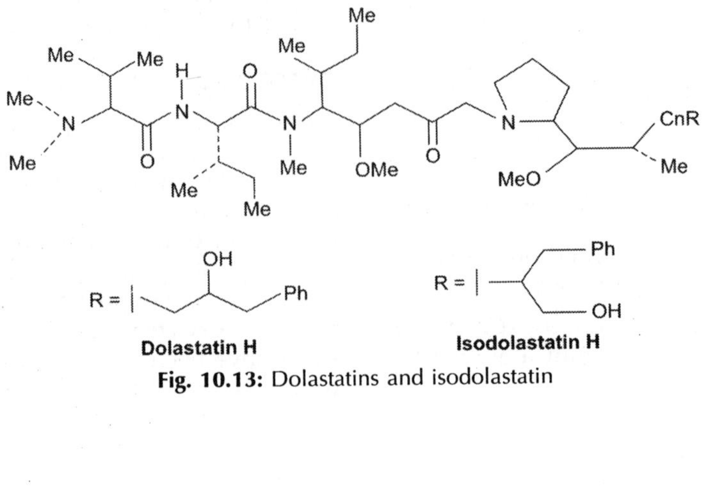

Dolastatin H   **Isodolastatin H**

Fig. 10.13: Dolastatins and isodolastatin

Eleutherobin is a compound obtained from a marine encrusting gorgonian *Erythropodium caribaeorum*. It is extremely potent for inducing *in vitro* tubulin polymerisation and is toxic to cancer cells with an IC-50 similar to that of taxol.

Xenia a novel diterpene called xenicane isolated from the soft coral *Xenia elongata*. This compound has shown some effectiveness in inhibiting mitochondria respiration in cancer cells.

Nephthea: The soft Coral Nephthea reported to contain a bioactive compound **Lemnabourside** which is 5 alpha-reductase inhibitor. It is quite active in prostate cancer cells, as they tend to be androgen dependent. The drug possess ability to inhibit the conversion of testosterone into more potent dihydrotestosterone.

Halimide: A low molecular pectin like molecule isolated from green algae *Helimeda opuntia*, used in the treatment of early stage cancer, particularly breast cancer resistant to current chemotherapy.

Ecteinascidin 743 (ET-743), a natural new product isolated from the Caribbean sea squirt. It is totally novel and different from existing anticancer drugs. ET-743 have shown high activity in cases of advanced sarcoma, that had relapsed or were resistant to conventional therapy.

Yondelis TM (ET-743): Yondelis TM is a new antitumour drug derived from the marine organism *Ecteinascidia turbinata* a 'Sea Squirt' or tunicate found in the Caribbean and Mediterranean sea. It is still at the stage of being an investigational drug and it has been suggested (USA) that drug is quite useful in the treatment of patient with advanced sexually transmitted diseases (STD) after failure of conventional chemotherapy.

Aplidine: Spanish biotechnology firm Zeltia, developed this drug from a marine organism, Mediterranean tunicate *Aplidium albicans*, against medullary thyroid carcinoma.

It is reported that Aplidin, a **novel antitumour** agent of marine origin undergoing phase II clinical trials, induces growth arrest and apoptosis in human MDA-MB-231 breast cancer cells at nanomolar concentrations.

Ara-C a potent inhibitor of tumour such as Sarcoma-180, Erlich carcinoma and L-1210 leukaemia in mice. It is also reported to be active against acute myelogenous leukaemia and human acute leukaemia. It is one of the standard drugs used in the treatment of **acute leukaemia**; both in children and adults.

Ara-C is a semi-synthetic drug originated from the Caribbean sponge, the basic compound was **spongothymidine**, which led to the synthesis of **1-α-D-arabinofuranosyl cytosine (Ara-C)**, developed and marketed by Upjohn Pharmaceutical Company as **Cytosar**.

Ara-A: It is another synthetic analogue to adenine arabinoside, of Ara-C compound. The reports says the compound to be effective for the treatment of *Herpes encephalitis*.

Asperidol: It is a non-lactonic cembranoid obtained from gorgonian coral, have **anti-cancer** activity.

Aplysistatin (LSV) an **antileukaemic** agent obtained from sea hare *Aplysia angasi*.

Dola-triol (LIV): Active **antileukaemic** agent possessing different diterpenoid ring system has been reported from the Indian Ocean sea hare *Dolabella auricularia* **Holothurin**. It is a toxic triterpenoid glycoside obtained from sea cucumbers belonging to phylum *Echinodermata* (*Actinopyga agassizi*) are reported to inhibit the growth of sarcoma-180 and adenocarcinoma in mice.

Thelothurin A and thelothurin B: These both are cytotoxic saponin obtained from sea cucumber *Thelenota ananas*.

Spongouridine isolated from Caribbean sponge *Cryptotethya crypta*, has shown promising **antiviral** and antitumour activities.

Tocotrienol (Lx): An antitumour compound, isolated from water soluble extract of *Sargassum tortile* (brown algae).

CARDIOVASCULAR AND NEUROPHYSIOLOGICAL AGENTS

Anthopleurin A is a heart stimulant possessing four times more activity than natural cardiac glycosides (digitalis and strophanthus). It is a polypeptide in nature, isolated from sea anemone *Anthopleura xanthogrammica*.

Eledoisin is a peptide obtained from posterior salivary glands of *Eledone* spp. *Eledone moschata* and related species. It is fifty times more potent than acetylcholine, histamine or bradykinin ion provoking hypotension. It is a potent vasodilator and hypotensive agent.

Eptatretin is a potent cardiac stimulant, having direct action on mammalian myocardium as produced by epinephrine and digitalis glycosides. It is obtained from aneural bronchial heart of the Pacific hagfish *Eptatretus stoutii*.

D-octopamine is an amine found in salivary glands of *Octopus* spp. *O. vulgaris*, *O. macropus* and *Eledone moschata*. It is a potent cardiotonic.

Laminin belongs to heterotrimeric glycoproteins and is obtained from marine algae *Laminaria angustata*.

It has potent hypotensive effect on mammals.

Tetrodotoxin is a toxin but possessing cardiovascular and neurophysiological activities. It is obtained from the skin and testis of Goby, *Gobius criniger*; and also from the skin of male and female Costa Rican frog, *Atelopus chiriquiensis*.

α-Conotoxin, ω-conotoxin, μ-conotoxin and κ-conotoxin

α-Conotoxin is obtained from *C. figulinus*. It is used in stroke, Parkinson's disease as muscle relaxant, antihypertensive agents and analgesic.

ω-Conotoxin is obtained from *C. geographus*. It is used to block neuronal calcium channels at pre-synaptic terminal of neuromuscular junction like nifidipine and nitradipine.

μ-Conotoxin is also obtained from *C. geographus* and used in ischaemia.

κ-Conotoxins blocks potassium channel and is used in hypertension, arrhythmia and asthma.

ANTI-INFLAMMATORY AGENTS
Pseudopterosins

These are the group of diterpene glycosides. The **pseudopterosins-1** and **seco-pseudopterosins-3** were isolated from *Caribbean octocorals* but are found in small quantity. Both have shown more potent anti-inflammatory activity in comparison to indomethacin.

Marine bi-indole

The bi-indole compound is obtained from *Rivularia firma* (Marine cyanobacterium) and is quite potent anti-inflammatory compound active in both, the carrageenan (Sulphated polysaccharide carrageenan) induced rat paw oedema and kaolin induced rat paw oedema (Non-immune inflammatory response).

Manoalide

It is a non-steroidal anti-inflammatory and painkiller compound obtained from marine sponge *Luffariella variabilis*.

Dendalone-3-hydroxy-butyrate

It is marine anti-inflammatory agent obtained from sponge *Phyllospongia dendyi* var frondosa.

Tetrabromo heptanone has been isolated from red algae.

ANTHELMINTIC
Kainic Acid ($C_{10}H_{15}NO_4$)

A valuable anthelmintic used clinically in Japan against parasitic roundworm, tapeworm and for the treatment of ascariasis. It is obtained from red algae (dried) *Digenea simplex*.

Domoic Acid ($C_{15}H_{21}NO_6$)

It is obtained from red algae **chondria armata**. It is also used in the treatment of ascariasis and is effective in expelling another parasite pinworm.

ANTICOAGULANTS

Acanthaphora from red algae contain Laminaran sulphate used as anticoagulant.

Carrageenan

Carrageenan isolated from species of *Chondrus*, *Eucheuma* and *Gigartina*, reported to have anticoagulant activity.

Laminarin

A highly sulphated laminarin (polysaccharide from marine algae) has been reported to have anticoagulant activity.

PROSTAGLANDINS

The term prostaglandin is often abbreviated as PG, PGE_2, denotes a prostaglandin of the E series with two double bonds.

Prostaglandins are a family of cyclic oxygenated, C_{20} fatty acid (prostanoic acid, (Fig. 10.14) derivative substances which consist of a cyclopentane ring with two side chains having 7 and 8 carbon atoms, respectively. The carboxylic group is present on C_7 chain and a C_8 chain with methyl terminus. Prostaglandins are biosynthesised from three essential fatty acids, $\Delta^{8,11,14}$ eicosatrienoic (dihomo-γ-linolenic acids), $\Delta^{5,8,11,14}$ eicosatetraenoic acid (arachidonic acid) and $\Delta^{5,8,11,14,17}$ eicosapentaenoic acid, which yield prostaglandins of the 1-, 2- and 3-series respectively known as PGE_1, PGE_2 and PGE_3 (Fig. 10.15).

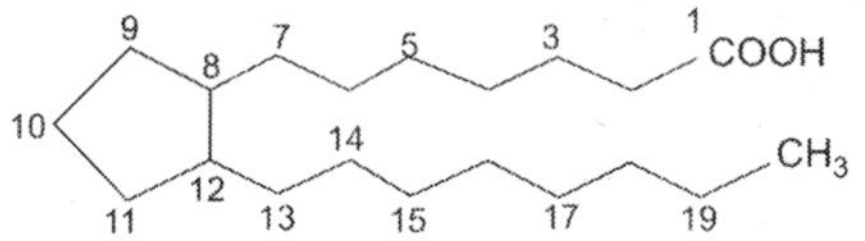

Fig. 10.14: Prostanoic acid

Name prostaglandins was given due to the fact that they were first discovered in seminal fluid, although later on, it was reported that they are not only produced in the prostate gland but occur practically in all mammal organs although in very small amounts. PGE_1 and PGF_1 were initially isolated from sheep seminal plasma but these compounds and PGD_2, PGE_2 and PGF_{2a} are widely distributed. Animal source cannot supply sufficient amounts for drug usage. The soft Coral *Plexaura homomalla* (sea whip) from **Caribbean** has been reported to have very high (2–3%) level of prostaglandin esters, predominantly, the C-15 epimer of PGA_2 (1–2%) with related structures. Prostaglandins of A-, E- and F-type (Fig. 10.16) are widely distributed in soft corals, especially *Plexaura*. Although some synthetic prostaglandins are also available, but it is reported that biological activity is effectively confined to the natural enantiomers; the Unnatural enantiomers of PGE_1 had only 0.1% of the activity of the natural isomer.

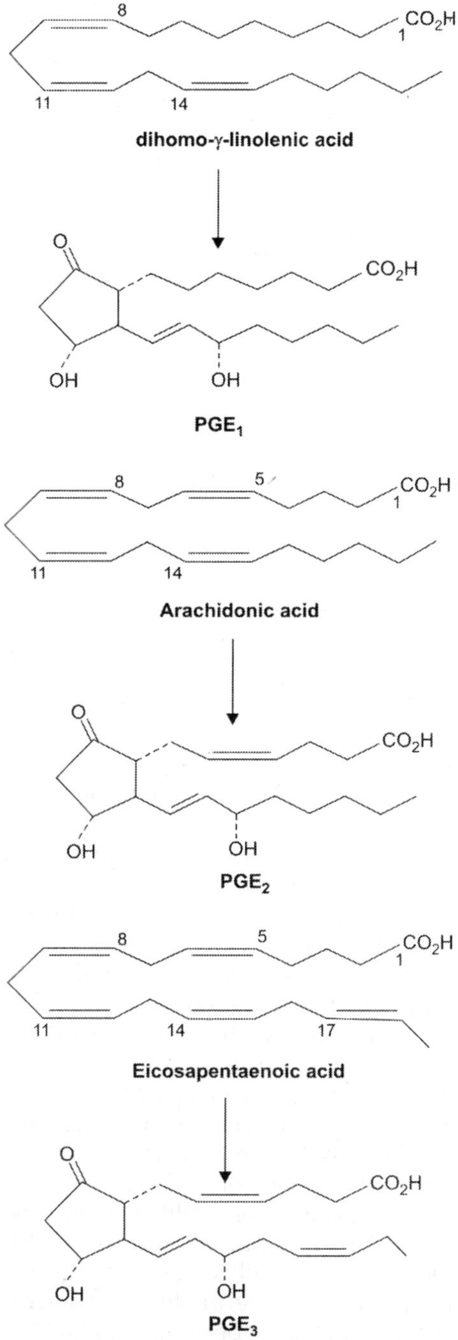

Fig. 10.15: Biosynthesis of PGE_1, PGE_2 and PGE_3

Prostaglandins constitute a group of biologically potent substances of wide spectrum

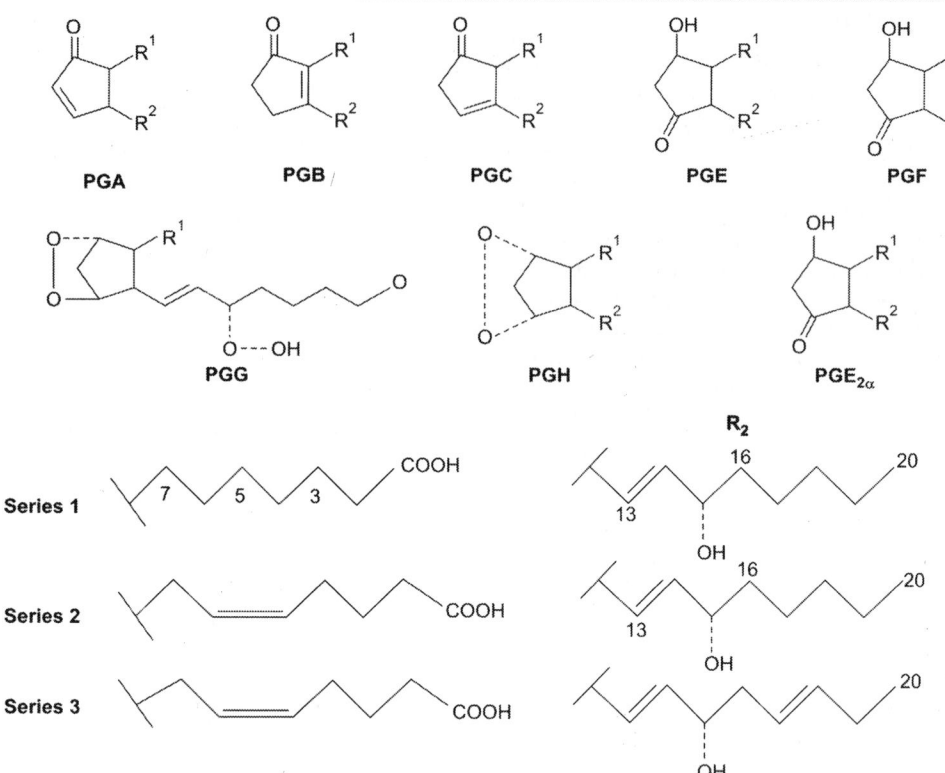

Fig. 10.16: Prostaglandins of A-, E- and F- type

activity. It causes contraction and relaxation of smooth muscle of the uterus, cardiovascular system, the intestinal tract and of bronchial tissue. They may also inhibit gastric acid secretion, control blood pressure and suppress blood platelet aggregation.

As such they are inactive but on modification, the inactive compounds become active. Six different series (A-E) produced by modification of the cyclopentane ring are now available as synthetic products. They can be useful in birth control, induced child birth, abortion, menstruation problem, peptic ulcers, treatment of asthma, regulation of blood pressure and tranquillising effect on CNS.

15-epi-PGA$_2$ acetate, methyl ester derivative, obtained from the caribbean gorgonial *Plexaura homomalla* in high concentration. **Some prostaglandins have also been isolated from red algae** *Gracilaria lichenoides*, i.e. PGE$_2$, which have antitumour activity. The inactive 15-epi

PGA$_2$ and its diester have been converted into useful prostaglandins (15s) PGA$_2$ and (15s) PGE$_2$. Active (15s) PGA$_2$ and (15s) PGE$_2$ identical to prostaglandins derived from mammalian sources has been isolated from *P. homomalla* collected from different location.

FURTHER READING

1. Costello MJ, Chaudhary C. Marine Biodiversity, Biogeography, Deep-sea Gradients, and Conservation. Current Biology. 2017;27(23):2051.
2. Evans WC. 2009. Trease and Evans Pharmacognosy, 10th edition, Elsevier, New York.
3. Kalia AN. Textbook of Industrial Pharmacogonsy. (2005). CBS Publishers and Distributors, New Delhi.
4. Mayer AMS, et al. Marine Pharmacology in 2012–2013: Marine compounds with antibacterial, antidiabetic, antifungal, anti-inflammatory, antiprotozoal, antituberculosis, and antiviral activities; Affecting the immune and nervous systems, and other miscellaneous mechanisms of action. Marine drugs. 2017; 29;15(9).

Index